HEALTH CARE FOR THE POOR IN LATIN AMERICA AND THE CARIBBEAN

Carmelo Mesa-Lago, Ph.D.
Distinguished Service Professor
  of Economics and
    Latin American Studies
University of Pittsburgh

A Joint Publication

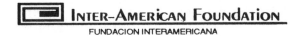
FUNDACION INTERAMERICANA

Pan American Health Organization
Pan American Sanitary Bureau,
Regional Office of the
World Health Organization
525 23rd Street, N.W.
Washington, D.C. 20037

Inter-American Foundation
901 N. Stuart Street
Arlington, Virginia 22203

PAHO Scientific Publication No. 539

1992

Also to be published in Spanish (1992) as:
Atención de salud para los pobres en la América Latina y el Caribe
ISBN 92 75 31539 6

Library of Congress Cataloging in Publication Data No. 061991
ISBN 92 75 11539 7

CONTENTS

PREFACE

The poor's lack of access to health care is part of the enormous social debt that has been accumulating for generations in the countries of Latin America and the Caribbean. The economic crisis of the 1980s aggravated that debt, plunging more people into poverty while simultaneously limiting the resources available to the social sectors. The situation seems to be a vicious circle: lingering economic problems lead to a lack of services that adversely affects the health of the population, but the countries need a healthy population in order to participate in economic and social development. Health is not only a by-product of development; it is an essential precondition without which people cannot lead normal lives, much less work and produce effectively. Consequently, it must be considered as a priority objective that is addressed through specific policies and that requires the countries' political will.

One key to resolving this dilemma is to learn to do more with the resources available. Greater efficiency is a goal of the Pan American Health Organization's technical cooperation with its Member Countries in health services development. The Organization also encourages the countries of the Americas to share experiences in this area, for while their societies may differ markedly given diverse historical conditions, cultural heritages, and political and economic systems, many of the basic questions they must address—how to improve access, increase efficiency, and guarantee equity—are the same, and the answers that work in one place can be instructive in another.

The impressive study undertaken by Dr. Carmelo Mesa-Lago, which was commissioned and supported by the Inter-American Foundation, represents a major contribution to the sharing of information. Focusing on the most socially vulnerable segments of the population, he provides an overview of the extent to which they are covered by the Region's health care systems, as well as the reasons for coverage shortfalls. Detailed analyses of health care provided for the poor by the public, private, and social insurance sectors in five countries offer lessons and a comparative basis for policy recommendations.

The Pan American Health Organization is pleased to join with the Inter-American Foundation in presenting the results of Dr. Mesa-Lagos's important work, in the hope that it will not only encourage further examination of this topic but also stimulate policy makers to seek innovative solutions for providing better access to health care to those groups who currently are the least served.

Carlyle Guerra de Macedo
Pan American Sanitary Bureau

1.

INTRODUCTION

In 1989, it was estimated that there were 183 million poor in Latin America, equal to 44% of its total population (ECLAC-CEPAL, 1990). There are no aggregate data on the poor in the non-Latin Caribbean, but if the above percentage is applied to the population of that subregion (6.5 million), an additional 3 million poor would bring the total to a staggering 186 million for the entire Region. The Director of the Pan American Health Organization (PAHO) has roughly estimated that 130 million poor (about 70% of the total) have no access to health care in Latin America and the Caribbean. If the grave economic crisis of the 1980s persists in the 1990s, the number of unprotected poor will rise dramatically. At the same time, PAHO considers that 30% of available health resources are currently wasted, and, if efficiently utilized, could help the poor. It is obvious that the World Health Organization's goal of health for all in the year 2000, launched in Alma-Ata in 1978, will not be fulfilled in most of the Region (Carlyle Guerra de Macedo, 1990). And yet, several countries have been capable of providing health care coverage to the poor.

This study has several objectives: to review problems confronted by the health care systems in Latin America and the Caribbean at the turn of the 1980s, analyze their current and potential capacity to provide adequate health protection for the poor, assess the public and private efforts of five countries to fulfill that goal, and offer recommendations for the Region.

Three sectors can be distinguished within the health system: public, social insurance, and private. The public sector is mainly represented by the Ministry of Health, which is charged by law with tending to the poor; in many countries, this sector's resources are grossly insufficient, leaving the poor unprotected in practice. The social insurance program of sickness-maternity normally does not offer any health services to the poor, but, in a few countries, "indigents" are protected through social welfare or other special programs administered by social insurance. (In this study, the term social security is used comprehensively to include all social-insurance programs that cover contingencies such as old-age, disability and death, sickness-maternity, employment injury, and unemployment.) The private sector includes prepaid plans; employer, cooperative, and community schemes; private hospitals, clinics, and medical personnel; and nongovernmental organizations (NGOs).

This study was done in a two-year period, from August 1988 to October 1990. It is divided into four chapters. The first identifies who are the poor in Latin America and the Caribbean, and explores the overall magnitude of poverty in the Region and its trends; urban/rural incidence of poverty; and characteristics of the poor such as geographical location, employment, income, and access to social services. This section does not intend to break new ground, but rather to summarize and integrate existing information in order to provide a basis for the rest of the study.

The second chapter reviews the Region's health care systems—their progress and problems—and the access of the poor to them. It provides systematic information on all 20 Latin American countries and occasionally on 14 non-Latin Caribbean countries (data on the Bahamas, Barbados, and Jamaica are systematically given). This chapter includes an overall analysis of the health care systems' administration, as well as their standards, facilities, inequalities, financing, and growing costs. Special attention has been given to an assessment of the currently protection of the poor, as well as to obstacles standing in the way of their coverage and the potential costs for reaching that goal under the currently predominant model of health care.

The third chapter analyzes in depth the cases of five countries: Uruguay, Costa Rica, Mexico, Peru, and the Dominican Republic. These countries were selected as representative examples of the Region, based on their size and geographical location, level of economic and social development, poverty incidence and size of the informal and traditional rural sectors, social insurance health coverage, and existence or lack of special programs to protect the poor. In each country we discuss the poverty situation, the current health care coverage of urban and rural poor and the reasons behind a low or high coverage, the financial viability of social insurance and the public sector to cover the poor, and the private alternatives that the poor have to get protected. In addition, in each country we focus on a health program that is or might be beneficial to the poor: in Costa Rica, the social-insurance and the Ministry of Health programs that provide health care to the urban and rural poor; in the Dominican Republic, the advantages and/or disadvantages for the poor of user fees in the public health sector and private HMOs; in Mexico, the social insurance health care program for the rural poor (COPLAMAR); in Peru, the communal organization of health services to protect the poor in a marginal town; and in Uruguay, the role of the mixed system of social insurance, Ministry of Health, and collective organizations in providing health care for the poor. In addition, some programs funded by the Inter-American Foundation (IAF) that care for the poor are evaluated in Mexico, Peru, and Uruguay.

The author conducted field research in the five countries between 1986 and 1989, and was aided by two researchers, Gerard M. La Forgia, who evaluated user fees in the Dominican Republic in 1989 and Margaret S. Sherraden who assessed Mexico's COPLAMAR in 1988–1989.

The fourth chapter summarizes the findings and lessons of the case studies and explores the possibility of replicating the successful programs elsewhere. It also offers some policy recommendations designed to reform the health care in Latin America and the Caribbean, in order to protect the Region's poor.

This study was commissioned and basically financed by the Inter-American Foundation (IAF). I am grateful for the opportunity, guidance, and support given by Charlie Reilly, Patrick Breslin, and Bob Sogge, as well as for the help of several IAF country representatives.

The Pan American Health Organization enthusiastically embraced this project and decided to jointly publish the work with IAF in both English and Spanish. I am indebted to the Director, Dr. Carlyle Guerra de Macedo, for his support.

Because the study involved three times more effort than anticipated, it took all my research time at the University of Pittsburgh in the summers of 1989 and 1990 and part of the fall of 1990, with support coming from Burkart Holzner, Director of the University Center for International Studies, and a sabbatical granted by Peter Koehler, Dean of the Faculty of Arts and Sciences and Kevin Sontheimer, Chairperson of the Economics Department. The study also benefitted from previous research I conducted in four of the five selected countries, for the Regional Program on Employment for Latin America and the Caribbean (PREALC), the World Bank, and the United States Agency for International Development (USAID). None of these institutions and individuals is responsible for what is said herein. My appreciation also goes to numerous people in the Region who graciously supplied data and/or accepted to be interviewed for this study, as well as to my secretary, Mimi Ranallo, who efficiently typed several versions of the manuscript, and to my research assistant Sarah Wheeler, who proofread the final version of the manuscript, and helped to assemble the bibliography. This study is dedicated to the poor in the region with the hope that it will contribute toward improving their health care protection.

2.

WHO ARE THE POOR IN LATIN AMERICA AND THE CARIBBEAN

Rather than advancing new knowledge on poverty in Latin America and the Caribbean, this chapter intends to summarize and consolidate existing literature, in order to provide a foundation for the subsequent analysis of health care protection of the poor.

Poverty has been defined as the inability to attain a minimum standard of living or to purchase the minimum basket of goods and services required for the satisfaction of basic needs; the poor, then, are those who fall under such a minimum level or "poverty line." This line could be uniformly fixed for all the world (or one region), thus establishing a "universal (or regional) poverty line" of "absolute poverty;" it also could be fixed within one country, according to its specific living standards or income—a "country-specific poverty line" of "relative poverty."

Among the poor, we can identify a poorest group of "extreme poverty" or "critical poverty," or "indigence," or "destitution." This group even lacks the means to buy food that would allow them to have a minimally adequate diet, much less to acquire other goods and services. "Poverty incidence" is the proportion of poor (however defined) in relation to the total population of the world or within a given region or country (Piñera, 1978, 1978a; Altimir, 1982; World Bank, 1990; ECLAC-CEPAL, 1990).

MAGNITUDE, TRENDS, AND INCIDENCE OF POVERTY

Poverty indicators can be direct or indirect; the former relate to measurements of purchasing power and income, and will be used in this chapter; indirect indicators are proxies such as infant mortality or life expectancy and will be used in subsequent chapters.

The measure of poverty in developing countries (including Latin America) has been occasionally undertaken by the International Labor Organization and the World Bank (Psacharopoulos, 1989; World Bank, 1990), and systematically for Latin America (excluding the non-Latin Caribbean) by the United Nations Economic Commission for Latin America and the Caribbean (ECLAC) (Piñera, 1978, 1978a; Molina, 1980; UN/ECLAC/UNDP, 1980; Altimir, 1982; ECLAC-CEPAL, 1990).

The pioneer study to measure poverty in Latin America was conducted by ECLAC using 1970 data and uniform criteria for eleven countries; the study covered 70% of the Region's population and GDP. Basically, it used consumer expenditure to measure regional absolute poverty and indigence, and income per capita (half of the national average per capita income) to determine relative poverty in each of those countries. Roughly, the line of indigence (in dollars) was about half the line of overall poverty, and there were twice as many indigents as overall poor. ECLAC has applied the same basic methodology retrospectively to 1960, and, later, to 1980 and 1990; there also is a projection for 1989. The ECLAC survey for the 1980s included ten countries that, combined, account for 91% of GDP and 85% of the population of the Region. All estimates are on absolute poverty: the overall poverty line was established based on the cost of a basket of goods plus additional nonfood basic needs; the indigence line was fixed by the costs of a basic food basket. In all ECLAC's studies, poverty calculations were made both for households and for the total population (ECLAC-CEPAL, 1990). To simplify the analysis, hereafter we will focus on the concept and measurement of absolute poverty.

Table 1 summarizes ECLAC's series showing magnitude, trends, and incidence (national, urban, and rural) of absolute poverty in Latin America in 1970, 1980, and 1986, as well as the projection for 1989. The number of poor (total population) increased from 110 million in 1960

Table 1. ECLAC estimates of absolute poverty and national/urban/rural poverty incidence in Latin America, 1970–1989.

	Households			Total population			
	1980	1986	1989[a]	1970	1980	1986	1989[a]
Population (millions)	69	87	94	283	331	396	416
Poor (millions)	24	32	35	113	136	170	183
Poverty incidence (%)[b]							
National	35	37	37	40	41	43	44
Urban	25	30	31	26	30	36	36
Rural	54	53	54	62	60	60	61
Poverty distribution (%)[c]							
National	100	100	100	100	100	100	100
Urban	49	58	59	37	46	55	57
Rural	51	42	41	63	54	45	43

Sources: Altimir, 1982; ECLAC-CEPAL, 1990.
[a]Projection.
[b]Percentages of national, urban, and rural populations under the absolute poverty line.
[c]Percentages of urban and rural poor over national poor population.

(not shown in the table) to 170 million in 1986. The annual average rate of increase in the number of poor was 0.3% in 1960–1970, 2% in 1970–1980, and 3.6% in 1980–1986. National poverty incidence (households) declined from 51% in 1960 (not shown in the table) to 40% in 1970, and to 35% in 1980, but, due to the economic crisis of the 1980s, it rose to 37% in 1986. When total population figures are used, the national poverty incidence steadily increased between 1970 and 1986, from 40% to 43%.

The World Bank estimated that in 1985, there were 70 million poor in Latin America and the Caribbean (about 100 million fewer than in ECLAC's survey) and a poverty incidence of 19% (compared to ECLAC's 43%). The reason behind the lower figures is that the Bank used a very low "universal poverty line" ($US370) to facilitate comparisons of Latin America and the Caribbean with poorer regions in the developing world. The Region's share of the world's poor is 6%, and yet the Bank noted that average per capita income in Latin America and the Caribbean is well above that of "middle income countries" and from five to six times the per capita income of other developing regions. Still, about one-fifth of the Region's population lives in poverty, partly due, according to the Bank, to the Region's exceptionally high income inequality (World Bank, 1990).

According to Table 1, the share of the urban poor in the total population of poor increased steadily from 37% to 55% between 1970 and 1986 (along with the increase in urbanization), while the share of the rural poor declined from 63% to 45% in the same period. Thus, while in 1970 the large majority of poor was rural, in 1986 it was urban. However, because of the relative decline in the Region's rural population,

poverty incidence in rural areas remained much higher (60% in 1986) than in urban areas (36%). In 1970–1986, poverty incidence declined slightly in rural areas (from 62% to 60%), but increased significantly in urban areas (from 26% to 36%). Therefore, the overall increase in poverty in the 1980s has concentrated in the urban areas, which have suffered more from the economic crisis than the rural areas. And yet, the rural population is still considerably more afflicted with poverty than the urban population; furthermore, critical poverty (incidence of indigence) is twice as high in rural than in urban areas (ECLAC-CEPAL, 1990).

Figures in Table 1 are regional averages, but variations among countries are significant, as Table 2 shows. In six of the ten countries, the national poverty incidence (households) declined in 1970–1980, but in four of those countries it increased in 1980–1986; in two countries for which we lack data for 1970, poverty incidence grew in 1980–1986; and in one country, that incidence steadily rose in 1970–1986. Only in three countries did poverty incidence decline in 1980–1986. National poverty incidence in 1986 (total population) ranged from 16% in Argentina to 73% in Guatemala, indicating that the level of development (roughly measured by GDP per capita) is inversely correlated with poverty incidence (ECLAC-CEPAL, 1990). As was seen in Table 1, the rural poverty incidence is substantially higher (in 1986 it ranged from 20% in Argentina to 80% in Guatemala) than the urban incidence (from 15% to 60% in the same countries). Poverty incidence among households is consistently lower than among individuals in the total population.

The ten countries surveyed by ECLAC are among the most developed in Latin America,

Table 2. ECLAC estimates of absolute poverty incidence (national/urban/rural) in selected Latin American[a] countries, 1970–1988 (in percentages).

	Households			Total population		
	National	Urban	Rural	National	Urban	Rural
Argentina						
1970	8	5	19	n.a.	n.a.	n.a.
1980	9	7	16	10	9	19
1986	13	12	17	16	15	20
Brazil						
1970	49	35	73	n.a.	n.a.	n.a.
1979	39	30	62	45	34	68
1987	40	34	60	45	38	66
Colombia						
1970	45	38	54	n.a.	n.a.	n.a.
1980	39	36	45	42	40	48
1986	38	36	42	42	40	45
Costa Rica						
1970	24	15	30	n.a.	n.a.	n.a.
1981	22	16	28	24	18	28
1988	25	21	28	27	24	30
Guatemala						
1970	n.a.	n.a.	n.a.	n.a.	n.a.	n.a.
1980	65	41	79	71	47	84
1986	68	54	75	73	60	80
Mexico						
1970	34	20	49	n.a.	n.a.	n.a.
1977	32	n.a.	n.a.	40	n.a.	n.a.
1984	30	23	43	37	30	51
Panama						
1970	n.a.	n.a.	n.a.	n.a.	n.a.	n.a.
1979	36	31	45	42	36	50
1986	34	30	43	41	36	52
Peru						
1970	50	28	68	n.a.	n.a.	n.a.
1979	46	35	65	53	38	80
1986	52	45	64	60	52	72
Uruguay						
1970	n.a.	10	n.a.	n.a.	n.a.	n.a.
1981	11	9	21	15	13	27
1986	15	14	23	20	19	29
Venezuela						
1970	25	20	36	n.a.	n.a.	n.a.
1981	22	18	35	25	20	43
1986	27	25	34	32	30	42

Source: ECLAC, 1990.

[a]The 1970 survey also included Chile and Honduras, but these countries were excluded in the 1980s survey, which added Guatemala and Panama.

with the exception of Guatemala. Out of the ten countries excluded, Chile and Cuba are fairly developed, but the remaining eight—Bolivia, the Dominican Republic, Ecuador, El Salvador, Haiti, Honduras, Nicaragua, and Paraguay—are among the least developed in the Region. Therefore, ECLAC suggests that the poverty incidence in these eight countries should be higher than that of those listed in Table 2. Unfortunately, we lack accurate data on these eight countries, which makes it extremely difficult to evaluate poverty in the Dominican Republic (one of our five case studies).

In its recent study on poverty, the World Bank (1990) provides some data on five of the same countries surveyed by ECLAC (not comparable because the Bank uses relative poverty lines, while ECLAC's survey is based on absolute poverty lines), but nothing on the eight excluded countries. Figures on 14 Latin American countries (including the eight not surveyed by ECLAC) are furnished in a previous Bank review on world poverty; unfortunately, it lacks information on definitions, method of calculation, sources, precise dates, and national poverty incidence; furthermore, rural incidence is not given for several countries, either (Psacharopoulos, 1989). That study's data on the Dominican Republic show an urban incidence of 45% (somewhere between 1977 and 1986) that is consistent with both that country's indicators of development and its ranking within Latin America. However, the Dominican Republic's rural poverty incidence is given as 43%, which is lower than the country's urban incidence and lower than ECLAC's rural incidence for five countries that are more developed than the Dominican Republic.

An ECLAC projection for 1989 (Table 1) indicates that the national poverty incidence in Latin America would have increased by one percentage point since 1986, reaching 44%; based on household data, the incidence was unchanged. On the other hand, the World Bank has projected a decline of 8 percentage points in the Region's poverty incidence for the year 2000, from 19% in 1985 to 11% in 2000. This forecast was based on optimistic assumptions: that the regional GDP would grow 4.2% annually (because the Bank predicted that the debt burden in Latin America and the Caribbean would cease to be a serious constraint on investment in the last five years of the century) and that GDP in industrial countries would grow 3% yearly, thus increasing the demand for and the prices of the Region's exports. However, if these assumptions fail to materialize, the Bank projects an increase of 5 percentage points in the poverty incidence, for a regional rate of 24% in the year 2000 (World Bank, 1990). It should be recalled that all World Bank figures are lower than ECLAC's.

To summarize, since 1980 both the number of poor and the poverty incidence have rapidly grown in Latin America. Although the number of urban poor is increasing faster than that of the rural poor, overall poverty incidence among the latter is about 70% higher than among the urban poor, and incidence of indigence is twice as high among the rural poor than among the urban poor. Poverty is inversely correlated with level of development—it is lower in the most developed Latin American countries (including three of our case studies, Uruguay, Costa Rica, and Mexico) and higher in the least developed countries (including Peru and, probably, the Dominican Republic).

CHARACTERISTICS OF THE POOR

ECLAC's initial surveys developed a "poverty profile" for Latin America that described the characteristics of the poor in terms of geographical location, demographics, educational level, employment, income, access to public services and markets, and degree of organization and participation. More recent information on some of these indicators has been compiled by the World Bank. The poor are concentrated in the countries' urban areas and least developed regions (mostly rural areas with a high percentage of Indian population). The urban poor often live in shantytowns and illegal squatter settlements. The poor have a very low education level, are afflicted with high mortality rates, have larger families, earn a very low income, have little or no access to social services, and often lack mechanisms of organization and active political and social participation. Women and children are particularly affected by poverty (Piñera, 1978, 1978a; Molina, 1980; World Bank, 1990).

The urban poor are victims of open unemployment, and even more so, of underemployment, which affects 70% of them. Most of the urban poor are salaried blue-collar workers in small businesses, or self-employed, or unpaid family workers, or domestic servants,[1] all of which are typical labor categories of the so-called informal sector. Although not all informal workers are poor, the available information suggests that most of them are, particularly if owners of informal enterprises as well as self-employed professionals are excluded. In 1970, 34% of urban employment in the eleven Latin American countries was in the informal sector, and from 70% to 80% of the urban poor were within this sector: 38% worked in services (mostly personal), 20% in commerce, 19% in manufacturing (mostly small enterprises, often underground or illegal), and the remaining 24% in construction, transportation, or non-specified jobs.

---

[1] Data on the distribution of the informal sector by labor force categories, from nine Latin American and Caribbean countries at the end of the 1970s, indicate that: from 54% to 80% was salaried; 13% to 26%, self-employed; 1% to 10%, unpaid family workers; 1% to 9%, domestic servants; and 1% to 6%, employers. Because these data were gathered in the metropolitan area or the most important cities, the percentage of salaried workers was probably higher than if all the urban sector in the nation had been used (Mesa-Lago, 1990a).

Most of the urban poor work, but earn a low income. In 1970, between 19% and 50% of urban workers' earnings in 13 Latin American countries were below the minimum wage (the lowest in Argentina and the highest in Paraguay), and in seven major cities, between 73% and 93% of those working below the minimum wage were employed in the informal sector (the lowest in Mexico City and the highest in Panama City). In 1980, the average income of an informal worker, vis-à-vis that of a formal worker, in eight capital cities of Latin America was: 28% in Peru; 36% to 40% in Chile, Colombia, El Salvador, and Paraguay; and 47% to 51% in Costa Rica, the Dominican Republic, and Mexico. Data from a few countries suggest that, among informal workers, by type of occupation, unpaid family workers and the self-employed earn the lowest income, followed by salaried workers; business owners earn the highest income. By economic branch, domestic servants and street vendors earn the lowest income, followed by repair shop workers.

Due to the economic crisis, in 1980–1985, non-agricultural employment in the formal sector declined by almost 8%, while employment in the informal sector increased by almost 4%; thus, total urban employment decreased by 4% and urban open unemployment rose in the same proportion. The urban groups most affected by the crisis are those suffering from open unemployment and the informal workers; 57% of the increase in poverty incidence is concentrated in the former and 39% in the latter (Tokman, 1980, 1987; PREALC, 1988).

We have seen that overall poverty incidence and indigence in rural areas are much higher than in urban areas. Average rural income, health status, education, and housing are always below national averages, and considerably worse than urban averages. Critical poverty in Latin America and the Caribbean usually is concentrated in arid zones or steep hill-slope areas that suffer from environmental degradation and that are economically vulnerable and physically and culturally isolated. In these areas, arable land is scarce, labor demand is highly seasonal, and labor productivity is extremely low. Landless peasants and poverty are highly correlated in rural Latin America and the Caribbean, and even when the poor have land, it is normally unproductive, of very low productivity, or organized in ineffective communal farms. Rural poverty is also correlated with race and ethnic background: in Bolivia, Ecuador, Guatemala, Mexico, and Peru, indigenous people are disproportionately represented among the poor.

Health conditions, too, are much worse among the rural poor than among the urban poor. Data on five Latin American and Caribbean countries for the mid-1980s show that infant mortality rates in rural areas in Panama and Mexico were from 27% to 172% higher, respectively, than in urban areas. Lack of access to safe water in rural areas ranged between 37% to 207% higher in Panama and Peru, respectively, than in urban areas. According to other data, ratios of urban to rural services are: physicians, five to one; hospital beds, four to one; and sewage, from five to twenty to one (World Bank, 1990; La Forgia, 1990).

In rural areas, most of the poor work in agriculture, mainly in small-scale farming; non-agricultural employment is in cottage industries, services, and commerce. In the rural sector, the self-employed and unpaid family workers represent the highest proportions among agricultural workers (and the poor). Data from a few Latin American countries in 1972 indicate that among poor heads of households, from 46% to 60% were self-employed. However, the self-employed and unpaid relatives are often partly engaged in salaried employment as temporary or seasonal workers. Increases in salaried work in agricultural enterprises come mostly from the hiring of temporary or casual labor. A significant part of the rural poor is unemployed: in the four months of lowest employment, from 25% to 60% of the agricultural labor force is unemployed. The number of family dependents per active worker in rural households is much higher than in urban households, hence aggravating poverty (León, 1980; World Bank, 1990).

This study will concentrate on the two major groups of the poor.

▪ In the urban areas, we will focus on the informal sector, particularly on the self-employed, unpaid family workers, and domestic servants. Informal salaried workers of small enterprises will be considered but, due to lack of data, it is almost impossible to disaggregate this subgroup from salaried workers as a whole. Small informal employers often have higher incomes than the other subgroups and most of them are not poor; data on this group also are very scarce.

▪ In rural areas, most of the poor are landless peasants, small farmers, the self-employed, and temporary/casual/seasonal workers. Disaggregate data on these subgroups are extremely difficult to obtain; hence, we normally shall deal with the rural poor as a whole.

Finally, whenever possible, we will consider the unemployed, whether urban or rural.

ACCESS OF THE POOR TO SOCIAL SERVICES

According to Altimir (1982), the welfare of low income groups largely depends on whether or not they have access to free or highly subsidized social services such as education and health care. In practice, inequalities in the access to these services among the population aggravate the incidence of poverty. In a rough attempt to measure the differences in probability of access among the population, he has argued that, "lowest income groups experience the greatest difficulties of access to available social services and their probability of access is therefore below the [national] average. . . . That probability diminishes even further the less extended a particular service is, since restricted conditions of supply tend to favor access by the middle and higher groups of the population" (p. 68).

Referring specifically to health care, Altimir argues that if national average population coverage is 60%, the poor have a 40% rough probability of not being covered. Comparing health facilities among different countries he comes up with a rough probability of the poor's access to such services. For instance, the ratio of hospital beds per 1,000 inhabitants is between 5.5 and 6.0 in Uruguay and Argentina, but between 1.0 and 1.3 in Paraguay, Honduras, El Salvador, and Mexico, which means that the poor have three times more probability of access in the first group of countries than in the second.

The World Bank, in its recent study on poverty, asserts that "no task should command a higher priority for the world's policymakers than that of reducing poverty" (1990:5). To fight poverty, the Bank recommends a strategy that combines efficient labor-intensive growth plus adequate provision of basic social services, among which health care plays a fundamental role. This study analyzes the lack of access of the poor to such services and alternative ways to solve that crucial problem.

3.

Overall Evaluation of Health Care and Access of the Poor

First, this chapter briefly describes health care systems in Latin America and the Caribbean, identifying their three major sectors (public, social insurance, and private) and analyzing the inadequacy of the resources assigned to the public sector, which normally is charged with caring for the poor. Second, it provides estimates of health care coverage of the population and its inequalities, as well as an analysis of current coverage of the poor, obstacles to achieving the poor's protection, and the high cost of providing it under the predominant model of health care. Third, it evaluates health standards and facilities in the Region, as well as their inequalities and the redistributive impact of health programs. Fourth, it discusses the sources of health care financing in Latin America and the Caribbean (both in the public sector and social insurance) and assesses the impact of the economic crisis on health care, particularly upon the poor. Finally, the chapter provides data on the size, distribution, and growing trends of health care expenditures in the Region, as well as on the causes behind the increase in health costs and the obstacles this increment poses for extending coverage to the poor. Each of the five sections of this chapter ends with a summary of major findings, emphasizing the relationship with poverty.

ADMINISTRATION OF HEALTH CARE: TRENDS AND PROBLEMS

In Latin America and the Caribbean, health care is administered by many providers, including ministries of health, social insurance institutions, the armed forces, trade unions, mutual-aid societies and cooperatives, charitable institutions (*beneficencias*), employers, insurance companies, health maintenance organizations (HMOs), and nongovernmental organizations (NGOs). These providers can be grouped into the three major sectors: public, social insurance, and private.

Public, Social Insurance, and Private Sectors

The most important provider within the public sector is the ministry of health, which is charged with two major functions: prevention and sanitation (e.g., immunization, environmental sanitation, control of endemic and epidemic diseases, health education, supervision of all health care, etc.) and curative services. In some countries, such as Argentina, states, provinces, departments, and municipalities also have their own health services independent from those of the federal or central government. Throughout Latin America (with the exception of Costa Rica, which has no army), the armed forces also have their own health services, and in some countries, certain autonomous public institutions do too. Charitable institutions can fall within either the public sector or the private sector.

In 20 out of 28 of the Region's countries for which we have information, most health services are supplied by the public sector, mainly by the ministry of health. The poorest segment of the population usually only has access to the services provided by the ministry of health (under the concept of social welfare), because this group is not eligible for social insurance and cannot afford private medicine. However, the ministry's facilities are normally insufficient to effectively care for the population assigned to them, and their services are often the worst in quality.

Social insurance has become the second major provider of health care in the Region (basically curative services), mainly through the sickness-maternity program and, to a lesser extent, through employment-injury and family-allowance programs. In some countries, the sickness-maternity program is not unified, but divided by labor force categories or occupations (e.g., private white- and blue-collar workers, civil servants, railroad workers, petroleum workers, electricity workers, banking employees). In eight Latin American countries, social insurance covers a larger population than the ministry of health. Such coverage focuses on the population's middle-income groups, with upper-low and lower-high income groups added in some countries (those covered claim a ''right'' to care). Consequently, the poor usually are excluded, save for in a few countries where social insurance provides health care to ''indigents.'' Social insurance facilities normally are better and there are more of them than those of the ministry of health.

The private sector is essentially devoted to for-profit or nonprofit curative medicine. It constitutes the smallest of the three sectors, with the possible exception of Brazil's, although it is rapidly expanding in many countries. Prepaid plans are still incipient and include insurance (individual and group policies), as well as employer, cooperative, and community plans. Most of these function in large urban areas, but some are found in small cities and agroexport areas (Gwynne and Zschock, 1989). In addition, there are private hospitals, clinics, and medical personnel that care for individuals not covered by any plan, as well as traditional medicine practitioners (curanderos, midwives, etc.). Finally, there are NGOs that provide some health services. Except for nonprofit NGOs, the private, for-profit sector covers the high-income group and part of the middle-income group, obviously excluding the poor. In general, access to private services is inversely correlated with their complexity and cost: there is greater access to lower-cost services such as outpatient consultations and child delivery and medicine, but considerably less access to complex diagnostic services and hospitalization, particularly high-tech medicine (PAHO, 1989). Although the quality of private services varies greatly among countries, they tend to be the best, except for some highly technical equipment and specialists.

Data on the distribution of health care services among the three sectors are scarce and often unreliable. According to Table 3, in five out of twelve countries in Latin America—Cuba, Ecuador, Colombia, the Dominican Republic, and Peru, in that order—the majority of the population is covered by the ministry of health; this also is true for the non-Latin Caribbean, although it is not shown in the table. In four countries—Costa Rica, Argentina, Mexico, and Panama—the majority of the population is covered by social insurance. In one country,

Table 3. Percentage distribution of population coverage on health care by sector in selected Latin American countries, circa 1985.

Countries	Ministry of Health & others[a]	Social insurance	Private	Total
Argentina	23	74[b]	3	100
Brazil	----------87----------		13	100
Chile	--------85–90[c]--------		10–15	100
Colombia	74	16	10	100
Costa Rica	14	81	5	100
Cuba	100	0	0	100
Dominican Republic	64	6	30	100
Ecuador	83	11	6	100
Mexico	30	60	10	100
Panama	42	58	n.a.	100
Peru	55	17	28	100
Uruguay	43	53[b]	4	100

Source: Mesa-Lago, 1989.
[a]Includes armed forces, other public institutions, and, in some countries, charity institutions.
[b]Includes mutual-aid societies, cooperatives, and union services.
[c]FONASA is a public agency that collects all contributions from the insured.

Uruguay, the percentages covered by the Ministry and by insurance (including mutual-aid institutions) are almost equal; in Brazil and Chile, it is difficult to separate the two sectors. Although there is no information on the remaining eight Latin American countries, all of them (except Venezuela) are the least developed and have a very small social insurance coverage, leaving the public sector responsible for covering the majority of the population in them.

Organizational Types and Systems of Health Care Services

Medical-hospital services in the Region are delivered through direct and indirect systems. Under the direct system, the most common one, the administrative agency owns the hospitals and other facilities and hires the physicians. This system requires a higher initial investment, but grants more control to the administrative agency and, theoretically, reduces operational costs. Under the indirect system (seldom found in a pure form in Latin America), the agency contracts with other providers, whom users can pay directly and then get a reimbursement from the agency, or whom the agency can pay according to a preestablished fee schedule for services or per user. This system does not require a substantial investment, but gives little control to the administrative agency and its costs might be higher (ISSA-AISS, 1982; Gwynne and

Zschock, 1989, argue that costs are lower). Many countries combine direct and indirect systems, because the administrative agency's own services are insufficient.

The considerable variety of organization of health services in Latin America and the Caribbean makes it difficult to develop a strict classification, but the following three major types can be identified (Castellanos, 1985): countries with a national health system that is basically operated by the ministry of health with its own facilities (non-Latin Caribbean, except Bermuda, as well as Cuba and Nicaragua); countries where social insurance (either with a single or several agencies) covers the majority of the population through direct or indirect systems, while the ministry of health covers the noninsured and provides other services such as prevention and supervision (Argentina, Brazil—where the indirect system through private facilities is a majority—Costa Rica, Mexico, Panama, Uruguay, and Venezuela; however, only in Costa Rica and Mexico does the social insurance agency provide most services directly); and countries where the ministry of health (which has insufficient facilities for that task) is expected to cover the vast majority of the population, while social insurance covers less than one-fourth of the population either directly or indirectly (Bolivia, Colombia, the Dominican Republic, Ecuador, El Salvador, Guatemala, Honduras, Paraguay, and Peru). Haiti has no sickness-maternity social insurance, and its ministry of health is grossly inadequate to cover the population.

The Inadequacy of Public Sector Resources

As has been said, in most of Latin America, the only health services available to the bulk of the population (including the poor) are those provided by the ministry of health rather than by social insurance, but the former receives a considerably smaller percentage of the national funds allocated to health care. Table 4 presents, for only six countries, the scarce data contrasting the percentage distributions of population covered by and national revenue for health care in the ministry of health and in social insurance in 1980, as well as the revenue/coverage ratio.

For instance, in the Dominican Republic, 91% of the population (outside of the private sector) is covered by the ministry and 9% by social insurance, but the respective proportions of revenues for each agency are 53% and 47%, respectively, resulting in ratios of 0.58 for the ministry and 5.22 for social insurance. Similarly unequal ratios are shown for Colombia, Ecuador, and Peru. (There seems to be a growing gap in the physical plant and care quality between the two sectors.) Conversely, the most equal ratios are registered in Costa Rica and Panama. Most non-Latin Caribbean countries have completely avoided that inequality because they usually have a single national health system.

Given the above-mentioned inequality, the ministry of health does not have the minimum resources needed to provide health care to the majority of the population, particularly to the poor. Furthermore, the unequal allocation of resources produces a negative distortion, because the ministry usually concentrates on primary health care (e.g., prevention, nutrition, sanitation, health education, infant and maternal care), while social insurance health care is typically curative and geared to the population's productive age bracket (which has a lower sickness incidence than infants and pregnant women) and the retired (which have a high incidence of illness and require complex and expensive care).

In the least developed Latin American and Caribbean countries, infant mortality rates are very high and the main causes of death are digestive and respiratory diseases that often affect

Table 4. Comparison of percentage distributions of health care population coverage and revenues, between the Ministry of Health and social insurance, in selected Latin American countries, 1980.[a]

Countries	Ministry of Health			Social insurance		
	Coverage	Revenue	Ratio	Coverage	Revenue	Ratio
Colombia	82	38	0.46	18	62	3.44
Costa Rica	15	22	1.47	85	78	0.92
Dominican Republic	91	53	0.58	9	47	5.22
Ecuador	89	59	0.66	11	41	3.72
Panama	45	34	0.76	55	65	1.18
Peru	76	50	0.66	24	50	2.08

Source: Mesa-Lago, 1989.
[a]Excludes private sector; the percentage distributions are based on coverage and revenue data for the ministry and insurance only, hence, coverage data in this table is different than in Table 3.

infants of low-income families. These diseases (and infant mortality) can be sharply reduced with a shift of health resources from social insurance to the ministry (and from productive and retired population groups to the infant and maternal groups), but these sectors' separation of budget makes this goal difficult to achieve (more on this in the section on "Predominance of Curative Medicine," starting on p. 49).

Integration or Coordination of Services

One of the most important problems in this field is the lack of coordination among the multiple providers of health care (particularly in the public and social insurance sectors), as well as the separation between preventive and curative services (PAHO, 1981; McGreevey et al, 1984; Mesa-Lago, 1985a; Ugalde, 1985a). In the last three decades, this problem has been discussed by regional and international organizations and by associations related to social security and public health, such as the ILO, the International Social Security Association (ISSA), CPISS, OAS, OISS, PAHO, and WHO, which have recommended the coordination or integration of health services.

There are three levels of integration. The highest is represented by countries with unified national health systems. The intermediate level is made up of countries that have a high degree of coordination between the ministry of health and social insurance, where some services have been integrated, and where there is a clear division of labor between the two agencies (Costa Rica is a good example). The lowest level is typical of countries that use standardized planning and normative systems in all agencies.

To be a successful solution, integration must be coupled with a change in emphasis towards primary health care and increased efficiency (Ugalde, 1985a). It has been said that in the 1970s, preference shifted from integration towards coordination, and that since the early 1980s, a new approach has been pursued that focuses on results (universal coverage), rather than on the method to achieve them (Castellanos, 1985).

Despite the importance of this topic, few serious studies are available on concrete experiences of integration in Latin America and the Caribbean, with the exception of a recent study on Panama. It shows that integration has led to an important reduction in urban-rural disparities in access to health care, but that it failed to curtail the curative and urban biases of the system or to increase efficiency (La Forgia, 1990).

Since the 1980s, a rapprochement between the ILO and WHO (also reflected in the domestic agencies of social insurance and ministry of public health) has aimed at coordinating their activities and promoting a coherent strategy for health care particularly at the primary level (PAHO/ILO/CPISS, 1986). However, despite advances, many problems remain. Although most countries have enacted legislation to establish national health systems (e.g., Mexico and Peru) effective progress has been slow, and coordination between the two major agencies, with few exceptions, is nascent and continues to be the subject of debate and friction. Coordination policies have not yet managed to incorporate both agencies in the decision-making process and service delivery. Furthermore, resilient barriers to the process of coordination remain, such as separate clienteles, different financing means, and resistance within the two bureaucracies (Castellanos, 1985). In a PAHO meeting held in 1987, these problems were confirmed, and it was acknowledged that despite the fact that there was consensus regarding the benefits of coordination, there was no agreement concerning the proper methods to achieve it—the who, what, and how (PAHO, 1987).

In 1990, PAHO appointed social security and health experts to an advisory committee that would counsel on the issues of coordination/integration and expansion of population coverage. A committee document recognized that the existence of multiple and diverse institutions needed to be accepted, and expressed a preference for functional rather than structural or administrative integration (unification). Further, it acknowledged both the potential of social *security* (not social *insurance*) and its advantages over public assistance for expanding health care coverage. Finally, the document stressed the need to define the responsibilities and areas of activity of the public and social security sectors and the importance of strengthening the political authority and coordination role of the ministry of health (PAHO, 1989).

This document suggests that given the significant financial constraints for reaching the goal of health for all, PAHO has decided to compromise with social insurance institutions in Latin America and the Caribbean based on the following three points: the ministry of health will maintain and increase its overall coordinating power; social insurance will gradually evolve to become social security, with expansion of coverage to currently excluded groups as a key element in such transformation; and both institutions will retain their separate identities but will promote functional integration on mutually agreeable terms.

Summary of Organizational Trends and Problems

The public sector (mainly the ministry of health) has been increasingly expected to provide both preventive and curative care for the noninsured (largely indigents and other low-income groups) under the concept of social welfare. The scanty data available suggest that the ministry of health, although it covers most of the population in the majority of countries, receives a considerably lower proportion of national health funds and has poorer facilities than social insurance. Those countries that have national health systems (mostly in the non-Latin Caribbean) are exceptions to this situation.

The social insurance sector, the second major health care provider in the Region, covers the majority of the population only in a minority of countries and only in two through a direct system of delivery, although the trend appears to be shifting from direct to indirect delivery. This expanding sector principally covers the middle-income segment of the population that has a "legal right" to health care. It receives a larger proportion of national health funds than the ministry of health—its physical plant and quality of services are better than that of the ministry, and this gap appears to be widening. Exceptions to this rule are countries which have been able to achieve fair integration between the two sectors, such as Costa Rica.

The private sector is the smallest of the three, and covers mostly the high-income and upper-middle income groups of the population. This sector is expanding (partly through contracting with social insurance), and its health facilities and quality of services are probably the best in most countries.

Without question, there is a need to integrate or efficiently coordinate the public and social insurance health services. However, despite agreement on the benefits of such a process among specialized international/regional agencies and legislation to that effect that has been enacted in several countries, there is no consensus on the means to achieve the goal, progress has been slow, and significant barriers remain.

ACCESS OF THE POOR TO HEALTH CARE

In Latin America, social risk coverage has outpaced population coverage, because priority has been given to vertical extension (risks covered), rather than to horizontal extension (population protected). Social insurance has gradually expanded risk coverage (such as occupational accidents and diseases, old age, disability and death, nonoccupational sickness and maternity, unemployment) either to a minority of the population or to a majority of salaried urban workers, practically always excluding the poor. The poor, even in the best of cases, only have access to social welfare services provided by the ministry of health and other government agencies.

Health Care Coverage of the Population

In any discussion of the health-care coverage of the population, a distinction should be made between legal and statistical coverage. The former is prescribed by law, but is not always in effect; the latter comes from estimates of the population protected, which are closer to reality, if not always trustworthy. We also could refer to "real" coverage, but unfortunately lack accurate and comparative data to measure effective access of the population to health services in the Region.

Legal Coverage

Table 5 provides a comparative view of when legal coverage began in Latin American and Caribbean countries and its current scope (persons entitled to legal coverage). The table separates the countries with social insurance from those with national health systems: in the former, social insurance grants benefits both in cash (payments to compensate for loss of income or additional expenditures) and in kind (medical and hospital services, medicines); in the latter, the national health system provides benefits in kind and social insurance grants cash benefits. The table excludes coverage of the public sector (ministry of health) in countries without a na-

Table 5. Legal coverage of health care benefits by national health systems and/or social insurance in Latin America and the Caribbean, 1987–1988.[a]

Countries	Initial law	All residents	Salaried employees All[b]	Salaried employees Part[c]	Poor groups Self-employed	Poor groups Domestic servants	Poor groups Rural workers[d]
Social insurance							
Argentina	1934M, 1944S		X		Xf	X	X
Bolivia	1949			X	X		
Brazil	1923S, 1931S			X	Xf	Xi	X
Chile	1924		X		Xf	X	X
Colombia	1938M, 1946S			X	Xf	Xf	X
Costa Rica	1941		X		Xf	X	X
Dominican Republic	1947			X		j	
Ecuador	1935			X		X	
El Salvador	1949			X	X		
Guatemala	1946S, 1953M			Xe			
Haiti	1967						
Honduras	1952			Xe	Xf		
Mexico	1943			X	Xf	Xf	X
Panama	1941		X		Xf	X	X
Paraguay	1943		X		Xf	X	
Peru	1936		X			X	
Uruguay	1958M, 1960S		X			X	X
Venezuela	1940		Xe			X	
National health system							
Antigua and Barbuda	1973	X	X		X		X
Bahamas	1972	X	X		X	X	X
Barbados	1966	X	X		Xh	X	X
Belize	1979	X	X				X
Bermuda	1970	X					
Cuba	1934M, 1963S	X	X				X
Dominica	1975	X	X				X
Grenada	1983	X	X		X		X
Guyana	1969	X	X			X	X
Jamaica	1979M	X			X	Xg	
Nicaragua	1955	X	X		Xf		X
St. Christopher and Nevis	1971	X	X				X
St. Lucia	1978	X	X				X
St. Vincent	1978	X	X				X
Suriname		X					
Trinidad and Tobago	1971	X	X			X	X

Sources: Based on U.S. Social Security Administration, 1987, and additional legal data collected by the author.

M = Maternity; S = Sickness

[a]In the non-Latin Caribbean, Cuba, and Nicaragua, there is a national health system (except in Bermuda that has a compulsory hospitalization private insurance), and coverage of all residents, as shown in the table, refers to benefits in kind. In addition, these countries usually have social insurance that grants cash benefits (these are shown in the table for salary employees, the self-employed, domestic servants, and rural workers). In the remaining countries, coverage refers to social insurance for both benefits in cash and in kind.

[b]Practically all countries exclude unpaid family workers and eight countries also exclude temporary workers.

[c]Normally covers permanent employees in industry, commerce, mining, transportation, communications, civil service, and public utilities. Usually excludes agriculture and domestic service, as well as temporary, home, and unpaid family workers.

[d]Refers to salaried work and, in some countries, to cooperatives, in Uruguay includes small producers, too. For self-employed in agriculture, see self-employed column. In Brazil, rural workers are covered under a special program; in Colombia, only some regions are covered; in Mexico, coverage is being gradually expanded to salaried work, coops, and small and communal farms; in Panama, excludes those employed less than six months; in Cuba, excludes private farmers.

[e]Coverage is geographically limited to capital city and large urban areas.

[f]Voluntary coverage; in Panama, members of trade unions are compulsorily covered; in Brazil, Chile, and Nicaragua, agricultural self-employed are not covered.

[g]Only in maternity.

[h]Voluntary continuation of coverage is available to those who shift from salaried work to self-employment.

[i]In-kind benefits only.

[j]Only those who work in business, not in homes.

tional health system, because they neither grant a "right" to benefits in kind (except in very few cases) nor any cash benefits at all.

Based on the first column of Table 5, we can distinguish three groups of countries according to when legal coverage was introduced. First, influenced by the 1883 social insurance sickness law enacted in Germany under Chancellor Bismarck, seven Latin American countries passed similar laws in the early 20th century: in the 1920s in Chile (sickness-maternity insurance for blue-collar workers) and Brazil (maternity insurance for female railroad workers), and in the 1930s in Ecuador and Peru (sickness insurance for blue-collar workers) and in Argentina, Colombia, and Cuba (maternity for female workers). Second, sparked in part by the example set by these seven pioneers but also influenced by the ILO and the Beveridge Report, eleven Latin American countries enacted sickness and/or maternity insurance laws in the 1940s (Venezuela, Costa Rica, Panama, Mexico, Paraguay, Argentina, Colombia, Guatemala, maternity only; the Dominican Republic, El Salvador, and Bolivia), followed by three other countries in the following decade (Honduras; Nicaragua; and Uruguay, law enacted in the 1960s).

Finally, in the 1960s and 1970s the non-Latin Caribbean nations, newly independent mostly from the United Kingdom, enacted laws that granted cash benefits under social insurance, but they had previously adopted the British model of a national health system. In this final group, Haiti in 1967 was the last Latin American country that passed a law on sickness insurance, but it has not been enforced yet.

With few exceptions, the most developed and urbanized countries that had powerful trade unions (the "pioneers"), were the first in enacting such laws, while the least developed and urbanized countries were the last. In Argentina, Cuba, and Uruguay, the introduction of sickness insurance was delayed due to the early development of health care through mutual aid societies, cooperatives, and unions.

The remaining columns of Table 5 roughly identify the segment of the population legally covered. In the 16 countries with a national health system (all the non-Latin Caribbean, plus Cuba and Nicaragua) all residents are covered for benefits in kind. In addition, in 13 of these countries, social insurance covers all salaried employees with cash benefits (at least three countries exclude temporary and unpaid family

workers); in Jamaica, only domestic servants are eligible for a sickness grant; Bermuda and Suriname do not provide cash benefits.

Among the seventeen Latin American countries with a social insurance system in effect (excluding Haiti), eight have laws that cover all salaried employees (both for benefits in kind and cash), but several countries exclude temporary workers. In Venezuela geographic coverage is limited to the capital city and major urban areas, and in Paraguay and Peru the rural areas are not covered in practice. In the remaining nine countries, legal coverage is limited to a portion of salaried employees, generally excluding agricultural workers, domestic servants, and temporary workers. In Guatemala and Honduras, coverage is limited to the capital and urban areas, although the former is expanding coverage to rural areas.

In all countries (except Ecuador) the law covers the dependents of the insured (spouse and children under legal age) for benefits in kind, but at least six countries have limitations (e.g., only maternity in kind benefits for the wife or pediatric care for infants are granted).

Table 6 summarizes legal coverage information by type of work where the poor are normally concentrated. In the non-Latin Caribbean, as well as in Cuba and Nicaragua, the poor (in all listed categories) are legally eligible for benefits in kind under the national health system; hence, the table's information refers exclusively to cash benefits. In Latin America, coverage refers to both cash and in-kind benefits, but in Chile and Costa Rica, the poor are legally eligible only for benefits in kind. In practically all the countries, neither the unpaid family workers nor the unemployed are covered. In about half of the countries, the self-employed, domestic servants, and temporary/casual/seasonal workers are legally excluded; if

Table 6. **Type of work (where the poor are concentrated) not legally covered by social insurance in Latin America and the Caribbean, 1987–1988 (number of countries).**

Type of work	Legally covered[a]			Legally excluded[b]	Total
	Mandatory	Voluntary	Total		
Self-employed	6	11	17	17	34
Rural	21[d]	0	21[d]	13[d]	34
Domestic servants	14[c]	2	16	18	34
Temporary/casual	16	0	16	18	34
Unpaid family	0	1	1	33	34
Unemployed	0	0	0	34	34

Sources: Table 5 and additional legal information gathered by the author.
[a]Coverage of cash benefits in countries with national health systems (all types of work are covered on benefits in kind) and of both cash and in kind benefits in countries with social insurance systems.
[b]In three Latin American countries, "indigents" have the right to welfare benefits in kind.
[c]In two only for maternity.
[d]Salaried employment; other forms of agricultural work (self-employment, small landowners, sharecropping, seasonal) usually excluded.

voluntary affiliation of the self-employed is also excluded, this group's lack of coverage increases to 82%.

More than one-third of rural salaried workers are not legally covered, but there are significant exclusions in four countries. It should be noted, however, that most agricultural work is not salaried and permanent, but rather done by self-employed, temporary/seasonal workers, and independent small farmers or under sharecropping or similar arrangements; all these activities are usually not covered in most countries. In all the above cases, when workers are excluded from coverage their dependents are logically excluded as well, and among the poor, the number of dependents is usually higher than among middle- and high-income families.

I have demonstrated in a previous work (Mesa-Lago, 1978) that in most of Latin America, social insurance coverage evolved in a gradual and stratified manner, largely as a result of the pressure of the most powerful occupational groups (e.g., the armed forces, civil servants, the ''labor aristocracy''), who were able to obtain coverage earlier, better benefits, and proportionally lower contributions. Conversely, the least powerful groups (the self-employed, domestic servants, and agricultural workers, where poverty is concentrated) either were the last to be covered or still lack legal protection and are entitled (if at all) to the worst benefits.

For instance, in Chile and Peru, separate health care institutions covered the armed forces, white-collar employees, and blue-collar workers. In Mexico, there were separate services for the armed forces, civil servants, private white- and blue-collar workers, petroleum workers, railroad employees, and electrical utility workers. In the 1960s and 1970s, several countries underwent a process of unification, but by the end of the 1980s, there were still separate health care services in ten countries (even without considering the armed forces, which have their own health services in all countries except in Costa Rica and Cuba).

Statistical Coverage

Estimates of statistical coverage in Latin America and the Caribbean are not always reliable. For instance, an ILO report on Brazil acknowledged that coverage data on health care were highly speculative: there was no registry for the insured and data on contributions were so flawed that they could not be used as surrogates for registration figures. In countries that have multiple managing agencies, it is nearly impos-

sible to estimate the total coverage, because although there are statistics on the large agencies, there are none on the small ones. Thus, in Mexico it is easy to obtain data from the two largest agencies (covering salaried employees in the private sector, IMSS, and in the federal government, ISSSTE), but extremely difficult to obtain them from the agencies that cover the armed forces, petroleum employees, and other minor groups.

Table 7 shows data on social insurance coverage on sickness-maternity. Data on national health systems or the public health sector could not be obtained (figures for Bahamas, Barbados, Cuba, and Jamaica refer to cash benefits under social insurance). The table provides fair total coverage figures for countries with multiple agencies that have been the subject of careful study (Chile, Colombia, Mexico, Peru, and Uruguay), but only gives coverage under the main agency in those countries where an in-depth analysis has not been done (e.g., Bolivia, Paraguay, Venezuela). Another problem occurs in countries where a high percentage of health services are provided by mutual-aid societies, cooperatives, and private clinics for which data are almost unavailable (e.g., Argentina, Uruguay).

Health coverage of dependents, which is extremely important because it involves the largest cohort of insured, is grossly estimated in many countries using a dependents/insured ratio; small changes in that ratio can induce sizable increases or decreases in overall coverage. Therefore, data on coverage of the economically active population (EAP) are generally more reliable than those on coverage of the total population. Finally, there are problems of comparability; for instance, for Cuba Table 7 presents estimates based on legal coverage, because there are no statistics on coverage. Countries in which a single agency manages the entire system provide statistics on total coverage (e.g., the Ministry of Health in Nicaragua); other countries, even those with highly integrated health systems, often report coverage of social insurance, but not of the ministry of health nor of the indigent population covered by social insurance.

Despite the above-mentioned flaws, Table 7 offers the most reliable data currently available for the Region on coverage by social insurance for sickness-maternity. Data are included for all Latin American countries (except Haiti) and for three non-Latin Caribbean countries. Based on EAP coverage in 1985–1988, the countries can be ranked as follows: 80% to 100% in Cuba, Bar-

Table 7. Total and economically active population covered by social insurance in Latin America and the Caribbean, 1960–1988 (in percentages).

Countries	Economically active population				Total population	
	1960	1970	1980	1985–88	1980	1985–88
Argentina	55.2	68.0	69.1	79.1[f]	78.9	74.3[f]
Bahamas	n.a.	n.a.	85.3	85.9	n.a.	n.a.
Barbados	n.a.	75.3	79.8	96.9	n.a.	n.a.
Bolivia	8.8[b]	9.0	18.5	16.9	25.4	21.4
Brazil	23.1	27.0	87.0	n.a.	96.3	n.a.
Chile	70.8	75.6	61.2	79.2	67.3	n.a.
Colombia	8.0	22.2	30.4	30.2	15.2	16.0
Costa Rica	25.3	38.4	68.3	68.7	81.5[h]	84.6[h]
Cuba	62.6[a]	88.7[i]	93.0[d,i]	n.a.	100.0	n.a.
Dominican Republic	n.a.	8.9	11.6	10.2	n.a.	4.2
Ecuador	11.0	14.8	21.3	25.8	9.4	13.4
El Salvador	4.4	8.4	11.6	n.a.	6.2	n.a.
Guatemala	20.6	27.0	33.1	27.0	14.2	13.0
Honduras	3.7	4.2	14.4	12.8[f]	7.3	10.3[f]
Jamaica	n.a.	58.8	80.9	93.2	n.a.	n.a.
Mexico	15.6	28.1	42.0	40.2	53.4	59.7[e]
Nicaragua	5.9	14.8	18.9	31.5	9.1	37.5
Panama	20.6	33.4	52.3	59.8	49.9	57.4
Paraguay	8.0	10.7	14.0	n.a.	18.2	n.a.
Peru	24.8[b]	35.6[c]	37.4	32.0[j]	15.7[j]	22.2[j]
Uruguay	109.0[g]	95.4	81.2	73.0	68.5	67.0[e]
Venezuela	11.9	24.4	49.8	54.3	45.2	49.9[e]
Latin America	n.a.	n.a.	61.2	n.a.	61.2	n.a.
Excluding Brazil	n.a.	n.a.	42.7	n.a.	42.7	n.a.

Source: Mesa-Lago, 1990.
[a] 1958.
[b] 1961.
[c] 1969.
[d] 1981.
[e] 1983.
[f] 1984.
[g] More than 100% due to multiple coverage.
[h] Includes coverage of the dispossessed ("indigents").
[i] Estimate based on legal coverage and population censuses.
[j] Corrected figures.

bados, Jamaica, Brazil, and the Bahamas; 60% to 79% in Chile, Argentina, Uruguay, Costa Rica (these four countries would show a higher coverage if welfare programs were included), and Panama; 40% to 59% in Venezuela and Mexico; 20% to 39% in Peru, Nicaragua, Colombia, Guatemala, and Ecuador; and 1% to 19% in Bolivia, Paraguay, Honduras, El Salvador, and the Dominican Republic. Ranking by coverage of the total population on sickness-maternity is as follows: 80% to 100% in Brazil and Costa Rica (although there are no statistics for the Bahamas, Barbados, Cuba, and Jamaica, these four countries probably are included in this rank); 60% to 79% in Argentina, Uruguay, Chile (if coverage of "indigents" and mutual-aid societies were taken into account, these three countries would show higher percentages); 40% to 59% in Mexico, Panama, and Venezuela; 20% to 39% in Nicaragua and Bolivia; and 1% to 19% in Peru, Paraguay, Colombia, Ecuador, Guatemala, Honduras, El Salvador, and the Dominican Re-

public. The highest coverage is found in the most developed countries, which also have the oldest programs (with the exception of the non-Latin Caribbean).

Table 7 shows declines in population coverage between 1980 and 1985–1988 in Argentina (total population), Chile (a fall in the EAP coverage in 1980 and a subsequent recovery), Guatemala (both total and EAP), Honduras (EAP), Mexico (EAP), and Uruguay (both). In Brazil, coverage of the manufacturing sector in the EAP decreased from 79% to 62% in 1978–1983, and, although it rose in 1984–1985, it did not reach the previous level (McGreevey, 1988). These declines probably stem from the economic crisis, which has brought about increases in open unemployment and in the informal sector; however, some decreases may have been the result of changes in the coverage calculations.

In the penultimate line of Table 7, an estimate is made of overall coverage in Latin America in 1980, which is put at 61% for both the EAP and the total population. Without doubt, in this respect the Region leads the developing countries; furthermore, a group of Latin American countries has reached levels similar to those of the developed world. Thus, in the pioneer countries, in a couple of other Latin American countries, and in the non-Latin Caribbean, coverage has been rapidly expanded, and, if we take into account the protection of the indigent by welfare programs for sickness-maternity, it has become almost universal.

However, in most of the countries of Latin America, social insurance coverage is very low and structural barriers hinder its expansion. A more detailed analysis of Table 7 shows that the total coverage of the Region is strongly influenced by the very high coverage in Brazil, a country which concentrates more than half of all the insured in Latin America. Given that Brazilian data require more precision, the Latin American global coverage figures may be overestimated. When Brazil is excluded from the calculations, as in the last line of Table 7, coverage in Latin America drops to less than 43% of the EAP and the total population. Moreover, in about half the countries, coverage is less than one-third and in seven countries is less than 25%. As will be seen in the section ''Coverage and Extreme Poverty,'' beginning on p. 25, the poor are not covered by social insurance, particularly in Latin America. Based on the average annual rate of growth in coverage of the EAP in 1960–1985/1988, it would take from 45 to 64 years in Mexico, Nicaragua, and Colombia; from 80 to 98 years in Peru and Ecuador; from 176 to 272 years in Honduras, Bolivia, Paraguay, Guatemala, and El Salvador; and 530 years in the Dominican Republic for the social insurance system to reach universal coverage—and, hence, to protect the poor.

Inequalities in Coverage

In addition to low overall coverage, most Latin American countries suffer from uneven coverage among occupational groups, economic activities, and geographical areas. Coverage tends to be positively correlated with income, the degree of labor skills, the power of pressure groups, urban residency, and the level of regional development.

Occupational Groups

Surveys carried out in Argentina, Chile, Costa Rica, Cuba, Mexico, Peru, and Uruguay show that the emergence of coverage for various occupational groups was largely determined by the power of pressure groups, and that there was a gap of almost 200 years between the first and the last groups to be covered by pensions: the armed forces and civil servants were covered first, while agricultural workers, domestic servants, and the self-employed were covered last (if at all). The gap in sickness-maternity insurance is narrower and the sequence of inception is different than that for pensions, but still, agricultural workers, domestic servants, and the self-employed were the last to be covered (if at all). It should be noted that in most surveyed countries all the groups are covered, although the degree of coverage varies substantially, despite measures taken in most countries to make coverage more universal, unified, and uniform. These differences are much more significant in the countries with low coverage, inasmuch as the majority of the population is excluded from the social insurance system. A recent analysis for Brazil also shows a positive correlation between coverage, on the one hand, and skill and income on the other, with the lowest coverage being found among the unemployed unskilled workers (especially those in agriculture and self-employment) and the lowest income group (Mesa-Lago, 1978, 1990; Isuani, 1985).

Economic Activities

A 1970 study of ten Latin American countries showed that, in seven of them, social security covered less than 2% of agricultural workers, who represented more than one-third of the EAP. Information from Chile, Colombia, Costa Rica, Ecuador, Mexico, and Peru on the degree of coverage of the EAP in 1979–1984, by economic branch, indicates that the highest level of coverage is to be found in the electricity, gas, and water industries (64% to 100%), manufacturing (40% to 90%), and transport and communications (32% to 71%, except for Ecuador); the lowest is in agriculture (4% to 59%), with the highest percentages being in Costa Rica and Chile, countries where coverage is almost universal. Separate information on Bolivia shows that in 1986, 78% of mining and 108% of petroleum workers were covered by social insurance (some by more than one agency), but only 0.2% of agricultural workers were (Mallet, 1980; Mesa-Lago, 1990; Schulthess, 1988).

Geographical Units

Finally, information from Argentina, Bolivia, Chile, Colombia, Costa Rica, Ecuador, Mexico,

Panama, Peru, and Uruguay on differences in the degree of geographical coverage in 1979–1986, proves that the most developed states, provinces, or departments (those that are industrialized, unionized, urbanized, or those that have the highest percentage of wage earners and the highest per capita incomes) are substantially better covered than the least developed states, provinces, or departments (agricultural, little unionized, and rural and with a high proportion of self-employed persons and lowest per capita incomes). The extreme range of geographical coverage varies between 6% and 100% in Argentina, 11% and 33% in Bolivia, 39% and 95% in Chile, 3% and 25% in Colombia, 54% and 100% in Costa Rica, 3% and 20% in Ecuador, 17% and 100% in Mexico, 11% and 75% in Panama, 3% and 27% in Peru, and 17% and 69% in Uruguay. With two exceptions, the province, state, or department where the capital city is located is the one with the highest coverage (Mesa-Lago, 1990).

Coverage and Extreme Poverty

In Latin American countries, persons living below the poverty line are not usually protected by social insurance, with the exception of those countries that protect ''indigents'' through social insurance, such as Chile, Costa Rica, Cuba, and several non-Latin Caribbean countries. As we saw in the second chapter, the poor are either unemployed or underemployed, are seasonal or temporary workers, or are unpaid family workers, and, therefore, are not employed on a permanent full-time basis. Even though they may be employed, they work in occupations that are not covered or that have low coverage in most of the countries, such as agriculture (especially self-employed or small farmers, sharecroppers, etc.), domestic service, and self-employment. We also have noted that in 1980, 33% of the Latin American population lived below the poverty line, and that this proportion increased to 39% in 1985.

According to Table 7, in 1980, 39% of the total population of Latin America was not covered by social insurance, and we have seen that, due to the economic crisis, coverage had not significantly increased in 1985–1988, and even had declined in some countries. Based on the rationale used by Altimir (discussed in Chapter 2) and the above analysis on the characteristics of the insured (income, occupation, geographical location), we conclude that the poor are not covered by social insurance and only have access to usually insufficient and underfinanced public health and social welfare services.

The Latin American and Caribbean countries with the highest degree of social insurance coverage also are those that have the lowest proportion of poor (e.g., Argentina, Chile, Costa Rica, Cuba, Uruguay—Brazil is an exception), but even in most of these countries the percentage of the uncovered population (15% to 30%) is greater than the percentage of those below the poverty line (8% to 24%). Part of the difference is made up by the highest income group, which is not covered by social insurance, but pockets of poor left without health care protection may remain in those countries unless the public health sector takes care of them. In the least developed countries, where the majority of the population is not covered by social insurance (63% to 94%), where public health services are grossly insufficient, and where poverty incidence is highest (45% to 65%), the poor obviously lack access to health care (Mesa-Lago, 1983, 1990b).

Most of the surveys on coverage inequality in the Region have been conducted in the relatively more developed countries; none have been carried out in the least developed countries where such inequalities would be worse. Furthermore, most of those surveys were done before the crisis of the 1980s, and little or no data are available on how that crisis affected these inequalities. Finally, the only study available on the lack of coverage of the most needy groups used data up to 1980, and, in the 1980s there should have been an increase in the extreme poverty population.

Several experts have pointed out that the Bismarckian model of social insurance, which finances social insurance through contributions from the worker and employer based on the worker's wages, has not been able to operate satisfactorily in most of Latin America, despite modifications introduced to the original model (Arroba, 1979). This is due to the fact that in the developed countries of Europe, most of the labor force consisted of wage-earning urban workers, while in many Latin American countries, the labor force is overwhelmingly composed of agricultural workers, the self-employed, and unpaid family workers. The self-employed often cannot afford to pay the employer's contribution, and agricultural workers have low incomes, are scattered, and are frequently migrant, often changing employer.

The first (left) segment in Table 8 shows that in the Region's most developed countries (Argentina, Barbados, Brazil, Chile, Costa Rica, Cuba, Panama, Trinidad and Tobago, Uruguay, and Venezuela), wage earners comprise from

Table 8. Percentage distribution of the labor force by occupational category and sector in Latin America and the Caribbean, between 1980 and 1983.

Countries	By occupational category[a]			By sector			
				Urban		Rural	
	Salaried	Self-employed	Unpaid relatives	Formal	Informal[b]	Modern	Traditional
Argentina	71.2	25.1	3.2	65.0	19.4	8.8	6.3
Barbados	78.2	9.8	0.8	n.a.	n.a.	n.a.	n.a.
Bolivia	38.2	48.9	9.2	17.9	23.2	5.2	50.9
Brazil	65.3	27.0	5.1	45.2	16.9	9.8	27.6
Chile	66.7	25.3	3.6	54.1	20.1	14.0	8.8
Colombia	53.5	--------- 42.5 ---------			42.6	22.3	15.8	18.7
Costa Rica	75.2	19.6	3.9	52.9	12.4	19.6	14.8
Cuba	94.1	5.7	0.2	n.a.	n.a.	n.a.	n.a.
Dominican Republic	51.3	36.5	3.3	42.6	16.0	16.7	24.6
Ecuador	47.6	37.3	5.8	22.7	25.4	13.7	37.9
El Salvador	59.2	28.2	10.9	28.6	18.9	22.3	30.1
Guatemala	46.9	42.2	6.7	26.7	17.8	22.3	33.1
Haiti	16.6	59.4	10.4	n.a.	n.a.	n.a.	n.a.
Honduras	45.4	33.3	14.6	25.6	17.2	24.4	32.5
Mexico	c	c	c	39.5	22.0	19.2	18.4
Nicaragua	n.a.	n.a.	n.a.	29.5	28.3	18.0	23.8
Panama	63.3	23.2	3.6	45.3	20.9	9.1	24.6
Paraguay	36.7	41.2	11.6	n.a.	n.a.	n.a.	n.a.
Peru	45.1	49.1	5.8	35.0	23.8	8.0	32.0
Trinidad and Tobago	80.1	14.6	3.5	n.a.	n.a.	n.a.	n.a.
Uruguay	69.4	23.8	2.0	63.3	19.0	9.5	8.0
Venezuela	64.1	26.5	3.1	62.6	16.4	4.4	15.1

Sources: PREALC, 1982; Mesa-Lago, 1990.

[a]Excludes a small percentage of nonclassified workers. Self-employed includes employers. Years do not correspond to 1980–1983 in Bolivia (1976), Honduras (1977), and Uruguay (1975). There are no figures available for the Bahamas and Jamaica.

[b]Includes domestic service.

[c]Results of the 1980 census are not reliable; they give a very high percentage (22%) of nonclassified workers.

63% to 94% of the labor force, and less than one-third of the labor force is either self-employed or works for a relative without pay; this explains why the Bismarckian model has been able to function and extend its coverage in these countries. On the other hand, in the least developed countries (e.g., Bolivia, Guatemala, Haiti, Honduras, Paraguay, and Peru), from 48% to 70% of the labor force is either self-employed or an unpaid family worker (and a similar proportion is engaged in agriculture). These countries are precisely those that have the lowest social insurance coverage, and extending coverage in them beyond the salaried labor force would be very difficult using the Bismarckian model.

In research conducted on the determinants of social insurance coverage of the EAP in all Latin American countries, several independent variables were tested, and the regression showed that the percent of the salaried EAP explained .622 of coverage. A dummy variable, "political commitment," was introduced, whose value was "1" when state initiative was present (e.g., through law and direct state action on social insurance) and "0" when it was absent. The best fit was obtained when the two variables—salaried EAP and political commitment—were

regressed jointly, and they explained .793 of coverage (Mesa-Lago, Cruz-Saco, and Zamalloa, 1990). These empirical findings prove what specialists have alleged for years.

Protection of the Informal Sector

Another way to approach the problem of universal coverage is to look at the size of the formal sector. The second (right) segment of Table 8 presents the distribution of the EAP by sectors: formal, informal, modern, and traditional.

When one compares the percentage of the EAP in the urban-formal sector (Table 8) with the percentage of the EAP covered by social insurance (Table 7), one finds a remarkable correspondence between both in most Latin American and Caribbean countries. A few countries have been able to extend coverage somewhat beyond the formal urban sector, either because they have a relatively modern and unionized rural sector (e.g., Chile and Costa Rica) or because, having a large traditional rural sector, they have created new methods of financing—the urban sector provides at least partial support for the extension of primary health care coverage to rural areas (e.g., Brazil) or the state and social insurance provides such coverage (e.g., Mexico). In Colombia and Venezuela, the percentage covered by social insurance is substantially lower than the percentage in the formal urban sector, indicating that these countries—particularly the latter, which has relatively abundant resources—could make a greater effort to expand coverage, even within the narrow limits of the Bismarckian model. Only in Brazil and Uruguay does social insurance coverage exceed the sum of the formal urban and modern rural sectors, which indicates the obstacles involved in expanding coverage to the informal urban and traditional rural sectors. In these two sectors we find the self-employed and unpaid family workers who are typically underemployed and have low incomes, making it difficult for them to finance their own coverage.

The possibility for rapidly expanding social insurance coverage seems remote for many Latin American and Caribbean countries. Between 1950 and 1980 (years of rapid economic expansion in the Region), the formal urban sector grew by more than 14%, but the modern rural sector shrank by almost 10%. The growth of the formal sector was insufficient to absorb the increase in the labor supply, the intense rural to urban migration, and the already existing levels of underemployment. (Production methods that emphasize capital vis-a-vis labor hamper labor absorption.) In the same period, the traditional and informal sectors in the Region declined by 4% (the traditional sector dropped by almost 10%, but the informal sector increased by almost 6%).

In order to reduce the informal and traditional sectors by one-third by the year 2000, it was calculated that an annual growth in GDP of 7.5% would be needed. However, due to the economic crisis of the 1980s, the Region has experienced an annual average negative growth rate: −8.3% in 1980–1989. Employment in the formal sector declined by 6% in 1980–1985, while employment in the informal sector increased by 5% and the rate of unemployment rose by 1% (ECLAC, 1989; PREALC, 1981a, 1988). According to Table 7, coverage of the EAP by social insurance declined in some countries, probably due to the above-mentioned causes.

Table 9 offers data on social insurance coverage of the informal sector in nine Latin American and Caribbean countries in 1980–1987. As a percentage of the EAP, the informal sector ranges from 20% in Chile to 55% in Peru. The percentage of coverage of the self-employed (a very important component of the informal sec-

Table 9. Statistical coverage of the informal sector by social insurance in selected countries of Latin America and the Caribbean, 1980–1987.

Countries	% informal sector over EAP[a]	% coverage informal sector[b]	% contribution over income paid by:	
			Salaried	Self-employed
Bahamas	n.a.	48.4	1.7–3.4	6.8–8.8
Barbados	n.a.	24.8	4.6–5.5	8
Chile	20.1[c]	11.9–17.5	20.6–28.5	19.4–27.4
Colombia	22.3[c]	0.6	4.5–6.2	15–20
Costa Rica	21.6	93.0	9	12.2–19.5
Jamaica	37.7	4.0	2.5	5
Mexico	30.9	0.8	3.75	13.57
Panama	20.9[c]	1.5	7.25	18–22
Peru	54.9	4.0	6	18

Source: Mesa-Lago, 1990a.
[a]Self-employed workers, plus domestic servants, plus unpaid family workers over EAP; excludes informal wage earners.
[b]Only self-employed.
[c]All the informal sector.

tor) ranges from 0.6% to 4% in Colombia, Mexico, Panama, Jamaica, and Peru; from 12% to 48% in Chile, Barbados, and the Bahamas; and reaches 93% in Costa Rica (due to coverage of ''indigents''). Although coverage of the self-employed is mandatory in Jamaica, only 4% of them are actually covered. One of the reasons for the low coverage of this sector is the heavy contributory burden. Table 9 shows that the percentage of contribution to be paid by the self-employed is from two to four times the percentage to be paid by the salaried worker; the only exception is in Chile where both percentage contributions are similar. This largely explains the low coverage of this group, as well as the high degree of payment evasion and delays in countries with mandatory coverage (Mesa-Lago, 1990a).

Unfortunately, there is no adequate data on salaried workers of small informal enterprises who could qualify as poor. A key question is whether these workers would join social insurance, to which they are often legally entitled, if they had a realistic option to do so. Scattered information suggests they would not, because the cost of joining the system would be too high for them. In any case, the informal employer, by saving in social insurance and other taxes, as well as by paying lower wages and offering fewer fringe benefits, reduces production costs and successfully competes with formal enterprises. This could lead to a shutdown of the formal sector, with labor transferring to the informal sector and, in turn, reducing social insurance coverage and revenue. And yet, forcing the informal employer to fulfill his obligations to social insurance (assuming enforcement is feasible, which it seldom is) would substantially reduce his small profit, potentially provoking the shutdown of enterprises and an increase in unemployment (Mesa-Lago, 1990a).

Given the growth of the informal sector in the 1980s, it is all the more imperative to explore conventional (social insurance) and unconventional (mutual aid societies, collective insurance policies with low premiums, solidarity groups) alternatives to protect this sector. Chapter 3 of this study reviews the approaches of Costa Rica, Mexico, and Peru.

Protection of the Rural Sector

Several countries have made great strides in extending health care coverage to the rural sector: in Cuba and Nicaragua through national health systems; in Chile (Castañeda, 1989) and Costa Rica through sickness-maternity insurance programs that protect the ''indigent'' as welfare cases; and in Panama through the process of integration and expansion of rural infrastructure for primary health care. In addition, Brazil, Ecuador, and Mexico have significantly extended coverage of peasants through innovative programs that deserve mention. Mexico's experience will be discussed in detail in Chapter 4; hence, the other two approaches will be explored here.

In Brazil, the social security system (SINPAS) extended coverage to rural areas in the 1970s through two programs: one of social insurance (FUNRURAL) and another of the federal Ministry of Health and states' health services (PIASS). FUNRURAL began independently in 1971, granting welfare pensions and health care to the rural population and towns with fewer than 20,000 inhabitants through a network of facilities (health posts and centers, polyclinics, and hospitals) developed through agreements with trade unions, states, municipalities, and private institutions. In 1977, FUNRURAL became part of the social insurance system, and was financed by three taxes: 2.4% on the payroll of urban enterprises (this tax generated 63% of total revenue in 1980); 2.5% on rural production, collected by the producer and paid by the buyer (35% of total revenue); and 0.036% paid by rural employers based on the value of agricultural production or the value of noncultivated farms (2% of total revenue).

From 1978 through the 1980s, the program operated at a deficit (11% of revenue in 1981) that resulted from an evasion estimated at between one-third and one-half of the potential revenue of the three taxes combined. To help finance the program, FINSOCIAL was created in 1982, with a contribution of 0.5% of the revenue of all the country's enterprises. In addition to its financial imbalance, FUNRURAL was basically a curative model that was not tailored to the sector needs; its resources were predominantly allocated to urban over rural zones and to developed over underdeveloped regions; its equipment was insufficient and deteriorated and its services were of poor quality; medicines were scarce; access to hospitals was restricted; and high user fees precluded the lowest income group from using the services.

PIASS was created in 1976 to provide primary health care to rural zones and small towns and rapidly spread nationwide, first under the Ministry of Health and later under the responsibility of the states. In 1979, the program suffered a serious financial crisis and was rescued by social insurance, but at a price—its approach became predominantly curative and with less community participation. At the beginning of the 1980s there was a plan to create a national health system that would consolidate all existing programs, including FUNRURAL and PIASS. The plan's features involved a twofold increase of the federal government financing, priority to primary health care, and an increase in the role of community assistants. Integration was achieved by the end of the 1980s, thus eliminating the special programs as such; since 1990 all health services came under the Ministry of Health and all pensions, under the Ministry of Labor and Social Insurance. Reportedly, the economic crisis of the 1980s did not affect the quantity of peasants covered, but it did affect the quality of the services provided (McGreevey et al, 1984; Rezende, 1983; Delyle Guerra de Macedo, 1990).

In Ecuador, the Peasant Social Security (SSC) began in 1968 as part of the Ecuadorian Social Security Institute (IESS), and was pushed forward in 1973 and 1981. Peasants (and their dependent family) who are organized in cooperatives and agrarian associations are eligible; in 1987, SSC covered 4.8% of the total population and 10% of the rural population. Emphasis is on primary health care at low cost, and the services are based on a rural post built on community land with a basic structure supplied by IESS and erected through community work. A traveling physician offers medical, maternity, and dental care at the post, while auxiliary permanent personnel provide prenatal care, health education, and immunization. Patients who cannot be treated at the rural post would be referred to more complex IESS facilities.

The program is financed with a 1% contribution from the payroll of all those insured at IESS (paid in equal parts by the insured, the employer, and the state), plus the equivalent of 1% of the minimum wage which is paid by the participating peasant (in 1985 the minimum wage doubled, making the peasant contribution very heavy). It is impossible to estimate SSC costs or its financial stability, but, being a part of IESS, it can be guessed that it operates with a deficit; scattered information suggests that hospitalization costs are high. Coverage has increased at a low rate in 20 years and there are indications of discrimination against the poorest, most isolated peasant population; a low number of referrals to higher levels of attention; and different treatment of peasants and of insured at IESS facilities. Furthermore, the SSC does not coordinate with the rural health system of the Ministry, its number of immunizations is small, and it only pays lip service to basic sanitation. The economic crisis of the 1980s harmed this program (Mesa-Lago, 1984, 1989b).

Despite the importance of the described programs, there are very few serious studies of their characteristics, effects, and potential for replication elsewhere.

The Cost of Universalization and Coverage of the Poor

The cost of extending social insurance coverage to all the population in Latin American and Caribbean countries using the current Bismarckian model would not be economically viable in many countries, even were they able to overcome the structural barriers. Table 10 shows how social insurance expenditures (all programs, not only sickness-maternity, because we lack separate data for that program on all countries) over GDP would increase in 22 countries if coverage were granted to the whole population under the current model. The estimates in the third column of figures in Table 10 were obtained by roughly extrapolating the expenditures for a 100% coverage, assuming that such expenditures would increase proportionally with coverage.

According to Table 10, only six countries would reach universal coverage with a relatively low percentage of GDP: Jamaica (0.5%), Bahamas (0.8%), Barbados (1.2%), Venezuela (2.9%), and Mexico and Brazil (5.4%). The three non-Latin Caribbean countries have the lowest

Table 10. Social insurance expenditures as a percentage of GDP in 1980 and extrapolated on the basis of universal coverage, in Latin America and the Caribbean.

Countries	Social insurance expenditures[a] as % of GDP (1980)	% of total population covered (1980)	Extrapolation of % of social insurance expenditures over GDP when 100% of population is covered
Argentina	11.9	78.9	15.1
Bahamas	0.7	85.3[b]	0.8
Barbados	1.0	79.8[b]	1.2
Bolivia	2.9	25.4	11.4
Brazil	5.2	96.3	5.4
Chile	11.0	67.3	16.3
Colombia	2.8	15.2	18.4
Costa Rica	7.5	81.5	9.2
Cuba	8.6	100.0[c]	8.6
Dominican Republic	0.7	4.2[d]	16.7
Ecuador	3.7	9.4	39.4
El Salvador	1.3	6.2	21.0
Guatemala	1.6	14.2	11.3
Honduras	0.9	7.3	12.3
Jamaica	0.4	80.9[b]	0.5
Mexico	2.9	53.4	5.4
Nicaragua	2.3	9.1	25.3
Panama	6.1	49.9	12.2
Paraguay	1.2	18.2	6.6
Peru	2.6	15.7	16.6
Uruguay	8.1	68.5	11.8
Venezuela	1.3	45.2	2.9

Source: Mesa-Lago, Cruz-Saco, and Zamalloa, 1990.
[a]Includes all social insurance programs.
[b]Economically active population covered by cash benefits; the total population is legally covered on health care by public health.
[c]Legal coverage.
[d]Only IDSS.

projected costs because they exclude public health care expenditures and because their pension programs are new; if the cost of health care had been included (to make it more comparable with social insurance sickness-maternity costs in Latin America), their extrapolated percentages would be more in line with that of Brazil. Mexico's and Venezuela's very high GDP, due to the oil boom, reduces the relative cost of their coverage; Venezuela also has one of the newest pension programs in the Region. Finally, Brazil and Mexico, as mentioned earlier, have significantly expanded coverage to the rural sector through innovative, relatively low-cost programs, and that partly explains the small extrapolated percentage in both countries.

Next, with higher extrapolated percentages, are Paraguay (6.6%, but there are serious questions about this country's quality of data), Cuba (8.6%), and Costa Rica (9.2%); the last two already cover all or practically all their populations. Another group of countries that already approximates universal coverage, but with ever higher extrapolated percentages, are Uruguay (11.8%), Argentina (15.1%), and Chile (16.3%). But these three countries, as well as Costa Rica, have either social insurance or public health programs for the dispossessed; hence, the extrapolation exaggerates the cost of universal protection.

In some of the least developed Latin American countries, the extrapolated cost (percentage) of universal coverage would be intolerable, such as in Ecuador (39.4%), Nicaragua (25.3%), El Salvador (21%), Colombia (18.4%), and Peru (16.6%). Extension of coverage in the Region (particularly in the less developed countries) cannot be attained with the current levels of benefit and administrative structure, because the financial burden would be intolerable, as has happened already in some of the pioneer countries (Mesa-Lago, Cruz-Saco, and Zamalloa, 1990).

Summary of Access of the Poor to Health Care

Information on both legal and statistical health care coverage of the population in Latin America and the Caribbean demonstrates that the poor are not protected in most countries. In those countries that have national health systems (mostly the non-Latin Caribbean), the poor appear to be legally covered by benefits in kind; this also is true in 4 out of 20 Latin American countries. But most labor categories where

the poor are concentrated are not legally eligible for cash benefits in the Region—unpaid family workers and the unemployed are excluded in practically all countries, as well as the self-employed, domestic servants, and temporary/casual workers in one-half of the countries, and rural salaried workers in one-third of the countries. Statistically, about 39% of the population of Latin America is reportedly not covered, but the proportion rises to 57% if Brazil is excluded; in about one-third of the countries, the proportion increases to 75%. At the 1960–1988 annual average growth rate of population coverage expansion, it would take eleven Latin American countries between 45 and 530 years to reach universal coverage.

The least developed, urbanized, unionized geographical regions of Latin America, as well as the primary economic activities and the least powerful occupations where the poor are concentrated (self-employment, domestic service, agriculture) are those with the lowest degree of coverage or a lack of protection altogether. The proportion of the Latin American population that is not covered roughly coincides with the proportion of that population living below the poverty line. A structural barrier to the extension of coverage is the Bismarckian model of social insurance financed with wage contributions. The most developed countries where the majority of the labor force is salaried have been able to reach or approximate universal coverage, but the least developed countries where the majority of the labor force is not salaried (self-employed, domestic servants, unpaid family workers, owners of microenterprises, small farmers, and peasants) cannot expand coverage beyond the small proportion in the urban formal and rural modern sectors. With the informal sector growth in the 1980s, the possibility of expanding social insurance coverage became more remote; statistical coverage actually even declined in some countries. Coverage of the self-employed (a key group in the informal sector) is extremely low, ranging from 0.6% to 25% in seven countries, and reaching 48% in the Bahamas and 93% in Costa Rica. Even the unconventional programs to cover peasants in Brazil, Ecuador, and Mexico either cover a small proportion of the population or have been harmed by the economic crisis of the 1980s, or both. The cost of reaching universal coverage, and, hence, protecting the poor, under the current model of social insurance would be unfeasible in many countries: from 11% to 39% of GDP in 13 of them.

HEALTH STANDARDS AND FACILITIES, AND THEIR INEQUALITIES

Health Standards and Facilities in the Region

Health standards in Latin America and the Caribbean are the highest in the developing world (see Table 11). In 1980, the regional average of infant mortality was 66 per 1,000 and life expectancy was 64 years among females and 60 years among males. These averages were considerably better than those of Africa, Asia, and the Middle East, and superior to world averages. Only the averages of industrialized countries and those of European countries at a middle stage of development surpassed those of Latin America and the Caribbean. The fact that the Region's countries are at an intermediate level of development (ahead of other developing areas of the world) probably helps explain why Latin America and the Caribbean lead in health standards. However, it is impossible to separate this variable from others such as social insurance and public health programs, education, and nutrition.

The Region's high world rank hides substantial variations in health standards and facilities among Latin American and Caribbean countries. As Table 12 shows, the most developed Latin American countries (Argentina, Chile, Costa Rica, Cuba, Uruguay, Venezuela), as well as those in the non-Latin Caribbean (not necessarily at the same levels of development as the others), have the best facilities and standards. Conversely, the least developed countries (Bolivia, the Dominican Republic, Ecuador, El Salvador, Guatemala, Haiti, Honduras, Nicaragua) have the worst facilities and standards. However, there are important exceptions. For instance, Argentina and, to a lesser extent, Brazil rank as the countries with the best and relatively good facilities, respectively, but have relatively high and very high infant mortality rates. Peru ranks in an intermediate level regarding the supply of physicians, but is among the four countries with the worst health standards. Conversely, Costa Rica has relatively few hospital beds, but is among the three countries with the best health standards.

Inequalities in Health Facilities and Standards

The averages in Table 12 hide significant disparities among population groups. The above-noted inconsistencies between health facilities and standards might be explained by the fact that such facilities are not allocated according to the population's most urgent needs, but respond to other factors. Table 13 shows the distribution of health expenditures among public, social insurance, and private sectors. As we saw with health revenues (Table 4), data in Table 13 indicate that countries where social insurance covers from 13% to 18% of the population (e.g., Colombia, Ecuador, Peru) spend from 38% to 54% of total health expenditures. In 1984, the ratio of per capita expenditure between social insurance and the ministry of health was 7 to 1 in Colombia and 5 to 1 in Ecuador and Peru. It should be recalled that the population covered by social insurance has a higher income than the population covered by the ministry.

Furthermore, the bulk of social insurance health expenditures goes to the population in productive age—the majority of the insured—

Table 11. Comparison of Latin American and Caribbean health standards with those in other world regions, 1980.

| | Industrialized countries | Developing countries | | | | |
		Europe	Latin America and the Caribbean	Asia, Pacific, Middle East	Africa	Total
Mortality rates						
General	9.5	10.1	8.7	10.2	17.7	10.7
Infant	15.8	25.1	66.2	80.7	121.1	66.7
Life expectancy						
Men	68.9	67.1	59.7	55.8	44.4	58.4
Women	76.6	73.4	63.8	57.5	46.6	61.9
Composite index	1.0	0.8	0.2	−0.2	−1.5	0.0
Number of countries	22	7	34	24	38	125

Source: Mesa-Lago, 1990.
Method: Factor analysis, based on regional averages weighted by population. The World Bank classification by regions was used.

Table 12. Health facilities and standards in Latin America and the Caribbean, 1980–1985.

Countries	Hospital beds per 1,000 inhabitants (1980–1985)	Physicians per 10,000 inhabitants (1980–1985)	Infant mortality (1985)	Life expectancy (1985)
Argentina	5.4	25.7	34	70
Bahamas	4.3	10.0	27[c]	69
Barbados	8.7	8.5	17[c]	72[c]
Bolivia	1.8	5.1	117	53
Brazil	4.2	7.8	67	65
Chile	3.5	9.7	20	69
Colombia	1.7	5.8	55	65
Costa Rica	3.3	10.0	18	74
Cuba	4.6	20.8	17	74
Dominican Republic	2.1	5.7	74	64
Ecuador	1.7	8.8	50	64
El Salvador	1.2	3.2	65	64
Guatemala	1.6	4.1	65	60
Haiti	0.9[a]	1.2	123	54
Honduras	1.3	4.0	76	62
Jamaica	2.8	3.4	27[c]	71
Mexico	1.2	9.0	39[c]	67
Nicaragua	1.6	6.7	69	59
Panama	3.2	10.3	25	72
Paraguay	1.0	6.2	43	66
Peru	1.7	8.7	95	60[c]
Trinidad and Tobago	4.5[b]	7.4	22	69
Uruguay	6.0	19.9	30[c]	71
Venezuela	2.7	12.0	37	70

Source: Mesa-Lago, 1989.
[a]Only in the Ministry of Health.
[b]1975.
[c]1984.

Table 13. Percentage distribution of health expenditures by sector in selected countries of Latin America, 1980–1986.

Countries	Public sector[a]	Social insurance	Private sector	Total
Argentina	29.6	36.6	33.8	100.0
Brazil	30.7	31.2	38.1	100.0
Colombia	41.3	54.3	4.4	100.0
Costa Rica	19.3	80.7	n.a.	100.0
Ecuador	62.2	37.8	n.a.	100.0
Mexico	15.0	85.0	n.a.	100.0
Peru	59.0	41.0	n.a.[c]	100.0
Uruguay	33.2	7.7	59.1[b]	100.0
Venezuela	25.0	75.0	n.a.[c]	100.0

Source: Mesa-Lago, 1989.
[a]Includes Ministry of Health, armed forces, autonomous agencies, etc.
[b]Includes mutual-aid societies, cooperatives, and similar organizations.
[c]De Ferranti reports 53% for Peru and 58% for Venezuela.

which has a lower sickness risk than the infant-maternal population. In 1985, 30% of the productive-age population was insured in Peru, but only 1.4% of the population below 14 years of age was covered. In Colombia in 1984, the proportions were 15% and 3.6%, respectively. Yet, these two countries have the third and tenth highest infant mortality rates among 24 countries of the Region. There are no data for the least developed countries (e.g., Bolivia, Honduras, El Salvador, Guatemala), but it is highly probable that they confront a similar or worse situation than that of the two countries cited. In all of these countries the infant mortality rate is very high, and this contributes to a low life expectancy. A shift in the allocation of health resources that gives a higher proportion to the public sector and places more emphasis on infant and maternal care, sanitation, vaccination, and health education would reduce infant mortality and increase life expectancy in those countries.

Table 14 notes other inequalities in the distribution of health facilities among institutions that cover various population groups in four countries: in two countries the best facilities are those of the private sector, and in another country, they are second only to those of the armed forces; the armed forces have from three to four times better facilities than the ministry of health; and social insurance has better facilities than the ministry, which has the worst. With the exception of care received from the private sector, the insured do not fully pay for the services. The armed forces and social insurance groups, usually in the middle-income bracket and enjoying good to excellent services, receive

Table 14.   Inequalities in health care facilities[a] among providers in selected countries of Latin America, 1980–1984.

Providers	Colombia (1984) Hospital beds	Ecuador (1983) Hospital beds	Mexico (1980) Hospital beds	Mexico (1980) Physicians	Peru (1982) Hospital beds	Peru (1982) Physicians
Social insurance	1.4	1.9	1.2–1.4[b]	11.8–24.9[b]	1.6	11.1
Ministry of Health	1.2	1.2	1.1	6.7	1.8	5.1
Armed forces	n.a.	5.6	4.1	23.8	2.3	20.4
Private sector	5.6	4.7	n.a.	n.a.	1.1	70.8

Source: Mesa-Lago, 1990.
[a]Hospital beds per 1,000 covered and physicians per 10,000 covered.
[b]IMSS, ISSSTE, Petroleum.

transfers from the lowest income group covered by the ministry, which has the worst services.

Inequalities in health care are not limited to occupational groups, but also exist among geographical units. Studies of ten Latin American countries (Argentina, Chile, Colombia, Costa Rica, Cuba, Ecuador, Mexico, Panama, Peru, and Uruguay), based on scattered 1979–1984 data (see Table 15), have measured extreme differences in hospital beds and physicians per population between the best and worst geographical areas (states, departments, provinces). Those differences are positively correlated with the previously discussed degree of population coverage, and show that the least developed, poorest, isolated, rural regions (with the highest concentration of Indian population) have the worst services. Conversely, the most developed, wealthiest, urban regions (where the capital city is located) have the best services. Extreme disparities were found in Peru for physicians (63:1) and in Mexico for hospital beds (8:1). An analysis conducted in several countries of the level of development of regions and health facilities they have, found a positive significant correlation coefficient between these two variables (Mesa-Lago, 1978, 1985a, 1988c). We should recall that coverage of social insurance is concentrated in the urban, most developed areas, while the ministry of health is expected to protect the bulk of the rural population, the marginalized urban population, and the least developed regions.

In part, the above-mentioned inequalities are explained by the natural concentration of high-level health services in urban areas, but they are too great to be exclusively explained by this—they respond to political and economic factors as well. For instance, in 1983 the city of Lima had 31% of the nation's population, but concentrated 70% of all the physicians, 68% to 75% of nurses and health technicians, 61% of outpatient consultations, and 67% of laboratory tests, which could help explain the inconsistency between a high supply of physicians and extremely poor health standards in Peru. A proper

Table 15.   Geographic inequalities in population coverage and health facilities in selected countries of Latin America, 1979–1986 (compares most and least developed geographical unit).

Countries	Coverage of total population (%)	Physicians per 10,000 inhabitants	Hospital beds per 1,000 inhabitants
Argentina (1980)			
Federal Capital	123.9[a]	46.8	8.4
Formosa	6.0[a]	8.1	4.3
Bolivia (1986)			
Oruro	32.8	n.a.	0.9
Pando	10.7	n.a.	0.2
Chile (1980)			
Magallanes	95.0[c]	5.3	4.8
La Araucania	39.3[c]	2.1	3.2
Colombia (1984)			
Atlántico	24.7	n.a.	n.a.
Choco	2.7	n.a.	n.a.
Costa Rica (1979)			
San José	33.9[b]	12.4	5.7
Guanacaste	15.2[b]	1.9	1.1
Cuba (1982)			
Havana	n.a.	41.2	11.2
Granma	n.a.	7.2	4.1
Ecuador (1986)			
Pichincha	20.8	14.4	2.8
Los Rios	5.3	4.0	1.6
Mexico (1980)			
Federal District	100.4	21.1[d]	3.3[d]
Oaxaca	17.2	2.4[d]	0.4[d]
Panama (1984)			
Panamá	75.2	10.7	5.2
Darien	10.8	4.0	2.7
Peru (1981)			
Lima	26.7	19.0	3.0
Apurímac	2.5	0.3	0.6
Uruguay (1984)			
Montevideo	68.7[e]	35.4	3.8
Rivera	17.0[e]	6.5	1.8

Source: Mesa-Lago, 1990.
[a]1960.
[b]Excludes family dependents.
[c]EAP.
[d]1970.
[e]Members of collective institutions (1986).

geographical deconcentration of health expenditures and facilities would improve health standards in the least developed regions, which have the majority of the poor and the most urgent needs.

Finally, a highly stratified health care system (i.e., many providers covering different population groups with diverse benefit packages) appears to generate marked inequalities in both the services and the health standards. Conversely, integrated health care systems or those that are highly coordinated tend to reduce such inequalities. Several non-Latin Caribbean countries have achieved exceptionally high health standards, despite the fact that they do not have developed economies. Although these countries' small size may partially explain this, their national health care systems seem to have played an important role, too.

The Redistributive Impact of Health Programs: Do the Poor Benefit?

Several experts agree that, within social insurance, the effect of health benefits in kind on income distribution is more progressive than that of cash benefits (Rezende, 1974; Green, 1977; Mesa-Lago, 1983a). The reason is that benefits in kind—medical-hospital care—are basically equal (although in stratified systems there are differences in access to and the quality of services), while cash benefits, not only for sickness-maternity but also for pensions, etc., are established according to income. Furthermore, the lower-income groups suffer a higher incidence of disease (due to poor nutrition and hygiene), and since private medicine is prohibitive for them, the poor use the health program more frequently than those with a higher income. The latter, although covered, normally prefer to use private doctors and clinics, and only resort to social insurance in extreme cases. However, by the same token, public health expenditures should have a more progressive impact on distribution than social insurance sickness-maternity expenditures, because the former benefit the poorest group of the population. Hence, there should be a more progressive distribution effect in those countries that have a national health system. The evaluation is more difficult in those countries that have both social insurance and a ministry of health.

A few country studies have been done in Latin America (none in the non-Latin Caribbean) on the distributive effect of social insurance (particularly the sickness-maternity program) and public health, as well as a five-country comparative study on the distributive impact of public health subsidies.

Table 16 summarizes the results of three pioneering studies: one on Brazil focused on all social insurances, but was limited to the urban sector, while the ones on Chile and Costa Rica dealt with social insurance sickness-maternity plus public health. The most progressive effect appeared in Brazil, where the two insured groups with the least income received benefits 23% higher than what they contributed, while the two groups with the highest income paid 21% more than what they received. (Excluded from the study were FUNRURAL, which should have had a strong progressive effect, and the armed forces and civil servants who probably received more than what they contributed.)

In Chile, the two lowest-income groups received 7% more than what they contributed (a

Table 16. Impact of social insurance and public health programs on income distribution in selected countries of Latin America between 1969 and 1978.

BRAZIL (1973)[a]		
Units of legal minimum wage	% distribution of contributions	% distribution of health benefits
Less than 1	17.2	32.4
1–1.9	14.2	22.2
2–2.9	21.1	22.5
3–3.9	12.9	9.5
4–8.9	23.1	10.1
9+	11.5	3.3
	100.0	100.0

CHILE (1969)[b]		
Units of legal minimum wage	% distribution of contributions	% distribution of health benefits
Less than 1	29.8	33.4
1–1.9	31.6	35.0
2–2.9	17.6	15.7
3–4.9	11.9	9.5
5+	9.1	6.5
	100.0	100.0

COSTA RICA (1978)[c]		
% of families in each income bracket	Percentage of family income	
	Before health benefits	After health benefits
20 (poorest)	2.8	4.0
20	8.0	8.7
20	13.0	13.4
20	21.2	21.0
20 (wealthiest)	55.0	52.9
100	100.0	100.0

Sources: Arellano, 1976; Briceño and Méndez, 1982; Rezende, 1974; and Rezende and Mahar, 1974.

[a]All social insurance programs, but limited to urban sector; excludes armed forces and civil servants.

[b]Social insurance sickness-maternity and public health programs.

[c]Social insurance sickness-maternity (includes attention to welfare cases), public health, and family allowance programs.

transfer from the three highest-income groups). A first study done in Costa Rica in 1973 (not shown in Table 16) showed a slightly progressive, almost neutral, impact of sickness-maternity social insurance (Green, 1977). A second study (shown in the table) that also included family allowances and the Ministry of Health was conducted in 1978, after population coverage had been notably expanded, salary ceiling contributions had been eliminated, and welfare programs had been added; hence, the progressive effect increased—2% was transferred from the wealthiest 20% to the poorest 40%.

Table 17 compares the results of the impact of public health expenditures (subsidies) on family income in Argentina, Chile, Costa Rica, the Dominican Republic, and Uruguay in 1980–1982. The comparison of the income distribution before and after receiving the subsidy (last two columns of figures) shows that Costa Rica has the most progressive effect—a transfer of 2.5% from the wealthiest 20% to the poorest 40%. Chile follows, with a transfer of 1.9% from the wealthiest 20% to the poorest 40%. Of the remaining three countries, there was a transfer of 1% from the wealthiest 20% to the poorest 20%.

Two recent studies have added valuable information. An analysis of the impact of social expenditures in Brazil found that the poorest 41% of the population received 18% of such expenditures, and that only 8% received social insurance benefits. Conversely, 57% of the population—with mid-level income—received 70% of social expenditures and 35% of social insurance. The conclusion was that state subsidies mainly helped the middle class (McGreevey et al, 1988a). In Uruguay, an analysis of transfers found that the largest proportion went to the rural workers and domestic servants (with a highly progressive effect) and the second largest share went to civil servants and teachers (with a regressive effect) (Davrieux, 1987). Unfortunately, none of the above studies include a country that has a national health system, which prevents us from testing the hypothesis that that health model has the most progressive effect on distribution.

Although not all the above studies are comparable, they suggest that Costa Rica, which has a fairly unified social insurance system with a social welfare component and universal coverage, is the country which generates the most significant progressive effect. Argentina, Chile, and Uruguay, although they have almost universal coverage, have stratified health care systems. The studies on Argentina and Uruguay are lim-

Table 17. Impact of public health expenditures (subsidies) on income distribution in selected countries of Latin America, 1980 and 1982.

Percentage of families in each income bracket	Percentage distribution of health subsidy	Percentage distribution of family income	
		Before the subsidy	After the subsidy
ARGENTINA (1980)			
20 (poorest)	51.2	7.5	8.5
20	17.4	11.7	11.8
20	18.8	16.1	16.1
20	8.3	22.5	22.1
20 (wealthiest)	4.3	42.3	41.5
Total	100.0	100.0	100.0
CHILE (1982)			
20	22.3	3.3	4.2
20	29.0	7.1	8.1
20	21.5	10.4	10.9
20	15.9	18.1	18.0
20	11.3	61.0	58.8
Total	100.0	100.0	100.0
COSTA RICA (1982)			
20	30.0	6.1	7.9
20	19.0	11.2	11.8
20	20.9	14.9	15.3
20	16.9	21.4	21.1
20	13.2	46.4	43.9
Total	100.0	100.0	100.0
DOMINICAN REPUBLIC (1980)			
20	41.3	5.1	6.2
20	16.1	9.1	9.3
20	20.1	13.4	13.6
20	13.5	19.7	19.5
20	9.0	52.6	51.4
Total	100.0	100.0	100.0
URUGUAY (1982)			
20	34.0	7.2	8.1
20	29.7	11.8	12.4
20	16.1	14.8	14.9
20	8.4	19.9	19.5
20	11.8	46.3	45.2
Total	100.0	100.0	100.0

Sources: Petrei, 1987; Rodríguez V., 1986.

ited to the public sector, which in the former covers 23% of the population and spends 30% of the national health bill, while in the latter covers 43% of the population and spends 33% (in both, the effect is slightly progressive). If the sector of mutual-aid societies, unions, and cooperatives were added in both countries, it would reduce the progressive effect of the public sector. The entire health system of Chile prior to the reform in the early 1980s had a progressive effect but, when disaggregated by groups, the effect diminished. After the reform, the public health sector continues to generate a marked progressive effect, but if the new private sector (IS-

APRES, which covers 9% of the population with relatively high income) had been included, the effect would be significantly reduced (Arellano, 1987). In the Dominican Republic, where the public health sector covers a vast majority of the population, there is little progressive effect. But if we add the social insurance sector, which covers a tiny fraction of the population but receives many more resources, the global effect probably would be regressive. Brazil is not comparable with the other five countries; the two studies conducted are different and their results appear to be contradictory.

Summary of Health Standards, Facilities, and Inequalities

The average health standards in Latin America and the Caribbean are the highest in the developing world, but there are substantial variations among countries: the most developed countries enjoy the best facilities and standards while the least developed endure the worst. Some inconsistencies between facilities and standards in some countries can be explained by uneven and irrational allocation of such facilities among population groups and geographical regions—most health resources go to the productive-age population rather than to the infant-maternal population that is at a higher risk for sickness. Private sector facilities are the best, closely followed by those of the armed forces, and then by those of social insurance (these providers care for high and middle-income groups); the worst facilities are those of the ministry of health, which is expected to protect the poorest population affected by a higher risk of disease. The best facilities are concentrated in the most developed, wealthiest, urban, and industrialized regions, and the worst are located in the least developed, poorest, rural regions (extreme disparities were systematically found between the most and least developed regions in several countries). A redistribution of health facilities according to need would shift more resources to the infant-maternal group, the ministry of health, and the least developed regions. Such redistribution would help reduce infant mortality rates and increase life expectancy.

Integrated or highly coordinated health care systems tend to reduce inequalities in health facilities and standards, while the opposite is true of highly stratified systems. Among social insurance programs, benefits in kind (particularly in sickness-maternity) appear to have a more progressive effect on income distribution than cash benefits, because the former are basically equal and used more by lower income groups of insured. Public health programs, being geared to the poorest sector of the population, should have an even higher progressive effect. Empirical studies conducted in several countries appear to confirm some of the findings on the impact of Latin American and Caribbean health care systems on income distribution.

FINANCING HEALTH CARE

This section analyzes the financing of the sickness-maternity program of social insurance and of the public health sector, as well as the relationship between the two and its implications for the poor.

Financing the Social Insurance Sickness-Maternity Program

Sources of Revenue

In Latin America, social insurances are mainly financed by percentage contributions on wages paid by the insured, the employer, the state as such, and the state as employer. In some countries, the state does not pay a contribution on the wage bill, but assigns taxes or covers some services or part of the system's deficit. Investment returns can be an important source of revenue in pension programs, but not in sickness-maternity, because this program does not accumulate substantial reserves.

Table 18 shows the percentage contributions on salary (or income, in the case of the self-employed), established by law for the social insurance sickness-maternity program in Latin America. Countries with national health systems are excluded from the table, as well as four countries with social insurance (Brazil, the Dominican Republic, Ecuador, and Paraguay) because their legislation does not separate the contributions for the sickness-maternity program from the overall contributions; Haiti is also excluded because its law is not enforced.

In the non-Latin Caribbean and Cuba, the national health system is financed through the state budget, but cash benefits for sickness-maternity insurance are paid out of the overall wage contribution (in Cuba, all enterprises pay 10% of the wage bill for all the cash benefits and the insured does not pay). In the 14 countries in

Table 18. Legal contributions to sickness-maternity and all social insurances in Latin America, 1987–1989[a] (in percentages of wages or income).

Countries	Insured			State[b]				Total[c]		
	Salaried	Self-employed	Employer	% of wages	Taxes	Covers deficit	Others[d]	Sickness-maternity	All social insurances	% sickness-maternity over all
Argentina	3.0	n.a.	4.5					7.5	54.8–57.6	13.0–13.7
Bolivia	2.0	n.a.	8.0					10.0	21.0	47.6
Chile	7.0	7.0	0			X		7.0	21.4–29.4	23.8–32.7
Colombia	2.33–4.0	7.0	4.67–8.0				X	7.0–12.0	19.0–24.0	36.8
Costa Rica	5.5	5.5–12.25	9.25	0.75	X			16.0	33.9	47.2
El Salvador	2.23–2.5	8.75	5.57–6.25				X	7.8–8.75	10.8–13.8	63.4–72.2
Guatemala	2.0		4.0	3.0			X	9.0	17.5	51.4
Honduras	2.5	n.a.	5.0	2.5				10.0	14.0	71.4
Mexico	3.0	7.87	8.4	0.6				12.0	21.0	57.1
Nicaragua	2.25		6.0	0.25				8.5	15.5	54.8
Panama	1.0	n.a.	8.0		X			9.8	20.9–23.2	42.2–46.9
Peru	3.0	9.0	6.0					9.0	22.0	40.9
Uruguay[e]	3.0	n.a.	4.0			X		7.0	34.0–35.0	20.0–20.6
Venezuela	2.0		4.25–6.25	1.5[f]				7.75–9.75	12.5–14.5	62.0–67.0

Sources: Compiled by the author based on U.S. Social Security Administration, 1987, and additional information.

[a]Excludes the countries with national health systems, as well as four countries with social insurance that do not have a separate contribution for sickness-maternity (Brazil, Ecuador, Paraguay, and the Dominican Republic).
[b]State contribution as such in addition to contribution as employer.
[c]Sum of percentage contribution of salaried insured, employer, and state.
[d]Covers, in different countries, care of welfare users, part of the cost of health services or administration, or population-coverage extension.
[e]Only sickness.
[f]Contribution to all social insurances.

the table, the share of sickness-maternity in the overall contribution to social insurance (last column) ranges from 13% to 72%. If we delete the pioneer countries (Argentina, Chile, and Uruguay) that first introduced social insurance in the Region and where the bulk of contributions goes to the pension program, the range becomes 41% to 72%, with a nonweighted average of 52%. If we assume that this average is representative of all countries, we can say that about half of the total contribution of social insurance goes to health care.

The total contribution to sickness-maternity ranges from 7% to 16%, with an average of 9% for the 14 countries, which is relatively high by international standards—compared to that of developed countries, it is higher than in Australia, Austria, Canada, Ireland, and Luxembourg, and similar to that of Belgium, Israel, and Sweden (United States Social Security Administration, 1987). A comparison of the percentage contributions of Latin American countries in 1980 and 1987–1988, shows that such percentage increased in ten countries, stagnated in six, and declined in four. The last include Chile, which, after the 1981 social security reform, gradually eliminated the employers' contribution (but the state subsidy to the old system has steadily risen), and Bolivia, which due to a substantial cut in the employers' contribution is edging toward financial disequilibrium. With the exception of Costa Rica, which has the highest percentage of both contribution and population covered, there does not seem to be a relationship between the two variables: countries with lowest population coverage have some of the highest contributions (e.g., Colombia, Honduras, Guatemala) and vice versa (e.g., Argentina, Chile, Uruguay). Because the latter countries have higher health standards than the former, such discrepancies might be explained by inefficiency and waste.

The percentage contribution assigned to the employer is considerably higher than that of the insured (except in Chile where the latter pays all): the average employer/insured contribution ratio is 2.6 to 1. The percentage to be paid by the self-employed (a significant proportion of which is poor) equals the sum of the percentages paid by the insured and the employer (7% to 12%), which partly explains, once again, why it is so difficult to extend coverage to this group. In six countries, there is a state contribution based on wages, and it is smaller (except in Guatemala) than the insured contribution. In seven other countries, the state is legally bound to pay part of the costs, to cover the deficit of the program, or to earmark special taxes to partly finance the program. In summary, according to the law, the insured should normally finance one-third or less of the cost of protection, while the rest is paid by the employer and the state. This raises the question whether the insured really has a "right" to the benefits based on the assumption that he or she pays for them.

The Impact of the Financial System on Income Distribution

Table 19 presents the percentage distribution of revenue of all social insurance programs by source in 28 Latin American and Caribbean countries in 1983. It should be noted that the state's actual share is underestimated and the other shares overestimated in the table, because, since 1978, the ILO series excluded care provided by the public health sector. This particularly affects non-Latin Caribbean countries with national health systems, which showed much higher state shares prior to the change.

According to the table, the insured contributed less than 25% of total revenue in 11 countries and from 25% to 33% in 11 countries; only in 5 did the insured contribute more than 33%. The employer and the state contributed 60% or more of total revenue in 11 countries and from 40% to 60% in 13 countries. Averages for the 28

countries show that the insured's share was 26.5%, while the combined employer and state share was 57%; the remaining 16.5% came from investment (mostly from the pension program) and other sources.

Disaggregated data on the specific distribution of revenue of the sickness-maternity program by source, available for seven countries only, confirm what was said above (see Table 20): about two-thirds of revenue comes from employers and the state (except in Chile) and about one-third or less comes from the insured.

In practically all countries, the percentage contribution paid by the insured does not increase with income, and 75% of the countries have a contribution ceiling that limits the potential payment of the highest salary brackets. According to the literature, the employer's contribution can either be paid directly or it can be transferred "backward" (to the insured) or "forward" (to prices and consumers). This issue has been greatly debated (Musgrove, 1985), but it appears that in the least developed countries, the employer's contribution is frequently charged to production costs, and so it is trans-

Table 19. Percentage distribution of revenue of social insurances plus family allowances,[a] by source, in Latin America and the Caribbean, 1983.

Countries	Insured	Employer	State & taxes	Investment	Others
Antigua and Barbuda	29.3	48.8	0.0	19.2	2.8
Argentina	34.5	27.2	36.0	2.0	0.3
Bahamas	23.2	38.0	5.2	33.6	0.1
Barbados	36.2	37.5	0.0	22.3	4.1
Belize	11.6	69.1	0.0	14.3	5.0
Bolivia	25.5	34.8	24.2	12.4	3.1
Brazil	15.6	74.0	8.2	0.0	2.2
Chile	31.1	2.1	48.9	15.9	2.0
Colombia	26.6	62.8	0.0	10.2	0.4
Costa Rica	28.4	47.0	18.6	5.3	0.8
Cuba	0.0	44.3	55.7	0.0	0.0
Dominica	27.3	45.6	0.0	26.2	0.8
Ecuador	38.6	38.1	1.3	22.1	0.0
El Salvador	23.7	55.8	0.0	20.0	0.6
Granada	48.2	48.3	0.0	3.3	0.2
Guatemala	29.5	51.0	3.6	13.2	2.7
Guyana	20.6	30.9	0.0	48.5	0.1
Honduras	25.9	47.9	7.2	16.8	2.2
Jamaica	24.3	29.7	7.4	38.5	0.1
Mexico	19.7	62.0	12.3	5.2	0.8
Nicaragua	22.8	59.9	3.2	12.9	1.2
Panama	28.8	44.6	3.3	13.3	10.0
Peru	29.4	59.0	0.0	10.3	1.3
St. Lucia	43.5	43.5	0.0	13.0	0.0
Suriname	23.9	9.7	66.4	0.0	0.0
Trinidad and Tobago	18.1	36.2	27.2	18.5	0.0
Uruguay	23.5	23.3	49.2	1.6	2.3
Venezuela	28.6	39.3	13.7	18.3	0.1
Region X̄	26.5	43.1	14.0	14.9	1.5

Source: Author's calculations based on ILO, 1988.

[a]Family allowances are available only in Argentina, Brazil, Chile, Colombia, Suriname, and Uruguay.

Table 20. Percentage distribution of revenue of social insurance sickness-maternity program, by source, in selected countries of Latin America, 1974–1985.

Countries	Contributions			Investment	Others	Total
	Insured	Employer	State			
Colombia	28.4	54.4	16.7	0	0.5	100.0
Costa Rica	36.8	46.7	3.0	0	13.5	100.0
Chile	27.9	0	48.7	6.5	16.9	100.0
El Salvador	26.8	66.9	3.8	1.4	1.1	100.0
Guatemala	36.8	63.2	0	0	0	100.0
Mexico	24.5	62.0	11.0	0.2	2.3	100.0
Venezuela	26.6	53.2	20.1	0	0.1	100.0

Source: Mesa-Lago, 1989.

ferred to the consumer (Mesa-Lago, 1989c). The state contribution is financed by taxes, often of a regressive nature (such as sales taxes). As previously stated, in 1983 employers and the state jointly generated more than twice the social insurance revenue as the insured paid; therefore, it is probable that the consumer, rather than the insured, carried the heaviest financial burden.

When a country has achieved, or is close to reaching, universal coverage, the above situation ceases to be a problem, because practically all consumers are insured (e.g., Chile, Costa Rica, Uruguay). However, in countries where only a small proportion of the population is covered, the regressivity of the financial structure worsens. For example, in Colombia only 16% of the population is covered, but the combined employer-state contribution is 63%; hence, through price and tax mechanisms, 84% of the population (not protected, including the poor) probably finances most of the cost of covering the minority. El Salvador and Honduras are in a similar extreme situation, as only 6% and 10% of their populations are covered, but the employer-state contribution is 56% and 55%, respectively.

We have already discussed how the Bismarckian model of social insurance financing, combined with a low proportion of salaried employees in the labor force, represents a barrier to the expansion of social insurance coverage. In addition, this section showed that the financial structure of the current system is regressive and inequitable in many countries, and that the assumption of the insured's ''right'' to benefits (based on the alleged payment of their costs) is questionable at best. That assumption has justified the discriminatory treatment given to social welfare recipients versus that given to users of social insurance, and it has stood in the way of extending coverage in those countries that have a small salaried labor force. Once the assumption is questioned, the way is open for replacing

financing based on wage-related contributions by financing through another type of tax (e.g., on income or on value added), which could make achieving universal coverage easier and might correct possible negative economic effects of the current type of financing upon employment and/or distribution (see Mesa-Lago, 1989c).

As has been seen, there are only a few countries (Brazil, Costa Rica, Ecuador, Mexico) where transfers from the state budget (or from urban employers) cover marginal groups who are ineligible for social insurance benefits. The next section will demonstrate that the current social insurance sickness-maternity program usually suffers from actuarial and financial disequilibria that tend to worsen with time and eventually lead to an overall crisis.

Persistent and Growing Deficits

The financing method used in the social insurance sickness-maternity program in Latin America is pure assessment or pay-as-you-go (International Social Security Association, 1982; Thullen, 1985). Under this method, the annual revenues must pay for the corresponding expenditures, since there is only a small reserve for contingencies (Table 20 shows that investment returns for this program are negligible). If the wage contribution cannot cover costs (maintain the equilibrium), the latter must be cut, the former increased, or a combination of both must be carried out.

We lack disaggregated data from Latin America and the Caribbean to comprehensively evaluate the long-term financial equilibrium of the sickness-maternity program. However, Table 21 offers estimates of the equilibrium of the entire social security system in 21 Latin American and Caribbean countries for 1970–1983, by showing its annual financial surplus or deficit (revenue minus expenditures) as a percentage of GDP.

Table 21. Deficit/surplus of social security system as percentage of GDP in Latin America and the Caribbean, 1970–1983.

	1970	1975	1978	1979	1980	1981	1982	1983
Argentina	n.a.	0.7	0.3	−0.0	0.4	−3.0	−2.2	−2.3
Bahamas	n.a.	n.a.	n.a.	n.a.	1.6	2.1	1.3	1.4
Barbados	−0.2[b]	−2.4	0.4	0.5	0.5	0.3	2.0	2.5
Bolivia	0.2[c]	0.3	0.0	0.2	−0.0	0.7	0.6	0.1
Brazil	n.a.	n.a.	n.a.	n.a.	n.a.	−0.3	−0.0	−0.4
Chile	−4.1[b]	−1.0	−1.7	−2.0	−2.0	−2.3	−7.7	−5.7
Colombia	0.2	−0.0	−0.2	−0.1	−0.0	−0.2	−0.6	−0.2
Costa Rica	0.7	1.6	1.4	1.2	1.0	0.8	0.8	2.5
Cuba	n.a.	n.a.	n.a.	n.a.	n.a.	−6.2	−6.4	−6.4
Ecuador	n.a.	0.6[d]	1.8	2.1	1.7	1.3	1.5	1.3
El Salvador	−0.0	−0.3	0.6	0.6	0.4	0.6	0.8	0.8
Guatemala	0.1	−0.0	0.4	0.5	0.4	0.4	0.3	0.3
Honduras	−1.2	n.a.	n.a.	n.a.	n.a.	0.3	0.1	0.2
Jamaica	−0.7	−1.7	0.3	0.3	0.3	0.7	1.0	0.6
Mexico	−0.4	−0.3[d]	n.a.	n.a.	0.4	0.4	0.5	0.1
Nicaragua	0.1	−0.0	0.0	0.5	0.9	0.7	0.6	0.8
Panama	0.1[c]	1.2	1.0	1.7	1.9	2.7	3.1	2.4
Peru	n.a.	n.a.	n.a.	n.a.	n.a.	0.4	0.0	−0.1
Trinidad and Tobago	0.8	0.4	0.3	n.a.	0.2	0.0	0.0	−0.5
Uruguay	n.a.	−1.2	−0.5	−0.3	−0.8	−3.7	−5.8	−4.3
Venezuela	−0.7	0.3	0.4	0.2	0.3	0.2	0.2	0.0

Sources: Mackenzie, 1988; and author's calculations based on ILO, 1988.
[a]Excludes contribution of state as such (not as employer).
[b]1971.
[c]1972.
[d]1974.

These estimates exclude the state contribution as such (they include the state contribution as an employer), because it implies a subsidy or transfer (Mackenzie, 1988). According to the table, in 1970 and 1975, approximately half of the countries suffered a deficit and, after some improvement in 1981–1982, there was a deterioration in 1983, when 43% of the countries carried a deficit.

Scattered data available on the sickness-maternity program for several countries indicate that its disequilibrium is greater than that of social security as a whole. The reason is that the pension program usually generates a surplus that compensates for and helps to reduce—through loans or transfers—the deficit of the sickness-maternity program. The following information *includes* the state contribution as such: in Mexico the sickness-maternity program has ended in deficit each year since its creation in 1943, except for three years; in Panama there has been a steady deficit since 1975, which reached $US196 million by 1986; in Peru there has been a deficit since 1977 (the cumulative deficit reached $US162 million by 1985); in Ecuador there was a steady deficit in 1980–1988 (a cumulative deficit rose to $US35 million by 1987); in Costa Rica, the cumulative deficit in 1977–1981 was $US44 million; in Uruguay the cumulative deficit in 1982–1986 was $US17 mil-

lion; in Bolivia there was an annual deficit in 1982–1986, except for one year; and in Colombia the cumulative deficit in 1981–1985 was $US13 million (Mesa-Lago, 1989, 1990; La Forgia, 1990). According to the former director of ILO's Social Security Division, such a deficit is higher than shown in the accounting books, because only current expenditures are considered in the calculations, but not capital expenditures such as land acquisition and construction of hospitals, buying of equipment, etc. (Tamburi, 1980).

The Causes of the Deficit

The deficit becomes even more serious when one recalls the very high percentage of contribution on the payroll for sickness-maternity and the greater allocation of health care revenues to social insurance as compared to the public health sector, despite the smaller population usually served by the former. The obvious explanation for the deficit is that expenditures have outpaced revenue, but the question is why. An analysis of the causes of increasing expenditures will be covered in the next section. Regarding revenues, the causes of the disequilibrium have been insufficient contributions mainly due to employers' evasion and payment delays and the state's failure to honor its obligations.

Insufficient Contributions

The contribution for the sickness-maternity program is normally insufficient to cover expenditures. For example, in 1977 it was estimated that in Mexico the contribution of the major institute (IMSS) had to be increased from 6% (the prevailing rate at the time) to 10% to balance the program by the end of the century. But, if the amortization of the loans from the pension program to the sickness-maternity program was considered, the contribution had to rise to 13% (it was 9% in 1989). In several countries, the contribution is already so high (e.g., 15.5% in Costa Rica) that it is difficult to increase it. Usually, the contribution is set by law, and a legal amendment in congress faces strong opposition by employers and trade unions.

Another problem is that the revenue actually collected with the current contribution falls below the potential revenue; the salary used as a base for the contribution is often the minimum wage and excludes fringe benefits, and the contribution ceiling also reduces the potential revenue from the high-salary group. The employer normally declares a salary that is lower than that actually paid, and the system of computerized bills prepared in advance by the social insurance agency based on past salary data fosters the employer's improper behavior.

Evasion and Payment Delays

Evasion (avoidance of registration) and late payments or *mora* (by those already registered) are serious problems. Gross estimates of these problems among employers in the mid-1980s were: Argentina 23% evasion; the Bahamas 19% of combined evasion and *mora*; Barbados 44% *mora*; Brazil 60% of both; Chile 30% *mora*; Guatemala 50% *mora*; Jamaica 44% *mora*; Peru 33% evasion; and Uruguay 27% evasion (among the self-employed, combined evasion and *mora* reached 52% in the Bahamas and 95% in Barbados and Jamaica). The cumulative debt for these causes in Colombia by 1985 (with only an official estimate of 8% to 12% *mora*) reached $US135 million. Galloping inflation has eroded the real value of such debt; for example, in Peru it declined from $US46 million to $US7 million in 1985–1988.

There are multiple causes for evasion and *mora*. The system of registration of employers and insured, and the processing of payments are extremely deficient in many countries: there is no up-to-date information on employers' addresses or for the number of employees and their salaries; very few countries have a unified ID system for employers and insured; payments are often processed manually and there are neither individual accounts nor a current list of delinquent employers. In an effort to correct such deficiencies, several countries have introduced computerization, but despite some progress, many inefficiencies remain and computers have introduced new problems.

Small enterprises (where informal workers are concentrated) are difficult to detect and control. A 1988 study of social insurance conducted in Lima, Peru, showed that 33% of enterprises had more than six workers, employed 90% of the insured, and paid 96% of total contributions, but the remaining 66% of enterprises had fewer than six workers, employed 10% of the insured, and paid 4% of total contributions. The cost of detecting, collecting, and controlling these small enterprises (mostly evaders) is enormous, and their number is growing due to the rapid expansion of the informal sector in that country. The excessive paperwork required for registration, payment, and monthly reports is a deterrent to small enterprises.

There is a scarcity of skilled inspectors, and their low salaries encourage them to enter into fraudulent deals with debtors. In addition, the poor services or benefits often given by social insurance lead workers to conspire with employers to evade registration. Denunciation of corruption in Colombia, rather than inducing the prosecution of delinquents and the creation of proper incentives, led to the elimination of the Inspection Department.

Where inspectors are diligent, and evasion and *mora* properly detected, the legal and judicial system for efficient collection and enforcement may fail. The prosecution and imprisonment record in Latin America and the Caribbean is appalling. For instance, in the Bahamas there has not been a single case of prison for debt or fraud since social insurance was introduced, and in Barbados there has been one case in 20 years. In many countries, the judicial system is overburdened, and delays in prosecution are considerable. Last but not least, when an employer is finally prosecuted, if the debt is so high that it can cause the enterprise's bankruptcy, trade unions and the state often exert pressure to pardon or postpone the debt in order to avoid unemployment.

Very high inflation rates (particularly in the 1980s), combined with low interest rates and fines for the debt, encourage employers to delay payment: they can make juicy profits by depositing the contributions in commercial banks and earning a higher interest rate. In the late 1980s, the interest (deflated) charged to the debt was negative in many countries—Bolivia, −668% in 1985; Peru, −134% in 1988; Ecuador, −52% in 1988 (Mesa-Lago, 1990).

The State Debt

In an increasing number of the Region's countries, the state is the principal debtor to social insurance, because it has not paid its contribution as an employer (in some countries its obligation as third party contributor also is outstanding), it has retained tax payments collected for social insurance, and/or it has not fulfilled its obligation to reimburse social insurance for health services provided to the dispossessed or to civil servants or the military. In the mid-1980s, the state cumulative debt was: $US73 million in Costa Rica, $US95 million in the Dominican Republic, $US170 million in Colombia (only to the civil servants' fund), $US194 million in Peru, $US572 million in Panama, and $US602 million in Ecuador.

In some countries, the state has signed agreements with the social insurance institution to pay the debt. However, both the debt and the interest rate have not been indexed to inflation, hence, payment is made with devalued currency and the real interest rate is often negative. As a result, the real debt has shrunk dramatically—in Peru it was cut by 99.8% in 1981–1988 and in Ecuador it declined by 75% in 1973–1985. The economic crisis of the 1980s has aggravated the situation because of multiple urgent demands on the state (e.g., to pay the foreign debt), plus escalating inflation. In fact, the increasing state debt has been a major factor in a liquidity crisis of social insurance in several countries.

In order to ameliorate the shrinkage of the state's real debt, some governments have entered into agreements with foreign countries for the provision of hospital equipment or medical supplies to the social insurance sickness-maternity program. In this way, the real value of the debt is protected while the state becomes directly responsible to foreign governments or suppliers. In other countries, the social insurance institution has accepted a reduction in future state obligations in exchange for a firm commitment from the government to adequately pay the debt. But in most countries, the state has been reluctant to renegotiate both the terms and interest rates of old payment agreements in order to adjust them to inflation (Mesa-Lago, 1990).

Coping with the Deficit

The countries have tackled the growing deficit of their sickness-maternity programs in two ways. The most common short-term approach, particularly in those countries where such a program was introduced late and that, hence, has fewer pensioners and high reserves has been to take loans from the pension program reserve. For example, in 1981, 31% of the total investment of Peru's pension fund (IPSS) was in the sickness-maternity program. And in 1985, without transfers from the pension fund, the main sickness-maternity social insurance program in Colombia (ISS) would have been $US13 million in the red. However, in the long run these loans cannot be amortized (nor are interests usually paid), and, as the pension program matures and the number of pensioners increases, it faces growing difficulties to fulfill its obligations because of the decapitalization of its fund. Early in the 1980s, social insurance agencies in Colombia, Costa Rica, and Peru prohibited the pension program from giving loans to the sickness-maternity program. However, in Peru the practice continued in 1988, disguised by obscure accounting transfers (Mesa-Lago and De Geyndt, 1987; Mesa-Lago, 1988b, 1988c).

In some countries, the state has temporarily rescued the sickness-maternity program by covering its deficits through different means, often at the expense of depleting health funds from other institutions that covered the rest of the population (Arroba, 1979). The economic crisis of the 1980s made it impossible to continue this practice, and the only alternative left has been to cut expenditures, as will be discussed in the next section. However, the only long-term solution is to reorganize the health system completely, following the guidelines in Chapter 5.

Financing the Public Health Sector

The sources for financing the public health sector are the state budget, sale of health care services to users with sufficient income, user charges or fees, and foreign aid. The state budget is based on general taxation and, in some countries, on lotteries. In Barbados, there is a wage tax ("health levy") that is collected by the social insurance agency and transferred to the ministry of health.

Regarding the sale of health care services, practically all public hospitals in the Region have areas reserved for patients who can afford to pay for services and who want private rooms.

In those countries where health care is provided free to the poor only, a means test is administered to determine who can pay for the services, but revenue from the sale of services tends to be small. Cuba, taking advantage of a surplus of physicians and hospital beds and equipment, has promoted "health tourism," whereby foreigners are provided specialized care at a reasonable price. Unfortunately, there are no available financial data on the profitability of this practice.

In the 1980s, the application of user fees in the public health sector increased, in some cases including low-income users. If these charges are low they do not worsen distribution inequalities and may reduce the unnecessary consumption of health care services, but they do not significantly contribute to the sector's financing. Conversely, if charges are substantial, they can be an important source of revenue and help to maintain and improve the services, but they may deepen distribution inequalities. In the latter case, lower income groups should be exempt, otherwise user fees would reduce access of the poor and provoke a regressive effect (PAHO, 1989); however, this approach brings on some administrative difficulties. Another approach involves exempting certain services such as prophylaxis, sanitation, and primary health care and charging for hospital services as well as medicine (De Ferranti, 1985a). Still another approach is to vary fees according to the type, complexity, and location of services, as well as to the user's socioeconomic status ("El financiamiento. . .," 1989). This study will analyze in detail the application of user fees in the public health sector of the Dominican Republic and its effect on the poor.

Several international and regional organizations (such as USAID, IDB, and PAHO/WHO) provide health care grants and technical cooperation, usually to the ministry of health, except in Costa Rica, where external aid has focused on the social insurance agency (CCSS), because it manages all hospitals. More recently, Guatemala's social insurance agency (IGSS) has received external aid to expand population coverage to a less developed region. In general, however, foreign aid is not a significant source of revenue.

In most non-Latin Caribbean countries, access to health services is free, at least for the poor or for people with very low incomes, and sometimes for certain services or age-groups regardless of income. For instance, in the Bahamas, all children below the age of 14 who attend school and senior citizens receive free care. In Jamaica, primary health care, diagnosis of contagious diseases, and care of pregnant women always are free. Finally, in 1985 the Bahamas established a special fund (with transfers from the social insurance programs of employment injury and short-term benefits) to improve the public health system and create a national health insurance.

The Impact of the Economic Crisis on Health Care

The economic crisis that began affecting Latin America and the Caribbean in the early 1980s is the longest and deepest since the Great Depression. ECLAC has estimated that in 1981–1989, GDP per capita declined by a cumulative 8.3% (in twelve countries the decline exceeded 15%), and some specialists argue that the entire decade has been lost in the Region in terms of development (ECLAC-CEPAL, 1989). Here we summarize the impact of the crisis on health care (both the public and the social insurance sectors), focusing on revenues, expenditures, financial equilibrium, population coverage, and quality of services.

Declining Revenues

The real income of social insurance sickness-maternity and other programs has declined in most of the Region due to several factors. Real wages decreased in the 1980s (in 1989, eight out of eleven countries reported by ECLAC had a lower real minimum wage than in 1980), provoking a fall in real contributions. Open urban unemployment dramatically increased in 1981–1989, as much as fourfold in some countries. Although this phenomenon began to abate in the mid-1980s, 10 out of 16 countries for which data are available still had higher unemployment rates in 1988–1989 than in 1980—those without jobs have ceased to contribute to social insurance. We also have seen that the informal sector grew in the 1980s, reversing the trend of the 1960s and 1970s. Since the self-employed and other groups in the informal sector usually are not covered by social insurance, the shift from formal to informal labor also has resulted in a decrease in contributions. Furthermore, because those in the informal sector usually do not pay taxes (including social insurance), they have an unfair competitive edge over the formal sector, contributing to the decline of the latter.

According to ECLAC, annual average inflation in Latin America and the Caribbean jumped from 56% in 1980 to 275% in 1985 and, although it declined in 1986, it steadily rose in 1987–1989, reaching a record 994% in the last year. Argentina, Bolivia, Brazil, Nicaragua, and Peru have had inflation rates from 1,000% to 33,600% (ECLAC-CEPAL, 1989). In the many countries that have a ceiling for wage contributions or where these contributions are fixed according to income brackets, the fast increase in inflation (without proper adjustments of ceilings and income brackets) has led to a decline in real contributions.

In addition, as has already been discussed, hyperinflation provides an added incentive for employers to delay payments to social insurance. The lack of indexation of employers' debts, combined with low interest rates and soft fines imposed on delinquent employers, has stimulated payment delays, and social insurance revenues have declined. Inflation also has devalued the state debt and, in a few countries, has practically made that debt almost disappear in real terms. Furthermore, under increasing external pressure to attend to more urgent demands, such as servicing the foreign debt, the state has failed to fulfill its obligation to social insurance as a third-party contributor and as an employer.

Revenues of public health programs have declined dramatically. External pressures on the state to service the foreign debt and the need to cut domestic deficits, have caused stabilization programs to reduce budgetary allocations to social services, including health care.

Increasing Costs and Demand

Prices of medicines and medical-surgical equipment have increased due to domestic as well as foreign inflation. In addition, where salaries of social insurance employees are adjusted to inflation, this expenditure, the largest component of total expenditures, has maintained or even increased its real level, while real revenues have declined (e.g., in Peru until the end of 1988).

In 1980–1985, the health share in public spending fell from 9% to 5.5%. Table 22 presents data on public health expenditures per capita by the central government (excluding social insurance) in 24 countries in 1970–1984; the figures show that such expenditures decreased in 22 countries: in 12 countries expenditures peaked in 1980–1981 and then declined; in 4 countries the peak occurred in 1983 and expenditures diminished in 1984; and in 4 countries there had been a declining trend since 1978 or 1979 (Musgrove, 1986).

In countries where social insurance provides free health care for "indigents" (e.g., Costa Rica), as more people become unemployed or

Table 22. Per capita expenditures of the central government in public health, excluding social insurance, in Latin America and the Caribbean, 1970–1984 (in $US dollars)

Countries	1970	1978	1980	1981	1982	1983	1984
Argentina	7.98	11.47	11.38	8.56	6.03	8.27	9.80
Bahamas	n.a.	257.19	220.71	231.34	210.43	215.27	224.38
Barbados	127.46	188.65	151.16	147.06	115.47	113.65	118.98
Bolivia	5.82	7.33	10.94	5.91	2.44	n.a.	n.a.
Brazil	10.66	23.34	23.89	24.07	27.34	n.a.	n.a.
Chile	21.16	21.61	27.08	28.49	25.99	21.12	20.64
Colombia	6.04	8.22	8.34	9.18	7.89	8.73	n.a.
Costa Rica	13.61	20.88	29.16	18.09	16.76	15.80	24.34
Dominican Republic	14.78	20.08	24.07	25.44	14.09	13.74	12.87
Ecuador	2.83	10.67	12.69	16.07	14.70	11.95	13.16
El Salvador	n.a.	12.47	12.90	12.70	10.81	9.22	8.72
Guatemala	n.a.	14.50	22.47	15.71	18.34	8.89	9.38
Haiti	2.44	3.03	2.70	2.62	3.81	2.98	n.a.
Honduras	8.97	15.42	15.44	15.27	15.74	15.99	13.09
Jamaica	49.72	60.18	64.63	65.10	64.10	59.53	52.70
Mexico	n.a.	8.24	8.16	n.a.	n.a.	n.a.	n.a.
Nicaragua	10.13	27.27	39.59	44.99	38.01	39.55	n.a.
Panama	n.a.	20.65	33.46	32.86	34.97	37.70	n.a.
Paraguay	3.83	6.18	6.36	8.63	13.51	13.52	10.83
Peru	n.a.	12.18	10.96	13.08	n.a.	18.58	17.58
Suriname	n.a.	n.a.	10.30	8.26	8.28	5.75	n.a.
Trinidad and Tobago	n.a.	42.89	41.58	47.65	80.15	81.58	70.41
Uruguay	n.a.	20.79	25.69	22.47	21.52	22.25	n.a.
Venezuela	34.93	48.93	32.31	40.05	38.22	31.32	n.a.

Sources: Musgrove, 1986, 1989a.

work in the informal sector, they stop contributing, but become entitled to such free care. Although the state is expected to reimburse social insurance for those welfare costs, it has partially or totally failed to fulfill that obligation. In those countries where sickness-maternity care is available only to the insured, persons who have lost insurance coverage become dependent on the public health system, whose budget has been severely cut. Those members of the middle class who no longer can afford to pay for private health care, gradually turn to social insurance and the public sector, both of which are overloaded.

A PAHO/WHO study on the impact of the crisis on health care conducted in five countries (Brazil, Ecuador, Honduras, Mexico, and Uruguay) for 1980–1986, found that resources for the public health sector diminished, on the average, in the same proportion as total spending. Budget cuts fell mostly on investment, somewhat sparing current expenditures, except for cuts in real wages of health personnel. It is not known, however, what part of current expenditures might have become ineffective for lack of investment (Musgrove, 1989a).

Worsening Disequilibria

The crisis has aggravated the financial deficit suffered by social insurance in some Latin American countries prior to the 1980s. Furthermore, the surplus enjoyed by most countries has turned into a deficit in several.

A recent study has analyzed the effectiveness of social insurance as an anticyclical mechanism in Peru. Contrary to the belief that social insurance has an automatic stabilizing effect (i.e., that in times of crisis it protects vulnerable sectors against income loss), the study reaches the opposite conclusion. An empirical analysis of the 1980s crisis shows that, because income generation in the Peruvian Institute of Social Security (IPSS) wholly depends on the economic cycle, the effect is actually procyclical: benefits and services decline in times of recession and increase in periods of recovery and boom (Petrera, 1987).

To cope with the crisis, several social insurance institutions have enacted emergency programs, the first in Costa Rica in 1983, and the most recent in Peru in 1988. These are geared to cut expenditures and, in some cases, to increase contributions; the latter, however, has been difficult to implement in the midst of the recession. The Costa Rican Social Security Fund (CCSS) has been successful both in increasing sickness-

maternity contribution and in cutting expenditures and, in 1988, enjoyed a financial surplus. In a few countries, ministries of health have tried to cope with budget cuts by reassigning scarce resources to most urgent needs; for example, infant-maternal groups have been targeted in Chile with positive results in terms of reduction of infant mortality (Castañeda, 1984).

Effects on Protection and Quality of Services

The above-cited PAHO/WHO study found that serious planning shortcomings crippled investment programs, wiping out plans to expand coverage, and developed difficulties in maintaining basic care; hospital admissions also were reduced due to cost cutting policies, but they were offset by expansion of outpatient care; and curtailment of resources in hospital services had induced a small decrease in the average length of stay. The hypothesis that a decline in the quality of care is part of the cost of adjustment was investigated, but available data could not answer that crucial question, nor was it possible to judge whether the crisis had actually improved efficiency. Moreover, some evidence of deterioration attributed to the crisis was found among vulnerable groups of the population and in specific conditions such as rising infant morbidity from diarrhea and increase (or slowdown in the decrease) of infant mortality rates (Musgrove, 1989a).

My own research, conducted in the second half of the 1980s in the Dominican Republic and Peru, showed evidence of deterioration of the health services, including a paralysis of investment in physical plant, equipment, and maintenance; severe cuts in medical supplies (patients often have to provide syringes, gauze, and other basic surgical materials); elimination and/or reduction of hospital meals; sharing of one bed by two patients (Mesa-Lago, 1986b, 1988c).

As has been seen, population coverage of social insurance in the 1980s declined or stagnated, or its rate of expansion slowed down. This phenomenon has been caused by increases in unemployment, growth of the informal sector, and evasion of insurance payments. In addition, the crisis has harmed programs designed to extend coverage to rural areas in Brazil, Ecuador, and Mexico. Finally, legal mandates to extend coverage to peasants and workers in the informal sector have not been implemented in some countries (e.g., Peru in 1985–1988) due to the severity of the crisis. An encouraging sign, however, is the expansion of Guatemala's social insurance sickness-maternity program to the southwest coast to protect salaried employees (Instituto Guatemalteco de Seguridad Social, 1988).

The crisis' only benefit may have been the realization, domestically and internationally (although not in all countries or all organizations), of the magnitude and seriousness of the problems in social security and health care. In the international arena, the World Bank, and more recently, IDB and IMF, have begun to conduct studies and provide technical assistance in these areas, thus strengthening the work of organizations such as ILO, AISS, WHO, PAHO/WHO, and CIESS. In the 1980s, USAID expanded the resources allocated to health care in Latin America and the Caribbean. The IAF has commissioned this study with the aim of improving grants for health care for the poor. Finally, the crisis has prompted some international organizations, with divergent clientele and philosophies, such as WHO and ILO, to try and work together (Castellanos, 1985; Gwynne and Zschock, 1989; IDB, 1989; McGreevey, 1990; PAHO/ILO/CPISS, 1986; PAHO, 1989; WHO, 1987).

Summary of Health Care Financing

About one-half of the revenue of social insurance programs in Latin America go to the sickness-maternity program; in the non-Latin Caribbean the proportion is much smaller, because social insurance only provides cash benefits. The program is basically financed by contributions on wages paid by employers, the insured, and the state as such (the reserve is very small). By the end of the 1980s, the combined percentage contribution on the payroll averaged 9%, higher or similar to that in many developed countries, despite the very low population coverage in many of the Region's countries. Both legal and statistical data confirm that the insured pays one-third or less of the total revenue, while the employer and the state finance the remainder, making the insured's "right" to benefits (based on the alleged payment of their costs) a questionable supposition. Such an assumption has justified the discriminatory treatment dealt to users of social welfare, and has increased the obstacles (in addition to structural ones) for extending coverage in countries that have a small employed salaried labor force. Once that assumption is questioned, the wage contribution can begin to be replaced by other types of financing that might facilitate extension.

The current financing system also appears to have a regressive effect on distribution: the percentage contribution paid by the insured is flat, and in 75% of the countries there is a contribution ceiling; despite no solid evidence, it appears that the employer's contribution is transferred to prices, while the state contribution often comes from regressive taxes; and, when a small proportion of the population is covered by social insurance, the unprotected majority (including the poor) may contribute to finance coverage of higher income groups through prices and/or taxes (this effect diminishes as population coverage increases). Despite its high percentage of contribution and the large share of health revenue it receives (both within social insurance and vis-a-vis the public health sector), the sickness-maternity program has been steadily deficitary in most Latin American countries, because its expenditures have grown much faster than its revenue. The causes of the disequilibrium in terms of income are: actual revenue that falls below the potential to be collected (due to such factors as contribution ceilings and exclusion of fringe benefits in computing contributions); significant and increasing evasions and payment delays (fluctuating from 19% to 60%), largely due to administrative deficiencies such as poor registration, inspection, fines, and legal/judicial procedures, but also due to the small size of enterprises and abundant self-employment; and substantial and increasing state debt which is shrinking in real terms due to inflation (true of private debt for evasion and/or *mora*, too).

Deficits in the sickness-maternity programs were traditionally covered with loans from the pension program, but the former could neither amortize them nor pay interest, hence contributing to the decapitalization of the pension fund. As pension programs matured and their expenditures increased, the surplus shrank and deficits emerged in the pension program as well, forcing a halt to the transfers to sickness-maternity which, in turn, found itself in crisis. The state cannot come to the rescue of the program due to the economic crisis.

Sources of financing for public health care are mainly the state budget and, to a lesser extent, the sale of services, user fees, and external aid. In countries that have national health systems (or in the public health sector in those that have social insurance) health care traditionally has been provided free to the poor (assuming they have real access to the services). Due to the economic crisis of the 1980s, budgets of public health programs have been cut in 90% of the countries, and there has been an increase in user fees. The latter, however, may further reduce the poor's access to health care. The economic crisis also has sharply cut the revenue of both social insurance (due to a growth in unemployment, the informal sector, and evasion, as well as declining real wages) and the ministry of health (due to stabilization programs that have cut social services, particularly investment). Population coverage under social insurance has declined or stagnated in many countries (extension programs to rural areas also have been harmed), hence increasing the demand for public health care. It could not be ascertained whether an increasing demand by the public sector (combined with cuts in funding, hospital admissions, and the average stay) has provoked an overall deterioration in the quality of public health care. Nevertheless, there is evidence of rising infant morbidity from diarrhea and an increase (or slowdown in the decrease) of infant mortality in five countries, as well as cuts in medicines and in medical and other supplies in two countries. One of the few benefits emanating from the crisis is the increased concern for and involvement in health care in Latin America and the Caribbean by international and/or regional organizations.

THE GROWING COSTS OF HEALTH CARE

Health Care Expenditures: Size, Distribution by Sector and Trends

There are practically no studies on the total costs of the three health care sectors for the entire Region. Most available information pertains to the social insurance sickness-maternity program and, to a lesser extent, to the ministry of health. Table 23 presents gross estimates of health care costs as a percentage of GDP in nine countries of Latin America, mostly for the social insurance and public sectors; information for the private sector is presented for four countries only. The highest total percentages (last column of the table) were registered in Argentina and Costa Rica (7%) and in Uruguay, Colombia, Cuba, and Brazil (5% to 4%); all of them, except

Table 23. Health expenditures (by sector and total) as percentage of GDP in selected countries of Latin America, 1985–1986.

Countries	Public sector	Social insurance	Private sector	Total
Argentina	2.1	2.6	2.4	7.1
Brazil[a]	1.2	1.3	1.5	4.0
Chile	--------2.6--------		n.a.	2.6
Colombia	1.9	2.5	0.2[c]	4.6
Costa Rica	2.1[d]	4.8	n.a.	6.9
Cuba[b]	3.6	0.7[e]	0	4.3
Ecuador	1.2	0.7	n.a.[f]	1.9
Peru[a]	1.8	1.2	n.a.	3.0
Uruguay	1.8	0.4	3.2[g]	5.4

Source: Mesa-Lago, 1989.
[a]1982.
[b]1980.
[c]Excludes the private non-institutional sector (the majority of the private sector).
[d]Includes sewer and employment injury.
[e]Only cash benefits.
[f]In 1983 it was reported as 47.2% of total health expenditures.
[g]Includes mutual-aid societies, cooperatives, etc.

for Colombia, are among the most developed countries in the Region. The total percentage in Chile (2.6%) is surprisingly low, but the table excludes the rapidly growing private sector. Less developed countries, such as Peru and Ecuador, show percentages of 3% and 2%, respectively. Scattered information from the remaining Latin American countries suggests that, with the exception of Panama, they have percentages of 2% or less (Zschock 1979; De Ferranti, 1985; PAHO/ILO/CPISS, 1986; PAHO, 1987). In three of the countries in Table 23 (Argentina, Colombia, and Costa Rica), social insurance has the highest percentage, while in three other countries (Cuba, Ecuador, and Peru), the ministry has the higher percentage; note that in Cuba, the ministry provides all health care, while social insurance only pays cash benefits. In Brazil and Uruguay, the highest percentage is in the private sector due to the subcontracting of social insurance with the private sector; in Argentina the percentages of social insurance and the private sector are similar.

The absence of data and changes in methodology make the historical trend in health care costs as a percentage of GDP even more difficult to track. For many years, the ILO has compiled three series of reports on social security costs that include health care expenditures of social insurance (both cash and in-kind benefits) as well as "public health services." Although valuable, the ILO series do not completely fill the existing information vacuum and make it difficult to estimate costs in both sectors.

To complicate matters further, starting in 1978

the ILO excluded health care expenditures in the public sector from its series, but included such expenditures in countries with national health services (often of a contributory nature) that are part of social insurance. This change has created comparability problems in the series before and after 1978. Furthermore, it makes it practically impossible to assess health costs in non-Latin Caribbean countries, because they have a public health system that is not part of social insurance, and consequently, since 1978 its expenditures for medical-hospital care are not included in the series (ILO, 1985a). After considering these problems, the ILO series on social security health expenditures as a percentage of GDP for ten Latin American countries in 1960–1980, shows a clear increasing trend in all but one, and in two countries (Costa Rica and Panama) it shows fivefold to sixfold increases in such expenditures (PAHO/ILO/CPISS, 1986).

Health expenditures in Latin America—the highest in the Third World—are relatively high by international standards, and exhibit a growing trend that follows a similar trend in overall social security expenditures (Mesa-Lago, 1990). Health cost percentages over GDP in Argentina, Costa Rica, and Uruguay are similar to those in the United Kingdom, which has one of the most comprehensive national health systems in the world. Nevertheless, it should be said that higher percentages of GDP devoted to health care do not necessarily mean better health standards. To avoid distortions in international com-

parisons, it would be necessary to homogenize a series of factors, or at least control existing differences in such factors as the quality of services, deflation in the cost of goods and services, administrative efficiency, and environmental variations (Zschock, 1979; Musgrove, 1987).

Table 24 reconstructs the ILO series (1965–1983) on the percentage of benefit expenditures of social insurances (plus family allowances) devoted to health (cash and in-kind benefits) in 17 countries of Latin America. All but four of the countries show a clear declining trend, because, when social insurance began, practically all benefit expenditures were in health, given that the pension program was incipient and there were very few pensioners. As the pension program matured, the percentage of benefit expenditure going to pensions increased, with the opposite effect in the percentage of health expenditures. Between 1965 and 1983, the regional average of benefit expenditures going to health care declined from 57% to 48%, while the average percentage going to pensions increased from 24% to 51%. Countries with the oldest pension programs (Uruguay, Chile, Ecuador, Argentina, and Brazil) have the lowest percentages in health, while countries with the newest pension programs (Honduras, El Salvador, the Dominican Republic, Venezuela, and Colombia) exhibit the highest percentages in health. As we have said, these trends have had a destabilizing effect on both the pension program and health

Table 24. Percentage of benefit expenditure of social insurances[a] assigned to the sickness-maternity program, in Latin America, 1965–1983.

Countries[b]	1965	1970	1975	1980	1983
Argentina	n.a.	n.a.	14.5	24.1	27.1
Bolivia	55.4	58.0	56.0	56.6	40.9
Brazil	n.a.	47.2	40.0	37.9	33.7
Chile	16.6	19.9	25.1	24.0	15.4
Colombia	63.3	56.5	65.2	55.4	62.9
Costa Rica	77.8	78.4	77.4	79.8	68.6
Dominican Republic	n.a.	66.6	72.0	73.2	73.1
Ecuador	18.9	n.a.	37.5	32.7	16.9
El Salvador	91.2	88.9	91.0	87.9	75.8
Guatemala	18.8	50.3	51.2	49.6	42.6
Honduras	96.3	97.4	n.a.	93.7	91.3
Mexico	73.3	71.8	68.0	69.3	67.0
Nicaragua	89.4	85.2	81.9	74.8	27.9
Panama	60.4	58.1	54.2	55.3	54.5
Peru	n.a.	n.a.	n.a.	60.0	58.7
Uruguay	n.a.	3.6	6.1	6.3	8.8
Venezuela	79.9	94.7	72.0	65.8	n.a.

Sources: ILO, 1981, 1985a, 1988; Mesa-Lago, 1989.
[a]Includes benefits in cash and in kind of social insurances and family allowances.
[b]Haiti does not have health insurance in effect, Paraguay was not included in the series, and Cuba was included but health care is not provided by social insurance.

care programs (see the section, "Coping with the Deficit," beginning on p. 42).

Non-Latin Caribbean countries were excluded from Table 24 for the above-mentioned methodological reasons. Since the social insurance program in these countries only pays monetary benefits for sickness and maternity (medical-hospital care is provided by the ministry of health), their percentage of benefit expenditures devoted to health as reflected in the ILO series is very small, despite the fact that these countries were the last in establishing social insurance in the Region. However, if the old ILO series on total social security benefit expenditures is used (which included health care expenditures in the public sector until 1977), these countries' proportion devoted to medical-hospital expenditures increases to two-thirds or more (ILO, 1981).

Causes of the Increase in Health Care Costs

The increasing costs of health care in Latin America and the Caribbean, as well as the resulting financial deficits in the social insurance sickness-maternity program, can be explained by universal causes and by peculiarities in the Region. Determining factors are both external (demographics, inflation) and internal (health care philosophy, level of population coverage, generosity of benefits, high administrative costs, hospital inefficiency).

Demographic and Epidemiological Profiles

The Region's most developed countries (e.g., Argentina, Cuba, Uruguay, and several non-Latin Caribbean countries) exhibit demographic features similar to those seen in industrialized countries—low population growth rates, high life expectancy, and an aging of the population. The rapidly increasing older population groups demand health services for longer periods, as well as increasingly sophisticated and costly treatment. The epidemiological profile of these countries also resembles that of developed countries: the main causes of death are "development diseases" (cardiovascular diseases, malignancies, traffic accidents) that are difficult and costly to treat. Despite its relatively young population, Costa Rica shares the same epidemiological profile, because of its rapidly expanding social security and high health standards.

However, in most of Latin America, a high population growth remains as the major problem, and it is expected to induce a twofold increase in the demand for health services in the next two decades (Castellanos, 1978; Malloy and Borzutzky, 1982).

The Region's less developed countries have young populations and an epidemiological profile characterized by the predominance of "underdevelopment diseases" (perinatal, malnutrition, digestive, respiratory, contagious). These diseases can be efficiently treated with simpler and cheaper techniques, such as immunization, sanitation, health education, and nutrition supplements, than can "development diseases." This would lead one to believe that the relative costs of health care should be lower in these countries. However, social insurance—which takes a large and growing share of the health pie—emphasizes curative medicine and concentrates its resources in the productive age groups and retired populations, thus inducing higher health costs.

Inflation

Persistent inflation has brought on long-term increases in the cost of medicines, medical equipment, construction, and salaries, and the record high levels of inflation suffered in Latin America and the Caribbean in the 1980s have aggravated this problem. Technological advances in medical-hospital equipment and drugs, and the fact that most of them are usually imported at high prices, have reinforced the increasing trend in health costs.

Predominance of Curative Medicine

As has been said, the priority assigned to costly curative medicine (particularly by social insurance institutions) over low-cost preventive medicine is an inefficient way to allocate health care resources. Emphasis is put on capital intensive services and high technology, on hospitalization instead of outpatient care, on physicians over paramedic personnel, and on the use of increasingly complex and costly equipment, surgery, laboratory tests, and treatment such as kidney dialysis, chemotherapy, organ transplants, heart surgery, and nuclear medicine. The 1979 Brazilian budget assigned more funds to these high-tech services for 12,000 people living in the developed southeast and south regions than to primary health services and disease control for 41 million people living in the underdeveloped northeast regions. In Costa Rica, the rural health program at the beginning of the 1980s did more, with a smaller budget, to reduce mortality and morbidity than the capital intensive services of social insurance. The exorbitant cost of adding sophisticated health care benefits for the few obstructs the extension of basic services for all.

The distribution of health funds between preventive and curative medicine can be an indicator of the efficiency in health administration, especially when it is abnormally skewed. The ratio of curative to preventive expenditures was 4 to 1 in Costa Rica in 1978; 6 to 1 in Brazil in 1982; 9 to 1 in Mexico in 1980; and 15 to 1 in Chile in 1981. Because curative medicine treats the disease without dealing with its causes, it becomes more expensive than prevention in the long run. Consequently, shifting emphasis toward preventive medicine could cut down costs, reduce morbidity and mortality, and be more efficient over time by making curative medicine less necessary (Castellanos, 1978; Selowsky, 1980; CCSS, 1981; McGreevey et al, 1984; McGreevey, 1987, 1990).

Extension of Population Coverage

The expansion of social insurance coverage also helps increase health costs (and generate deficit). Once the urban-salaried sector, which has higher levels of income and health, is covered, then the incorporation of the informal and rural population, with lower income and health standards, is costlier; the latter group (in the few countries where it is protected) contributes nothing or relatively little, but uses health services more. In those countries where social insurance cares for ''indigents'' (Costa Rica, Chile) or partly finances programs for the rural sector (Brazil, Mexico), health care expenditures are higher than contributions plus state subsidies (when the latter are paid).

Generosity in Benefits

Benefits and entitlement conditions in sickness-maternity insurance in Latin America tend to be generous. According to Table 25, five countries do not require a qualifying period of work or contribution for paid sickness leave, requiring only that the person be employed; this also holds true for maternity benefits in four countries. Six countries require a qualifying period of only four to six weeks to receive paid sickness leave. Furthermore, in three countries, sickness leave is paid at a rate equal to 100% of the salary, and in two additional countries, at a 90% rate; in ten countries, maternity leave is equal to the salary. In the non-Latin Caribbean, however, there is always a qualifying period that is usually longer, with one exception for sickness, and

paid leave averages 60% of the salary (two countries do not grant this benefit). Finally, in most of the Region there is no qualifying period for medical-hospital benefits.

These conditions encourage workers to simulate sickness and collect paid leave (a problem reported in several countries), significantly increasing the costs of this program. In countries where the only conditions are to be insured or to have paid a few contributions, evaders frequently have access to costly health care treatment by simply registering or paying a small sum, and thereafter stopping their contributions.

It also should be recalled that, in Latin America, the insured's dependents (spouse and children and, in some countries, parents and siblings as well) are entitled to medical-hospital benefits. Some countries provide, at least until recently, expensive benefits such as contact lenses and orthodontics, as well as the cost of travel and treatment abroad when the required health care treatment is not available at home (e.g., in Ecuador, Peru, Costa Rica until 1982, and Colombia until 1986). In 1982, the cost of treating 131 insured Peruvians abroad was $US5 million, or $US38,168 per capita (Mesa-Lago, 1989).

Generous and lopsided social insurance benefits in the Region have had a perverse demonstration effect, have contributed to escalating costs, impeded universalization of coverage, provoked actuarial and financial disequilibria, and eventually have led to the deterioration in the quality of health care. Privileged benefits only partly financed by the insured also have had a regressive impact on income distribution. In the pioneer countries, the privileged programs covering the most powerful pressure groups were at the beginning easy to finance through subsidies (directly paid by the state, special taxes, and/or price increases), because those groups were relatively small and the state was capable of transferring part of the financing to other groups. These programs, however, served as models which were eventually imitated by larger, less privileged groups. Increasing trade unionism, combined with state intervention (to co-opt some groups) and concessions by political parties competing for electoral votes, played a key role in the so-called ''massification of privilege'' (i.e., gradual expansion of some generous benefits and entitlement conditions to an increasing number of insured). But, what was financially viable for a minority of insured (although unjustifiable under an equity viewpoint) could not, in the long

Table 25. Entitlement conditions for sickness-maternity benefits of social insurance in Latin America and the Caribbean, 1987.

Countries	Monetary benefits						Medical-hospital benefits	
	Sickness			Maternity				
	Contribution weeks	% of salary	Length (weeks)	Contribution weeks	% of salary	Length (weeks)	Contribution weeks	Length (weeks)
Latin America								
Argentina	a	100	26	42	100	12	a	
Bolivia	9	75	26–52	17	75	12	4S, 17M	26
Brazil	52	70–90	g	a	100	12	13	
Chile[d]	26	100		26	100	18	a	
Colombia	4	50–66.6	26–52	12	100	8	4	26–52
Costa Rica	4	50	26	26	50	17	4S, 26M	52
Cuba	a	50–90		11	100	18	b	
Dominican Republic	6	50	26	30	50	12	1S, 15M	26
Ecuador	26	66–75	26	26	75	8	26	
El Salvador	8e	75	52	12	75	12	8e	26–52
Guatemala	a	66	26	a	100	11	a	
Honduras	5	50–66	26–52	11	66	12	a	
Mexico	4–6	60	52–78	30	100	12	a	52–104
Nicaragua	8	60	26–52	16	60	12	a	
Panama	26	70	26–52	39	100	14	a	26
Paraguay	6	50	26–52	6	50	9	a	26–52
Peru	13	100	49	39	100	13	13	52
Uruguay	13	70	52–104	a	100	12		
Venezuela	a	50–66.6	52	a	66.6	12	a	52
Non-Latin Caribbean								
Antigua and Barbuda	26	60		26	60	13	b	
Bahamas	40	60	26	50	60	13	b	
Barbados	13e	66.6	26	30	100	12	b	
Belize	50	60	11	50	60	12		
Bermuda	h	h	h	h	h	h	c	
Dominica	13	60	26	26	60	12	b	
Grenada	a	60	26	30	60	12	b	
Guyana	50	60	26	15	60	13	b	
Jamaica	h	h	h	f	f	f	b	
St. Christopher	26	60	26	39	60	13	b	
St. Lucia	26	60	26	30	60	13	b	
St. Vincent	26	60	26	30	60	13	b	
Trinidad and Tobago	10	66.6	52	10	60	13	b	

Source: Author's compilation based on U.S. Social Security Administration, 1987.
S = Sickness; M = Maternity
aThe only condition is to be insured or be currently employed.
bNot supplied by social insurance but by the national health system or public health sector. Usually residency (or citizenship) is the only needed condition.
cResidents, with a waiting period of 39 weeks.
dOld system. In the new system the insured can freely select the provider; conditions and benefits are considerably different among providers.
eFor the unemployed; there are no conditions for those employed.
fFor domestic servants only.
gFor all the necessary time.
hThis benefit is not available.

run, work for the mass of insured (Mesa-Lago, 1978).

High Administrative Costs

Administrative expenditures for social security in Latin America are among the highest in the world. Because there are no disaggregated statistics on costs and employment in health programs, the first column of figures in Table 26 refers to all social security programs; however, the sickness-maternity program is the one with the highest administrative costs. In 1983–1986, the percentages of administrative expenditure over total expenditures in Latin America and the Caribbean ranged as follows: 3% to 5.9% in Argentina, Barbados, Costa Rica, and Uruguay; 6% to 8.9% in Brazil, Panama, and Chile; 9% to 11.9% in Peru, Colombia, and Guatemala; 12% to 14.9% in Jamaica, El Salvador, and Bolivia; 15% to 17.9% in Mexico, Venezuela, and Honduras; 19% to 22.9% in the Bahamas, the Dominican Republic, and Ecuador; and 23% to 32% in Nicaragua and Trinidad and Tobago. With very few exceptions, these percentages increased in 1977–1980, but in 1980–1983 they increased in only half of the countries and stagnated or declined in the other half. In contrast

Table 26. Indicators of administrative efficiency of social insurance[a] in Latin America and the Caribbean, 1980–1987.

Countries[b]	% of administrative expenditure over total expenditures (1983–1986)	Employees per 1,000 insured (1980–1987)
Argentina	3.4	n.a.
Bahamas	21.8	3.8
Barbados	5.0	2.4
Bolivia	14.5	6.7
Brazil	6.8	n.a.
Chile	8.2	n.a.
Colombia	11.6	7.4
Costa Rica	5.0	13.0
Dominican Republic	22.0[f]	20.5
Ecuador	22.5	13.2
El Salvador	13.7	13.5
Guatemala	11.8	7.4
Honduras	17.8	n.a.
Jamaica	12.8	0.6
Mexico	17.1–17.3[c]	8.9–10.4[c]
Nicaragua	28.0	4.5
Panama	7.7	11.7
Peru	11.4	7.0/10.5[e]
Trinidad and Tobago	32.4[d]	n.a.
Uruguay	5.4	n.a.
Venezuela	17.6	4.1

Source: Mesa-Lago, 1990.

[a]Includes family allowances or programs for civil servants in seven countries.

[b]There are no data for Cuba, Haiti, or Paraguay. In most countries, coverage by social insurances only; other countries include family allowances and/or pensions for civil servants and/or noncontributory pensions.

[c]In the largest two funds (IMSS and ISSSTE); IMSS data for 1985 are from Wilkie, 1989.

[d]8.7% if all programs (including social welfare) are taken into account.

[e]The lowest is the official figure and the highest is the figure adjusted in 1988 to correct overestimation of population coverage.

[f]41% in 1988.

with Latin America and the Caribbean, the percentages of administrative expenditures in industrialized countries of North America, Europe, and Asia are much lower, from 2% to 4% (ILO, 1981, 1985a, 1988).

In those countries where social insurance was introduced recently (as in the non-Latin Caribbean), a high percentage of administrative expenditures can partly be explained by the need for minimum personnel, equipment, and physical plant to operate the system, combined with low initial benefit expenditures; as the latter increase, the proportional cost of operation will be greatly reduced. However, Table 26 shows divergent percentages among the four non-Latin Caribbean countries, and these differences cannot be explained solely by the short time that the program has been in operation, but rather by a given country's administrative frugality

(5% in Barbados) or prodigality (22% in the Bahamas).

In countries that have multiple administrative agencies and/or low population coverage, administrative expenditure percentages tend to be higher (e.g., Dominican Republic, Ecuador, Honduras, Bolivia, Colombia) than in countries with universal coverage that began relatively unified or subsequently undertook processes of unification and standardization (e.g., Argentina, Brazil, Costa Rica, Uruguay, and Panama). Usually, administrative expenditures of privileged agencies are higher than those of the general agency; for example, in Bolivia, the petroleum institute spends six times per insured the amount spent by the general agency. In some countries the law fixes a percentage for administrative costs, but this norm, rather than restraining those expenditures, often becomes an incentive to spend up to the allowable ceiling (Thullen, 1985; Schulthess, 1988).

Economies of scale may reduce costs, thus explaining the lower administrative expenditures in industrialized countries (as well as in Latin American and Caribbean countries with the largest and most unified programs). However, Denmark, Ireland, and Norway, all small industrialized countries, have lower percentages of administrative expenditures than do countries in the Region, except for Costa Rica (Mackenzie, 1988).

Escalating Costs of Personnel and Medicines

Personnel represents the bulk of expenditures among administrative costs; the second column in Table 26 measures its importance in 15 Latin American and Caribbean countries through a ratio of employees per 1,000 insured. In some countries, the percentages are underestimated, because personnel data exclude temporary employees, which could account for a sizable percentage of the total number of employees. In addition, because population coverage data are often overestimated, the ratio of employees per 1,000 insured is underestimated.

The enormous bureaucracies in the Dominican Republic, El Salvador, and Ecuador, demonstrated by ratios of 13.2 to 20.5 employees per 1,000 insured, may explain the high administrative costs in these countries. And yet, although Costa Rica and Panama have ratios of 13.0 and 11.7, respectively, they have relatively low percentages of administrative expenditure, which could be explained by these countries' better health services and higher health standards, combined with greater efficiency in other administrative aspects. The ratios for the Bahamas (3.8), Barbados (2.4), and Jamaica (0.6) are the lowest in the Region; the Bahamas' highest ratio among the three countries possibly accounts for its higher administrative costs.

In the social insurance and ministry of health budgets, the highest line item is always personnel, particularly physicians, who not only have the highest salaries but also enjoy exceptional fringe benefits often gained through strikes. Social insurance personnel usually has a higher set of benefits (by collective agreement) than that of the insured, and is exempted from contributing to the sickness-maternity program. In some countries, the surplus of physicians exert pressure to be hired and to perform services that could be done at a lower salary by paramedic personnel. Salaries in the ministry of health are normally lower than in social insurance. In Costa Rica in 1982–1985, the cost of personnel in the former declined from 62% to 48% of the budget, while in the latter it increased from 53% to 57%. In Peru, the cost of personnel in social insurance increased from 38% to 50% in 1982–1985, while in Uruguay the corresponding cost at the ministry of health declined from 61% to 55% in 1983–1984 (DETEC, 1987; Acuña et al, 1987; Mesa-Lago, 1988b).

In some countries, stabilization programs introduced in the 1980s have targeted their overlarge bureaucracies; "emergency plans" have frozen employment and promoted early retirement. For instance, in Colombia the employee/insured ratio was reduced from 10.9 to 7.4 in 1975–1985, and in Argentina, 36% of the employees were dismissed between 1980 and 1986 (Mesa-Lago and De Geyndt, 1987). Political and social pressures, however, are very strong, and trimming the leafy bureaucracy is a formidable task. Social security agencies have often become a major source of employment that alleviates open unemployment but neglects its principal objective which is to cover the population, particularly those in need, against social risks.

The next highest item in health budgets in Latin America and the Caribbean is materials and supplies—between 22% and 34% in Argentina, Chile, Colombia, Costa Rica, Peru, and Uruguay in the 1980s. In this category, the most important expenditure is medicines, whose costs have gradually increased partly due to such factors as overprescription, unnecessary diversification, sale promotions that induce users to demand specific brands, and new discoveries that make the existing stocks obsolete

(International Social Security Association, 1982).

Hospital Inefficiencies

The lack of integration or, at least, of coordination among the various providers of health services, particularly between social insurance and the ministry of health, promotes duplication of physical plants and costly equipment, as well as low percentages of hospital occupancy. For instance, in Sucre, Bolivia, in 1986 the social insurance hospital had an occupancy of 30% and, nearby, there was a railroad hospital with 15% occupancy. Primary and secondary level services are often inadequately staffed and supplied; hence, the users, particularly of outpatient consultations, skip these levels and go directly to tertiary (specialized) hospitals, creating jams and depleting resources from these more complex services. Once again, a more rational allocation of resources (i.e., investing more at the primary level) could resolve or ameliorate these problems (Castellanos, 1985; PAHO, 1978, 1981, 1987).

Table 27 compares national averages of hospital occupancy and length of stay among eleven Latin American countries. Although figures are rough and not always comparable (e.g., they deal with different institutions), they show that hospital occupancy was 60% or below in three countries, under 70% in six, and above 80% in only three. Furthermore, with the exception of

Table 27. Indicators of hospital efficiency in selected Latin American countries, 1979–1985.

Countries	Sector	% of hospital occupancy	Days of stay
Argentina (1980)	Public	60.6	7.5–26.9[e]
Chile (1985)	Both	75.3	8.5
Colombia[a] (1984)	Public	56.2	5.4
Costa Rica (1985)	Insurance	81.0	6.3
Cuba (1980)	Public	81.0	9.6
Dominican Republic (1985)	Insurance	51.7	10.4
Ecuador[b] (1979)	Both	58.0	8.2
Mexico[c] (1982)	Insurance	67.0	4.6
Panama (1984)	Both	67.0	7.0
Peru (1985)	Insurance	70.4	11.7
Uruguay[d] (1984)	Public	81.8	13.3

National averages of

Source: Mesa-Lago, 1989.
[a]The social insurance sector had averages of 61% and 7.3 days.
[b]Within social insurance, in 1981, averages were 82.7% and 9.3 days.
[c]IMSS; the ISSSTE averages were 70% and 5.7 days.
[d]Montevideo (excludes chronic patients); outside of Montevideo, the averages were 51.2% and 7.9 days.
[e]Extreme variation among provinces.

Costa Rica, those countries with the highest occupancy also have an abnormally high average of length of stay. If the latter were reduced, the percentage of occupancy would decline as well. For instance, the occupancy percentage in Montevideo (81.8%) would have declined to 41% if the average days of stay had been cut from 13.3 to 6.6; in addition, outside of the capital city, occupancy averaged 51.2% with a still high average days of stay of 7.9. Although it is true that tertiary-level hospitals are concentrated in the capital city and some users must travel long distances and, consequently, need more days at the hospital for diagnosis and postoperative care, the average days of stay still are too high by international standards (Rodriguez Grossi, 1985).

National averages presented in Table 27 hide extreme variations among regions and individual hospitals. For instance, Ecuador's national average of hospital occupancy was 58%, but in seven out of twenty provinces it was below 40%; Peru's national average was 70%, but in three out of eight regions it was below 50%. The low population coverage in these two countries makes these inefficiencies all the more serious. Low occupancy usually is the result of either excessive hospital capacity (often there are two hospitals, the ministry's and social insurance's, in the same location), poor quality of the hospital, or cultural barriers that impede proper use. Better integration, planning, allocation of resources, and education could overcome most of these problems (Mesa-Lago, 1984, 1988c).

Other Managerial Inefficiencies

There is a universal trend in Latin America and the Caribbean toward an increased use of computers in social insurance and health administration, either through ownership or rental of equipment. Computerization usually is viewed as a panacea for multiple problems such as evasion, payment delays, and processing of benefits. Although this is a positive move, problems remain. For instance, lack of skilled personnel and software often result in serious underutilization of computing equipment: in Ecuador in 1984, costly rented equipment was used once a month by the budget department, but calculations were done manually and then entered into the computer only for printing purposes. Furthermore, computerization alone cannot solve problems that require follow-up actions; for example, up-to-date records on employee payments should be followed by a dynamic collection enforcement of delinquent accounts.

Financing data often are divided among several departments—accounting, budget, investment, treasury—and either are not integrated or are plagued with errors and contradictions. Budgets are commonly constructed by program (such as sickness-maternity or pensions), rather than by function or budget category; this makes integration difficult or impossible, a problem that is compounded by obscure transfers within programs. In other cases, data are not disaggregated, making it impossible to evaluate the financial status of each program. In some countries, accounts do not provide the necessary basis for establishing the links between contributions and benefit payments within one program. In a few countries, accounting records have lapsed for relatively long periods; Peru, for example, has no records for 1968–1978. In some cases, external consultants have been hired to study accounting problems, and their recommendations have been ignored by an incoming administration that, in turn, has hired new consultants to study the same problems.

In some countries that have an indirect system of health care, contracts with private institutions lack proper controls and have led to higher costs in services due to unnecessarily long hospital stays, prescription of unnecessary surgery or laboratory tests, overprescription of medicines, and charging for services which were not actually delivered. These flaws have been studied in Brazil and Peru.

Last but not least, are the corruption and irregularities in the administration. In Peru, a congressional commission investigating social security in 1973–1982, documented cases of fraud, illegal activities, and negligence. In Panama, social insurance lost $US40 million at the beginning of the 1980s due to fraudulent operation in housing programs. In the Dominican Republic, 40% of the health services of social insurance in 1986 was illegally provided to noninsured patients with political connections, and another 10% to 15% of patients were treated for "scientific interest" (McGreevey et al, 1984; Mesa-Lago, 1984, 1985a, 1986b, 1987a, 1988a; Rezende et al, 1982; La Forgia, 1990).

Summary of the Growing Costs of Health Care and their Impact on the Poor

Despite their serious deficiencies, available data indicate that total health care expenditures as a percentage of GDP in Latin America and the Caribbean are relatively high by international standards—they are the highest in the Third World and, in some cases, approximate those of developed countries. Health care expenditures are growing, but, within social insurance, the share of the sickness-maternity program over total benefit expenditure is declining (as the pension share increases), with negative consequences for the financial stability of that program and for social insurance in general.

Causes for these increases in health care costs are both external and internal. In the Region's most developed countries, an aging population and an epidemiological profile similar to that of the world's developed countries have pushed costs up; in the least developed countries, a young, growing population, combined with a misallocation of health resources (not aimed at the diseases of "underdevelopment"), has resulted in relatively higher costs, while mortality and morbidity rates have not been significantly reduced. Another cause is the overwhelming preference (particularly in social insurance) for high-cost curative medicine, often geared to a minority of the population, over low-cost preventive medicine that could benefit the majority and be more efficient in improving health standards in the long run. Expanding population coverage also increases costs, because as the lower income groups become incorporated, they pay lower contributions and use health services more. Benefits and entitlement conditions of the sickness-maternity insurance program in Latin America (not so in the non-Latin Caribbean) are excessively generous and costly, often fostering simulation of sickness to collect paid leave, have a perverse demonstration effect, and contribute to financial disequilibria. Administrative expenditures of social insurance health programs are among the highest in the world, well above those of industrialized nations. A major reason for this is excessive personnel with relatively high salaries and fringe benefits. Escalating inflation, particularly since the 1980s, has increased personnel, medical supplies, and medicine costs. A multiplicity of health care providers (mainly in social insurance and in the ministry of health) and a lack of integration/coordination promote duplication of physical plant and equipment and low hospital occupancy, while the average length of stay is abnormally high. Other causes of rising costs include managerial inefficiencies and corruption.

The current model of health care in Latin America is extremely expensive, inefficient, and unfair. Because of its high, and rising, costs, in most cases this model cannot extend coverage and effective protection to the poor. In fact, the model's high cost has stood in the way of universalization of coverage. Even in those few countries that have achieved such universalization, increasing health care costs threaten that gain and may eventually cause decline in the quality of care. Obviously, there is a need for an urgent, global reform of the current model to reduce its costs, increase its efficiency and financial viability, and make it capable of extending its coverage to all the population, including the poor.

4.

FIVE CASE STUDIES

THE SELECTION OF THE COUNTRIES

Five countries were selected for an in-depth analysis of health care protection of the poor: Costa Rica, the Dominican Republic, Mexico, Peru, and Uruguay. The countries were selected so as to have representative examples from the Region; their inclusion followed four criteria: size and geographical location of the country; level of economic and social development (the latter with emphasis on health standards); poverty incidence and size of the informal sector and the traditional rural sector; and social insurance health coverage and existence or not of special programs for protection of the poor (see Table 28).

The five countries were ranked from best to worst based on 16 variables in the table, such as lowest territorial size and population, highest development, lowest poverty incidence, smallest informal/traditional rural sectors, highest social insurance coverage, and best special programs. Uruguay and Costa Rica tied for the highest ranking, Mexico placed in the middle, and Peru and the Dominican Republic tied for the lowest positions. Given that Uruguay has older welfare programs than Costa Rica and that Peru has older programs than the Dominican Republic, we decided to present the analysis of the five countries in that order, without implying a ranking of their health care coverage of the poor.

Uruguay, a small South American country both in territory and population, has the highest GDP per capita and urbanization ratio and the second best health standards of the five countries. Among them, Uruguay has the lowest poverty incidence, the smallest traditional rural sector, and the third smallest informal sector. Social insurance health coverage, both legally and statistically (except for overall population coverage) is the second best, but there is no special health program to protect the poor.

Costa Rica is a small Central American country both in territory and population. It has the third highest GDP per capita and the best health standards of the five selected countries. It is the least urbanized country of the five, which partly explains the lowest informal sector. Despite having the largest rural population, it has the second lowest traditional rural sector, and its poverty incidence is the second lowest. Social insurance legal health coverage is the best for the rural sector and better than Uruguay's for the informal sector because it includes the self-employed. Finally, it has a comprehensive social insurance welfare program to protect "indigents," the highest overall and informal sector statistical coverage by social insurance, and the third highest for the rural sector; however, if coverage by the Ministry of Health and indigent programs are added, its rural coverage also ranks first.

Mexico located in North America, is one of the largest countries in the Region in territory and population, and the largest of the five under study. It has the second highest GDP per capita and degree of urbanization, but ranks third in health standards, poverty incidence, size of the traditional rural sector (it has the second largest informal sector), and social insurance legal coverage. However, it is the second best on overall social insurance coverage and the best on coverage of the rural sector, due to a special health care program for peasants.

Peru is one of the largest South American countries both in territory and population, and the second largest of the five selected. Among them, it ranks fourth in GDP per capita and in urbanization, but has the worst health standards and the highest incidence of poverty and largest informal sector and traditional rural sectors. Its social insurance health program is

Table 28. Characteristics of the five countries selected as study cases, 1986–1988.

Countries	Area (thousand Km²)	GDP p/c ($US)	Infant mortality (x1,000)	Life expectancy (years)	Population Total (millions)	Population Urban (%)	Population Rural (%)	% of population in poverty Total	% in poverty Urban	% in poverty Rural	% of EAP, 1980, in: Informal sector[a]	% of EAP, 1980, in: Traditional rural sector	Social insurance coverage — Legal[b] Informal	Legal[b] Rural	Statistical[c] Population	Statistical[c] Informal	Statistical[c] Rural	Special health program to protect the poor
Uruguay	176	2,470	24	71	3.1	89	11	20	19	29	19.0	8.0	Mandatory (partly)	Mandatory	57.7	53.3	55.2	None except public health
Costa Rica	51	1,690	18	75	2.7	45	55	27	24	30	12.4	14.8	Mixed	Mandatory	83.1	100.0	48.8[f]	Social welfare for indigents
Mexico	1,973	1,760	46	69	83.7	71	29	37	30	51	22.0	18.4	Voluntary	Mixed	64.8[e]	0.8	56.0[e]	Primary health care for peasants
Peru	1,285	1,300	86	62	20.7	69	31	60	52	72	23.8	32.0	Mixed	Voluntary	19.3	4.0	5.5	None except public health
Dominican Republic	49	720	65	66	6.9	59	41	49[d]	48[d]	54[d]	16.0	24.6	None	None	4.2	0.0	0.0	None except public health

Sources: Author's compilation based on: UN/ECLAC/UNDP, 1980; ECLAC, 1990; World Bank, 1990; Mesa-Lago, 1990a; and Tables 2, 5, 7, 8, 9, and 12 of this study.

[a] PREALC classification, 1980; author estimates for mid-1980s (excluding wage earners) give much higher percentages: 21.6% in Costa Rica, 30.9% in Mexico, and 61.9% in Peru.

[b] Coverage of population according to law but not necessarily enforced. The column of informal refers to the self-employed and domestic servants. Mixed means that some are covered mandatorily (domestic servants in Uruguay, Costa Rica, and Peru) and some voluntarily (self-employed in Costa Rica, Mexico, and Peru) or are not covered (in Uruguay, the self-employed without a fixed place of work). Excludes unpaid family workers and wage earners. The column of rural refers basically to salaried workers in agriculture; self-employed rural workers abide by rules of the informal column.

[c] Percentage of population covered by social insurance sickness-maternity program according to official statistics; excludes coverage by public health sector; in Uruguay, includes collective institutions of medical aid. The first column refers to total population (includes workers and their dependents); the column of informal refers to self-employed only except for Uruguay which includes employers also. The column of rural refers to labor force in agriculture.

[d] Not from the ECLAC series but from various rough estimates.

[e] Includes COPLAMAR.

[f] If effective coverage by the Ministry of Health is added, the percentage increases to 56.9%.

fourth in legal and statistical coverage, and it has no special program to protect the poor.

The Dominican Republic is a small Caribbean country; it is the smallest in territory and the third in population size among the five selected countries. It has one of the lowest GDP per capita in the Region and the lowest among the five case studies; among them, it ranks fourth in urbanization and health standards. Poverty incidence probably is the second highest among the five cases, but there are no comparable data. It has the second highest traditional rural sector but the second lowest informal sector. The country's social insurance health program has the worst legal and statistical coverage, and it lacks a special program to protect the poor.

URUGUAY

POVERTY: SIZE, TRENDS, AND CHARACTERISTICS

In ECLAC's 1986 survey on poverty in ten Latin American countries, Uruguay had the second lowest poverty incidence among the total population (after Argentina): national 20%, urban 19%, and rural 29% (see Table 2). In 1981–1986, the national poverty incidence (households) apparently increased from 11% to 15%; among the total population, poverty incidence seems to have risen from 15% to 20%. There are no data available for 1970, except for urban households (see below). The number of poor increased by 45% in the same period; in 1986, there were 608,500 poor in Uruguay (one-fourth of them indigents); 82% lived in urban areas and 18% in rural areas (ECLAC-CEPAL, 1990).

Under the military government's neoconservative policies, the country's economy grew at a fair annual rate of 4.2% in 1974–1981, but with significant social costs: the real average wage declined 45% in the period and pensions decreased by a similar proportion; open unemployment increased, peaking in 1976 at 12.8% (but declined to 6.7% in 1981); public social expenditures were cut and income distribution became more regressive; and inflation averaged 63% in the period (although it decreased to 29% in 1981). The economic crisis, the worst in the country's history, struck hard in 1982 and continued through 1984: GDP declined 17% in the period, the real wage fell an additional 28% (real pensions dropped 31%), unemployment hit a record 15.5% in 1983 (plus 15% underemployment); the informal sector expanded; and inflation increased again in 1984 to 66%.

The restoration of democracy in 1985 brought new policies that tried to offset some of the wage losses, stimulate growth and employment, and stabilize the economy. They were largely successful: GDP growth increased 13% in 1986–1987 (but stagnated in 1988–1989), real wages almost recuperated the 1981 level, and open unemployment gradually declined to 9.2% in 1989 (underemployment was down to 7.5% in 1987). However, inflation peaked at 83% in 1985 and, although it was somewhat reduced in 1986–1988, it returned to the 1985 level in 1989 (Cobas, 1986; Giral et al, 1986; Davrieux, 1987; ECLAC, 1989).

Given these economic trends, it is safe to assume that poverty peaked in Uruguay at the time of the crisis (1982–1984) and declined with the vigorous economic recovery of 1986–1987. The ECLAC surveys, therefore, measured poverty in the year prior to the crisis (1981) and in the first year of strong growth (1986), missing the poverty peak in between.

A study on poverty conducted in Uruguay by the Division of Statistics and Census (DGEC) in cooperation with ECLAC, provides information for 1984 (towards the end of the crisis) and 1986, but it used a different methodology than the ECLAC surveys, and preliminary results are limited to Montevideo, the capital city. The study combined two dimensions: income (measured by a poverty line) and nonfulfillment of basic needs (measured by indicators on education, housing, water and sewage, and family size). Unfortunately, health and nutrition indicators were not included because such data was absent from the 1985 census. Four household groups resulted from the combination of the two dimensions: chronic poor (those below the poverty line who also have a deficiency in at least one indicator); circumstantial or recent poor (those who have fallen below the poverty line but who still can fulfill their basic needs); nonpoor with inertial deficiencies (those who are above the poverty line but cannot fulfill at least one basic need due to cultural problems shaped by a previous condition of poverty); and nonpoor who meet all their basic needs. Measurements to be discussed subsequently (although not strictly comparable with the ECLAC survey), indicate that poverty incidence in 1984 was much higher than in 1981, and that it declined in 1986 as a result of an increase in employment, real wages, and pensions (DGEC/ECLAC, 1989).

The Urban (Informal) Sector

Uruguay is either the most urbanized or the second most urbanized country in the Region (after Argentina). According to the 1985 census, 89.3% of the population was urban; based on World Bank data, 85% was urban in 1988. The process of urbanization was rapid: by 1965, 81% of the population was already urban. In 1985, 44% of the total population lived in Montevideo, 45% in other urban areas, and 11% in rural areas (DGEC, 1989a; World Bank, 1990).

According to ECLAC, urban poverty incidence (households) slightly declined from 10% in 1970 to 9% in 1981 (the year prior to the crisis), but had increased to 14% in 1986 (the first year of recovery). Data on total population indicate a poverty incidence of 12.8% in 1981 and 19.3% in 1986 for all urban areas; 8.8% and 13.4%, respectively, for Montevideo. About one-fourth of the urban poor were indigents; the incidence of urban indigence increased from 3.3% to 4.3% between 1981 and 1986, from 2% to 2.6% in Montevideo (ECLAC-CEPAL, 1990).

The above-mentioned DGEC study estimated a household poverty incidence in Montevideo of 20.5% in 1984, declining to 16.4% in 1986; the proportion of households that did not meet at least one basic need declined from 11.1% to 10.2% in the same period. Once again, these figures are not strictly comparable with those in the ECLAC survey, but they suggest that the peak in poverty was reached during the crisis, that poverty incidence declined in 1986, and that poverty incidence in 1986 (at least in Montevideo) was higher than estimated in the ECLAC survey. This study distributed the

population in 1984 as follows: chronic poor, 7.5%; recent poor, 13% (these two groups combined result in the estimated 20.5% poverty incidence); nonpoor with inertial deficiency, 3.6%; and nonpoor who met all basic needs, 76%. In 1986, the corresponding distribution was 6.7%, 9.7%, 3.5%, and 80.2%. The latter figures indicate a significant increase in the nonpoor; a significant decline in the recent poor (these two groups benefited from the economic recovery); a small decline in the chronic poor (the effect of the recovery on this group was marginal); and practically no change in the nonpoor with inertial deficiency. Despite the economic recuperation, the latter group did not improve its fulfillment of basic needs (DGEC/ECLAC, 1989).

As a percentage of the EAP, the informal sector grew little in 1960–1970, from 15.6% to 16.8%, but then jumped to 19% in 1980 (PREALC, 1982). In that year, Uruguay had the eighth largest informal sector in Latin America, placing its magnitude slightly above the regional median (Table 8). All experts agree that during the crisis of the 1980s, the informal sector grew due to the increase in open unemployment and underemployment. A 1984 household survey that covered 65% of the metropolitan area was conducted in Montevideo working-class neighborhoods, and this survey estimated that 69.5% of the heads of household were employed in the formal sector (65.8% full time and 3.7% part time) and 30.5% were employed full-time in the informal sector (20.1% were workers and 10.4% employers with at least one employee). The percentage of individuals engaged in the informal sector was slightly smaller: 28.4%, of which 21.9% were workers and 6.5% employers.

The survey focused on working-class neighborhoods, so we can assume that had all city areas been included, the proportion engaged in the informal sector would have been somewhat smaller. PREALC estimates for 1980, which include all urban areas and are, therefore, not strictly comparable, put Montevideo as having 44% of the total population and about one-half of the urban population. With these caveats, the 1984 survey suggests an increase in the informal sector from 19% for all urban areas in 1980, to 28.4% in working-class areas of the capital city in 1984, still during the crisis. The survey also detected an increase in the informal sector (from 5 to 10 percentage points, depending on the estimate) within the survey population between 1980 and 1984 (Portes, Blitzer, and Curtis, 1986).

PREALC (1982) data show that the percentage of salaried workers in the EAP increased from

76.4% in 1970 to 79.6% in 1979, while the combined percentage of self-employed, employers, and unpaid family workers declined from 20.8% to 18.1%. Comparable PREALC data are not available for the 1980s, but the 1985 census reported the salaried EAP at 70.8% (declining from 1979) and the nonsalaried at 27.3% (increasing by more than 9 percentage points since 1979, another indication of a growing informal sector in the 1980s). The vigorous economic recovery of 1986–1987, which did reduce poverty incidence, may not have diminished the informal-sector growth: in 1985, the nonsalaried urban EAP was 21.9%, but had increased to 24.1% in 1987; self-employment rose from 16% to 18% in the same period, and unpaid family workers, from 1% to 2% (DGEC, 1989, 1989a).

Characteristics of the informal sector in Montevideo are available from the 1984 survey. Women were twice as likely as men to be employed as informal workers, but only one-third as likely to be informal employers. Contrary to findings in other Latin American and Caribbean countries, the average age of those in the informal sector was three years older than of those in the formal sector. Between 75% and 79% of informal workers had no elementary and secondary education, as compared with between 28% and 30% among formal workers. The distribution of informal employment by occupational category was as follows: 47% were self-employed; 36%, salaried workers; and 8%, unpaid family workers and others. By economic branch, 39% of informal workers were in personal services; 30% in trade and hotels; 20% in construction and manufacturing; and the remaining 11% in other activities. Informal employers were concentrated in hotels and trade (33%), manufacturing (21%), and personal services (17%). Informal workers' earnings were half those of the average among formal workers, but informal employers' earnings were at least twice those of formal workers (Portes, Blitzer, and Curtis, 1986; Fortuna and Prates, 1989).

The 1985 census did not gather information on the health status of the population, just on sanitary housing conditions. Only 3.3% of urban homes lacked piped or well water in 1985, 2.5% did not have a toilet, and 5.5% had neither a toilet nor a latrine (DGEC, 1989). A study conducted in 1975 proved that infant mortality rates were universally correlated with better potable water and excreta disposal facilities. For instance, in Montevideo the population with inside plumbing and toilets had infant mortality rates of 34.5 and 35.7 per 1,000 live births, but

the rates increased to 64.8 and 71.8 among the population who lacked any facilities. The 1984 DGEC study on poverty found that in Montevideo, 63% of the homes that lacked piped or well water and 72% of those that lacked toilets or latrines were poor; the proportions for other urban areas were 68% and 80%, respectively (DGEC/ECLAC, 1989).

The authors of the 1984 survey of the informal sector in Montevideo speculated that 30% of the employed EAP (mostly salaried workers), being informal, probably lacked social insurance protection, although legally they were entitled to it. And yet, the survey found that only 6% of heads of households who had jobs covered by social insurance lacked real access to health and maternity services. One footwear factory owner who employed homeworkers reported that he did not cover his employees under social insurance to save taxes and reduce costs (Portes, Blitzer, and Curtis, 1986; Fortuna and Prates, 1989).

The Rural Sector

Uruguay's rural population in 1985 was only 10.7% of the total population. In 1986, 17.7% of all poor were in rural areas, as well as 28% of all indigents; rural poverty incidence was 28.7% and indigence incidence was 11.6%, compared with respective incidences of 19.3% and 4.3% in urban areas (13.4% and 2.6% in Montevideo). Therefore, although in absolute terms poverty was concentrated in urban areas (mainly outside of Montevideo), the tiny rural zone proportionally suffered more poverty. In 1980, the traditional rural sector in Uruguay was the smallest in Latin America after Argentina's. Recent data on income distribution were limited to the urban zone, impeding any comparison of income distribution with the rural zone (ECLAC-CEPAL, 1990).

Standards of living in Uruguay are among the highest in the Region and differences in such standards between urban and rural zones, albeit significant, are small in comparison with other Latin American and Caribbean countries. What follows are rural averages compared with urban averages (in parentheses): illiteracy, 8.2% (3.7%); lack of any formal education, 8.1% (4.3%); homes without piped or well water, 28.6% (3.3%); and homes without sanitary facilities for excreta disposal, 14.3% (2.5%) (DGEC, 1989). The 1984 study on poverty did not provide data on sanitary conditions among the rural poor.

Differences in health facilities and standards among departments are significant, but less dramatic than in other countries; however, these differences appeared to widen in the 1980s. The least developed departments tend to have the worst health resources and health standards. For instance, in 1984, Montevideo had 5.5 times more physicians and twice as many hospital beds per inhabitants than the Department of Rivera; the latter had the highest infant mortality rate, while the former had one of the lowest. In 1983–1985, the range in average infant mortality rates among the 19 departments was 21.1–34.6 (in Colonia and Rivera, respectively) with an interval of 13.5; in 1986 the range had expanded to 14.8–44.8 (in Flores and Durazno) with an interval of 30.0 (Ministerio de Salud, 1987).

HEALTH CARE COVERAGE OF THE URBAN (INFORMAL) AND RURAL POOR

Administrative Structure and Legal Coverage

The health care structure in Uruguay is one of the most complex in the Region and, although it went through a partial unification and standardization in the mid-1970s, it remains a mosaic of many institutions and programs. Four sectors can be distinguished: social insurance, mutual-aid societies and cooperatives, public, and private (Acuña et al, 1987; Saldaín, 1988; Mesa-Lago, 1989; Marquez, 1989).

The social insurance sector is currently managed by the Social Insurance Bank (BPS) and includes two major programs for private salaried workers—sickness insurance and maternity-infant care. Although Uruguay's social insurance pension program was one of the first in the continent, sickness-maternity insurance developed late (due to the early vigorous development of mutual-aid societies and cooperatives); when it emerged, the two branches operated separately. Maternity and infant care was introduced in 1958 as part of family allowance funds that rapidly proliferated, totalling at least sixteen by the mid-1970s. Sickness insurance also evolved in a fragmented manner (with independent funds protecting some 16 occupations); it began in 1948, but did not expand until 1960–1972. From 1973 to 1979, the military government intervened in all family-allowance

and sickness-insurance programs, unified and standardized them, and placed each of the two as separate branches of a state agency that deals with social insurances (maternity became independent from family allowances) and that manages unified pension and unemployment branches. In 1984–1986, coverage on sickness and maternity became legally mandatory to all the private salaried sector, including domestic servants (with some exceptions), rural workers, small agricultural producers, owners of micro-enterprises (with no more than one employee), homeworkers, newspaper street vendors, spouses of rural employers who do not hire more than two employees, and the unemployed while they receive BPS compensation. The last three groups and most BPS pensioners are entitled to maternity-infant care, but not to sickness care. Most of these occupational groups include poor people, but other occupations with a high incidence of poverty are excluded, such as the self-employed without a fixed workplace and unpaid family workers (when they are not protected as dependent family of the insured). Public sector employees (including the armed forces) are covered by their own agencies; banking and public notary employees, as well as university graduate professionals also have independent programs.

Sickness insurance provides the following benefits to the insured: preventive, full curative (medical, hospitalization, medicine), and rehabilitation (the only exclusions are highly specialized treatments such as organ transplants and dialysis) and paid leave for sickness and maternity. The maternity-infant program covers the insured female worker and the noninsured female whose children are beneficiaries of family allowances; the latter are covered too. This program provides full health care for pregnant women and for infants up to 3 months old; primary health care for children under 6 years old; dental care for children up to 9 years of age; and treatment for childhood congenital malformations up to 14 years of age.

BPS operates one maternity hospital and five clinics, and all but one are located in Montevideo; these facilities have less than one percent of all hospital beds in the country. All remaining health services (including maternity-infant care outside of Montevideo) are provided through Collective Institutions of Medical Aid (IAMCs). The insured may join one IAMC and can freely change from one to another. BPS collects all contributions for sickness insurance (maternity-infant services are financed by the state), reimburses the IAMCs on a capitation basis, and pays sickness maternity leaves to the insured directly. IAMCs also offer supplemental coverage on curative medicine for infants after three months of age, as well as for noninsured spouses for treatment other than maternity (BPS, 1989).

The IAMC sector consists of about 50 mutual-aid societies and cooperatives of physicians similar to HMOs; the IAMCs offer different plans, but all must provide prevention, inpatient and outpatient care, and diagnosis and rehabilitation services subject to minimum standards set by the Ministry of Public Health. They operate about 17% of all hospital beds, mostly in clinics. The IAMCs cover all those insured by BPS (except those under collective labor agreements) who, in addition to their monthly contributions to BPS, must pay user fees to the IAMCs. The latter also provide care for noninsured voluntary members who pay the full cost of the services, and public employees.

The public sector is mainly represented by the Ministry of Public Health, which is in charge of all the noninsured who are citizens or residents for one year and who lack economic means. Those who pass the means test receive free care (72% in 1983); the remainder pay fees ranging from 20% to 100% of the cost of service, depending on their income. Most health facilities in Uruguay are operated by the Ministry of Public Health, including 60 hospitals and 200 clinics and health centers (63% of all hospital beds); in places where IAMCs lack facilities, the insured can use the Ministry's. The University Hospital of Montevideo also falls within the public sector; it operates 5% of all hospital beds and provides free third-level, specialized care to the poor. Many of the country's 19 departments operate their own clinics and health centers, focusing on primary health care and tending to the poor.

There are other health care institutions within the public sector, but they basically do not protect the poor—the military and the police have one hospital each in Montevideo (3% of all hospital beds) that covers these two groups and their families and pensioners; some autonomous institutions operate their own services or contract with IAMCs to cover their employees; and the State Insurance Bank manages the employment injury program (which practically excludes all the poor) and has a specialized hospital in Montevideo. As has been said, civil servants are covered through their agencies; most of these probably are affiliated with IAMCs or use private facilities.

The private sector includes institutions of highly specialized medicine that receive some government financing and provide highly technical hospitalization services for BPS-IAMC affiliates. About 60 large enterprises have signed collective agreements with unions, covering their employees (about 60,000, who earn salaries above the national average) with special health packages; therefore, they are not covered by BPS. These enterprises lack facilities, and they contract with IAMCs. There are a few private hospitals and clinics, and most of their services are contracted by IAMCs and public institutions; they also provide care for a small number of high-income individuals. Health insurance and similar arrangements are a recent development and, so far, of little significance. The private sector operates about 10% of all hospital beds in the country.

This complex juxtaposition of health institutions theoretically is supervised by the Ministry of Public Health. In 1985, a Basic Public Health Law charged the Ministry with setting policy for the sector and defining programmatic goals and strategies, but its authority over other providers remains very limited (Márquez, 1989). In 1987, the Administration of State Health Services was created to coordinate the public, BPS, and IAMC sectors, but little has been accomplished so far. The head of BPS believes that integration is impossible in Uruguay, but that some type of coordination, particularly between the Ministry and BPS is feasible given adequate planning (Saldaín, 1988).

In summary, the poor in Uruguay (mainly self-employed, unpaid family workers, seasonal rural workers, unemployed not receiving benefits, etc.) are legally entitled to coverage by the Ministry of Health, the University Hospital, and departmental services. The portion of the poor who are insured at BPS (e.g., domestic servants, rural workers and small producers, owners of urban microenterprises) are covered by the IAMCs and by BPS's own maternity-infant facilities. The latter also covers other groups of homeworkers and newspaper street vendors.

Statistical Coverage

Given Uruguay's level of development and the country's tradition as a welfare state and pioneer of social security in the Western Hemisphere, adequate statistics on population health care coverage should be expected. However, because of the multiplicity of institutions and pro-

Table 29. Rough estimates of population coverage on health care in Uruguay, 1981–1987 (in thousands and percentages).

	Total population (1)	Coverage social insurance (BPS)[a] (2)	Reported coverage noninsured			Total covered (6)	% of population covered				
			IAMCs[b] minus BPS (3)	Ministry of Public Health (MSP)[c] (4)	Others[d] (5)		BPS (2/1)	IAMCs (3/1)	MSP (4/1)	Others (5/1)	Total (6/1)
1981	2,927	293	1,000	827	400	2,520	10.0	34.2	28.2	13.7	86.1
1984	2,990	266	955	900	386	2,507	8.9	31.9	30.1	12.9	83.8
1985	3,012	393	897	850	400	2,540	13.0	29.8	28.2	13.3	84.3
1987	3,057	484	943	830	424	2,681	15.8	30.8	27.2	13.9	87.7

Sources: Author's compilation based on Meerhoff, 1986; Acuña et al, 1987; Saldaín, 1988; DGEC, 1989a; Márquez, 1989.

[a]Sickness insurance that covers the worker plus maternity-infant program that covers pregnant women and children of insured.

[b]Total IAMCs coverage minus those insured on sickness at BPS; those in the column are civil servants and private individuals.

[c]Available estimates vary widely: 1.1 million in 1984 and 1985, 596,000 in 1987, and more than one million in 1989; includes University Hospital.

[d]Mainly armed forces, banking, and professionals and employees in other public institutions, as well as collective agreements and other private arrangements.

grams and the lack of a strong central agency, this is not the case.

Rough coverage estimates are presented in Table 29. The most accurate data in the table are for those insured at BPS and for IAMC affiliates; there is a statistical series for both. BPS figures are mainly for the insured in the sickness program; in addition, there is a small number (declining from 20,000 in 1981 to 11,500 in 1987) of pregnant women and infants covered by the maternity-infant program. The IAMC figures are a subtraction of those affiliates insured at BPS from the total number of IAMC affiliates; the figures in column 3, therefore, constitute the affiliates from public institutions or individuals. (Until 1980, the IAMCs compiled information on the characteristics of the affiliates, but no longer do.)

The Ministry of Public Health coverage is speculative, because no statistical series is available, only very rough estimates. The latter fluctuate widely—more than one million people were reported under coverage in 1984–1985, but only slightly more than one-half a million were reported in 1987. A Ministry official and scholar assured me in 1989 that all of the population not covered by other institutions have actual access to Ministry services, and that the longest travel time between a given population cluster to a Ministry hospital is two hours, and considerably less for Ministry health centers (Arán, 1989). If this is correct, Ministry coverage in the table should exceed one million.

The "others" column includes the remainder of the public sector (mostly the armed forces and autonomous institutions and departments), as well as part of the private sector (collective agreements, prepaid plans, insurance). My educated guess is that this group is probably underestimated in the table. Figures on total coverage must be taken with extreme caution, since about one-third of that coverage is reported under the Ministry of Public Health. For instance, if the low Ministry coverage figure for 1987 is used, total coverage that year declines by eight percentage points, but if the high figure for 1989 is used, coverage increases by six percentage points.

With the above caveats, Table 29 indicates that total coverage of the population probably peaked in 1981 (prior to the crisis) at 86%, declined to 83.8% during the crisis (1984), and surpassed the 1981 level with the economic recovery, reaching 87.7% in 1987. Coverage by sickness insurance declined from 10.3% in 1981 to 8.9% in 1984, during the crisis, but rose significantly thereafter, reaching a record 15.8% in 1987. This was partly brought on by the economic recovery that reduced unemployment and increased real wages and enterprise profits, which, along with better tax control by the government, helped to curtail evasion. But the most important cause was the expansion of sickness insurance to 128,400 new workers in 1985, and subsequent increases in 1986–1988, which resulted from the new coverage expansion policy that incorporated rural workers, small agricultural producers, domestic servants, and owners of urban microenterprises (see below), among others.

The number of noninsured affiliated with IAMCs declined in 1981–1985 (from 34.2% to 29.8% of total coverage), and, although it increased in 1987 (to 30.8%), it was still below the 1981 level; the economic crisis and financial difficulties faced by the IAMCs have been partly responsible for this trend (see the section on "Financial Viability of Social Insurance, IAMCs, and the Public Sector to Cover the Poor," beginning on p. 72). Another factor is that some of those who were affiliated with IAMCs as private individuals in 1984, later became insured at BPS; consequently, total affiliation with IAMCs in 1985 recovered its 1981 level (1,275,000),

Table 30. Percentage of population covered in Montevideo and the rest of the country by health care providers/services, Uruguay, 1987 (in thousands and percentages).

	Montevideo		Rest of country		Total	
	No.	%	No.	%	No.	%
Total population	1,345	44.0	1,712	56.0	3,057	100.0
Health care coverage						
Sickness insurance (BPS)	277	58.7	195	41.3	472	100.0
IAMCs minus BPS	686	72.7	257	27.3	943	100.0
Total IAMCs	963	68.1	452	31.9	1,415	100.0
Birth coverage by BPS maternity						
Total births	22.8	42.7	30.6	57.3	53.4	100.0
Covered by BPS	3.7	32.2	7.8	67.8	11.5	100.0

Degrees of coverage (%)[a]	Montevideo	Rest of country	Total
Sickness insurance (BPS)	20.6	11.4	15.4
IAMCs minus BPS	51.0	15.0	30.9
Total IAMCs	71.6	26.4	46.3
Births covered by BPS	16.3	25.6	21.6

Source: Author's estimates based on Saldaín, 1988; DGEC, 1989a; BPS, 1988–1989.
[a]Percentage of the population (Montevideo, rest of country, total) covered by various providers, and percentage of births in each area covered by BPS.

reaching a historical peak in 1987 (1,415,215) that, however, was mainly due to the dramatic increase in the number of insured affiliates.

Coverage by the Ministry of Public Health should have increased during the crisis (from 28.2% in 1981 to 30.1% in 1984), because many who were previously insured at BPS or affiliated with IAMCs and lost that coverage, had to resort to the free Ministry services—in 1983, for example, the number of free-care IDs granted to the Ministry increased 3%. However, while Ministry coverage expanded, its financial resources shrank. The share of government expenditures in public health steadily declined from 8.1% to 3.8% in 1974–1982, and the Ministry's share in public health expenditures decreased from 94.7% to 66.2% in the same period; the share of the armed forces and autonomous institutions increased proportionally (Apezechea, Prates, and Franco, 1984). As coverage by most sectors recovered in 1986–1987, the population served by the Ministry of Public Health possibly declined to 27% in 1987; a lower estimate for that year sets it at 19.5%, but a higher estimate for 1989 sets it at 35%. Coverage by other public institutions and the private sector was steadily above 13% in the period, but decreased somewhat during the crisis.

In 1987, there were approximately 376,000 people apparently without institutional coverage, or 12% of the total population. Part of this group had medium or high income and could pay for health care in private institutions, IAMCs, or the Ministry, but a portion could have been poor who lacked protection. Let us assume that the latter represented roughly 6% to 7% of the population. In 1986, ECLAC esti-

mated that 19% of the total population were poor and that 5% were indigent; therefore, most of the poor should be covered, but the indigent and a small proportion of poor may not be protected.

We lack precise data on poverty, the informal and rural sectors, occupational categories of the labor force, or specifics about the population covered by health care to be able to undertake an in-depth analysis of the urban and rural poor covered in Uruguay. Because the 1985 population census did not gather information on health care, and both the DGEC and BPS annual statistical yearbooks do not provide the needed data on income of those covered, what follows is a general overview of the subject.

Coverage of the IAMCs is highly concentrated in Montevideo. Table 30 shows that although 44% of the total population lives in the capital city, 68% of all IAMC affiliates are in Montevideo. The total IAMC coverage of the population of Montevideo is 71.6%, compared with only 26.4% for the rest (the interior) of the country. However, when IAMC affiliates are disaggregated by BPS insured and noninsured, the Montevideo-interior gap narrows considerably, with the capital's degree of coverage at 20.6%, contrasted with 11.4% for the interior. The explanation is, of course, that Montevideo has almost three-fourths of the IAMC noninsured affiliates (public employees, individuals), for a degree of coverage of 51%, compared with 15% in the interior. The capital concentrates most of the public bureaucracy and its population income is higher than in the rest of the country (31% higher than in other urban areas excluding the countryside), so its population can afford a higher degree of coverage. Most of the 28% of Montevideo's population that is not affiliated to IAMCs probably is covered by the Ministry's or the armed forces' health services, by collective agreements, or by the private sector. Therefore, only a small proportion of the population in Montevideo should lack protection.

The situation in the country's interior is different—three-fourths of its population is neither insured against sickness nor affiliated with IAMCs. In 1987, lack of coverage in the 18 interior departments was inversely correlated with a given department's degree of urbanization and development, ranging from 81% in Rivera to 61% in Colonia (DGEC, 1989a). However, the interior population used the BPS maternity services for child delivery much more than did that in the capital: 25.6% of all births in the interior were attended at BPS maternity services versus 16.3% in Montevideo, because the latter were referred to other IAMC public and private facilities (Table 30). By the same token, Ministry services were much more utilized in the interior than in the capital—33% versus 11% in 1981.

Furthermore, the least urbanized, poorest departments had the highest proportion of Ministry coverage in 1984 (e.g., 52% in Treinta y Tres, 41% in Flores, 40% in Rivera, and 39% in Cerro Largo), while the most developed, urbanized departments with the highest coverage by IAMCs, had the lowest Ministry coverage (e.g., Montevideo 10.5%). It should be noted that the poorest departments, such as Rivera, suffer the highest infant mortality rates, while the most developed, such as Montevideo and Colonia, enjoy the lowest (DGEC, 1986; Mesa-Lago, 1989c).

The coverage extension of BPS sickness insurance in 1984–1988, led to a twofold increase of its protected population, most of whom are workers and small employers who could be poor. Table 31, segment A, shows that in that four-year period, 136,200 of these potential poor became insured, accounting for more than half of the 261,800 incorporated. In 1988, 27% of the total number of insured were potentially poor: 16.6% were in the rural sector (workers and owners of small enterprises with no more than two employees) and 10% were in the urban sec-

Table 31. Coverage of the EAP by social insurances (BPS), Uruguay, 1984–1988 (thousands and percentages).

A. POTENTIAL GROUPS OF POOR COVERED BY BPS						
	1984		1985		1988	
	No.	%	No.	%	No.	%
Total coverage BPS	250.1	100.0	378.5	100.0	511.9	100.0
Groups of potential poor	0	0	74.3	19.6	136.2	26.6
Rural	0	0	54.9	14.5	85.1	16.6
Workers	0	0	39.5	10.4	49.6	9.7
Owners of microenterprises	0	0	15.4	4.1	35.5	6.9
Urban	0	0	19.4	5.1	51.1	10.0
Domestic servants	0	0	4.7	1.2	13.7	2.7
Owners of microenterprises	0	0	14.7	3.9	37.4	7.3

B. ESTIMATES OF OCCUPATIONAL GROUPS COVERED BY BPS (1987)[a]				
	EAP	Insured	Covered (%)	Not covered (%)
Private sector	1,000.1	609.6	61.0	39.0
Salaried	728.5[d]	517.3	71.0	29.0
Industry and commerce	431.7	383.6	88.9	11.1
Rural	208.4	115.0	55.2	44.8
Domestic servants	88.4	18.7	21.1	78.9
Nonsalaried	271.6	92.3	34.0	66.0
Self-employed with fixed place of work[b]	130.7⎫	92.3	53.3	46.7
Employers	42.5⎭			
Self-employed with no fixed place of work[b]	77.9	0	0	100.0
Unpaid family workers	20.5	0	0	100.0
Public sector[c]	201.9	201.9	100.0	0
Totals	1,202.0	811.5	67.5	32.5

Sources: Segment A, author's calculations based on BPS, 1989; segment B, author's recomposition based on BPS, n/d.
[a]Refers to jobs rather than individuals in order to adjust for double employment.
[b]The BPS refers to "independientes con o sin local de trabajo" (self-employed with no fixed place of work).
[c]Covered by BPS on pensions but not on sickness insurance.
[d]Includes banking and university professionals not covered by BPS but by independent insurance.

tor, including domestic servants and owners of microenterprises with no more than one employee (according to the survey of the informal sector in Montevideo, the latter are not poor).

Segment B of Table 31 offers rough estimates of the number of jobs insured under BPS, without differentiating between sickness and pension programs. The public sector has universal coverage, while the private sector is covered by 61%; within the latter, there is a significant difference in coverage between salaried employees (71%) and nonsalaried persons (34%). Coverage is highest among industry and commerce employees (89%, the 11% not insured probably are employed in the informal sector), but drops to 55% among rural wage earners and to 21% among domestic servants. Within the nonsalaried group, the combined number of employers and self-employed with a fixed place of work have 53% of coverage, but the rest of the group is totally excluded from insurance. Only 36% of the combined number of employers and self-employed (the latter constitute 83% of this group) is covered.

Although Uruguay has achieved one of the highest health care coverage percentages in the Region, there are still some groups of poor that might be underprotected. Children older than three months are not entitled to curative care under the BPS and, if their parents cannot afford IAMC supplemental coverage, their only option is the Ministry of Public Health services. One expert estimated that in 1987, only 49% of the population up to 14 years of age was covered, 37% by the Ministry and 12% by BPS, which limited its coverage to infants younger than 3 months of age for curative care and, later in life for prevention and dental care (Saldaín, 1988). Poor nonworking women lack coverage on sickness insurance and cannot afford affiliation in IAMCs, so they basically depend on Ministry services. Poor pensioners, whose number has probably increased in the 1980s due to the erosion in the value of real pensions, lack sickness insurance coverage; ironically, they are entitled to maternity-infant care, a service that they probably do not need. Insurance and IAMC coverage in Montevideo is the highest in the country, and coverage in the rest of the urban areas is probably higher than in the countryside. The occupational groups with the worst coverage on BPS sickness insurance are those where poverty is concentrated—the self-employed without a fixed place of work and unpaid family workers are completely excluded, as are four-fifths of domestic servants, about one-half of rural workers, and the remainder of the

self-employed and employers (the latter may include a few poor). The poor in those groups cannot afford affiliation in the IAMCs and their only access to health care is through the Ministry and a few other public institutions (departments) and NGOs. Unfortunately, we lack data to accurately assess Ministry of Public Health coverage.

REASONS FOR THE HIGH COVERAGE OF THE POOR AND REMAINING OBSTACLES TO UNIVERSALIZATION

The previous section indicates that at least some two-thirds of the poor (and perhaps all of them) are covered by health care in Uruguay. This achievement can be explained both by general factors and by social security policies.

General Factors

Uruguay is the smallest South American country, and is basically flat without any significant topographical barriers. Its small, ethnically homogenous, population shares the same language and the same basic cultural traits; its literacy rate is the second highest in Latin America. The country's highway network and communication system are excellent, and there are no isolated population groups. These features have facilitated access to health care.

Throughout the 20th century, the nation has enjoyed solid democratic institutions, except for about a decade of military intervention in the 1970s and the first half of the 1980s. The two major political parties have alternated power, and both have supported social policies, often in competition for electoral votes. Trade unions are strong and have a long tradition of struggle for social gains. Political commitment to social security and health care has been a key factor in its universalization.

In 1986, according to ECLAC, Uruguay had the second lowest poverty incidence among ten of the most developed Latin American countries, which means that it also holds that rank in the Region as a whole. Uruguay is either the most or the second most urbanized country in Latin America and the Caribbean; almost half of the urban population lives in Montevideo, the capital. And yet, the size of its informal sector is only slightly above the regional median, much lower proportionally than in other less urbanized countries such as Mexico and Peru. The salaried labor force as a percentage of the EAP is the sixth largest in the Region, the proportion of self-employment is the sixth lowest, and that of unpaid family workers the third lowest. The tiny rural area (12% to 15% of the total population) has the second largest modern sector in the Region. These structural factors have facilitated the expansion of social insurance.

Income per capita in Uruguay is the third highest in Latin America and the Caribbean. Available data in 1963, 1976, 1981, and 1983 indicate that income distribution was one of the most equitable in Latin America, despite some concentration in the 1970s. Although there are no recent data on overall income distribution or of that in the rural sector, the ECLAC survey found that in 1986, income distribution in the capital city was the second most equitable among eight of the most developed countries in the Region. There are relatively small differences in standards of living between urban and rural zones (Davrieux, 1987; Mesa-Lago, 1989c; ECLAC, 1989a, 1990).

Social Security Policy

Uruguay is a pioneer in the establishment of social insurance in Latin America and the Caribbean, and is considered a typical Western Hemisphere welfare state. And yet, although pension and employment-injury insurance programs were introduced early in the century, sickness and maternity insurance programs did not emerge until the late 1950s or 1960s, considerably later than in countries with more recent social insurance programs such as Costa Rica

and Mexico. Furthermore, those programs did not significantly expand until the 1980s. The reason for this phenomenon was that in Uruguay, mutual-aid societies and medical cooperatives engaged in health care services developed early and vigorously.

These institutions began to be established in the 19th century by groups of immigrants such as Spaniards and Italians who wanted to have better health care than the poor. Later, broader associations (not based on ethnic membership) were developed by physicians or businessmen. With the possible exception of Argentina (and including union-managed programs in this country), Uruguay is the Latin American and Caribbean country that has the largest sector of its population (almost half) receiving health care through these types of providers. In fact, BPS, except for a few maternity-infant facilities, relies on IAMCs for the delivery of health care to the insured population.

With the return to democracy in the second half of the 1980s, sickness insurance and the maternity-infant program rapidly expanded to occupational groups, a portion of which may be poor. Yet, despite a legal mandate and a twofold increase in BPS coverage, the majority of these groups remains uninsured for reasons that will be explored below.

Table 32 shows that the percentage contribution on wages for sickness insurance is the same for all covered groups, 3% for the insured and 4% for the employer. The percentage paid by the insured is the same as in Mexico and Peru, and about one-half that of in Costa Rica; furthermore, because the employer's contribution is the smallest in these four countries, the combined insured and employer percentage contribution in Uruguay is about one-half of that in Costa Rica and Mexico, and two-thirds that of in Peru. In addition, the base for contributions (for

Table 32. Contributions to social insurance sickness program among different occupational groups in Uruguay, 1989 (percentages of salary or income).

Programs	Salaried			Rural			Domestic servants[a]			Home workers		
	I	E	T	I	E	T	I	E	T	I	E	T
Sickness[b]	3	4	7	3	4	7	3	4	7	3	4	7
Pensions	13	13–20[d]	28–33	10–13[e]	f	f	12	13	25	13	42	55
Total[c]	16	17–24	35–40	13–16	f	f	15	17	32	16	46	62

Source: BPS, 1989.

I = insured; E = employer; T = total.

[a]Applied on 85% of national minimum wage.

[b]Maternity-infant program financed out of general revenue.

[c]Excludes employment injury; the premium is fixed according to risk, and averages 5%; includes family allowances and unemployment.

[d]Industry and commerce, 13%; education, 15%; and civil service, 20%. The last two groups do not contribute to BPS sickness insurance as they are covered by their agencies.

[e]According to salary.

[f]Fixed according to size and productivity of farm (the more productive, the lower the rate) and the number of owners.

both employers and insured) in domestic service is only 85% of the national minimum salary, more beneficial than in Costa Rica and Mexico (less than in Peru). Finally, the maternity-infant program is fully financed by the state, so it does not require any contributions from the insured. These factors should foster the insurance of domestic servants and other informal and rural groups, yet between one-half and four-fifths of them are not actually covered.

One of the main reasons for this significant evasion is the extremely high contribution required for the pension program, which is one of the highest in the Region; however, because the BPS administers both programs, becoming insured in one, in practice leads to becoming insured in the other. For private salaried workers, the total percentage contribution for pensions ranges from 28% to 33%; the total percentage for domestic servants is smaller (25%), but is still four times that of Mexico and about three times those of Peru and Costa Rica. The percentage contribution that the insured have to pay for pensions in Uruguay is slightly reduced to 12% for domestic servants and to as low as 10% for rural workers, but it is still between four and six times higher than in the other three countries. Employers of homeworkers in Uruguay must pay 42%; due to the heavy contributory burden, employers and workers conspire to evade registration. Moreover, calculating the employer's contribution in the rural sector is extremely complex and a disincentive for registration. The high contributions to pensions are the result of the program's maturity, the large percentage of the retired population (a ratio of one pensioner for one active contributor in the labor force), and the excessively generous entitlement conditions. Unless entitlement conditions are restricted and the percentage contribution for pensions reduced for the most economically vulnerable groups, the heavy burden on pensions will continue to be a barrier for joining sickness insurance.

BPS appears to have given up on detecting, registering, and collecting from current evaders except for salaried workers in industry and commerce. Furthermore, the Bank's actuaries estimate that the cost of effectively incorporating uncovered domestic servants, rural workers, and the self-employed without a fixed place of work would be extremely high, and because of the low income of these groups, the cost of providing benefits to them would be higher than their potential contributions and would aggravate BPS's financial disequilibrium. Finally, BPS authorities believe that pure coercive methods to fight evasion would not be effective without a drastic reform of social insurance, particularly of the pension program (BPS, n/d).

The uninsured poor cannot join the IAMCs because these institutions' monthly premiums are unaffordable to them. The premiums were frozen by the military government as part of its anti-inflationary policy until 1979; thereafter, they began to increase gradually and, since 1984, have been determined by supply and demand (Arán, 1986).

Premiums skyrocketed in the 1980s, making it even more difficult for the poor to join the IAMCs. But even for those poor who are already insured in BPS and affiliated to an IAMC, the user fees charged by the IAMCs for their services might be yet another obstacle to their real access to health care. To the best of my knowledge, these fees have to be paid by all affiliates, regardless of their income.

The Ministry of Public Health is, therefore, the basic option for the uninsured, and it covers from 20% to 35% of the population according to various estimates. The Ministry also charges user fees for its services; in the past, these were very low, but they have slowly risen in the 1980s, narrowing the gap with IAMC user fees. Still, by 1986 they were relatively low: for outpatient consultation, $US2 to $US3; child delivery room, $US22; intensive care room, $US67 (daily); minor surgery, $US18; and major surgery, $US67. The Ministry classifies users into four groups according to their income and number of family members: those who are poor receive all services free; those who earn from $US80 to $US253 pay 20% of the fees; those who earn from $US100 to $US327, pay 40% of the fees; and the rest pay 100% of the fees. In 1952, user fees represented only 3% of all Ministry costs and 1% of the University Hospital costs. Free service for the poor has assured their access to the Ministry's health care (Arán, 1986; Meerhoff, 1986; Acuña et al, 1987; Davrieux, 1987).

FINANCIAL VIABILITY OF SOCIAL INSURANCE, IAMCs, AND THE PUBLIC SECTOR TO COVER THE POOR

At most, one-third of the poor are not covered in Uruguay, or between 6% and 7% of the total population, but even this group may be protected by the Ministry. In this section, we analyze the capacity of social insurance (through the IAMCs) and the public sector to continue expanding and fully universalize health care coverage for the poor.

Social Insurance (BPS) and IAMC Viability

Because BPS has very few facilities and relies on those of the IAMCs, both sectors need to be assessed. The overall BPS deficit (all programs) reached 95% of revenue and 45% of expenditures in 1982 (the worst year of the crisis); the deficit declined in 1983–1988, and in the last year it represented 16% of revenue and 14% of expenditures. Despite this decline, in 1988 the deficit represented 1.4% of GDP, and the government subsidy was 2.7% of GDP and 15% of government expenditures. In 1988, expenditures of sickness insurance and maternity-infant care (plus family allowances) were 16% of total BPS expenditures; the bulk of expenditures (76%) went to the pension program. The latter's deficit (and BPS's overall deficit) is expected to sharply increase in 1990 because of a constitutional amendment approved in 1989 that mandates that pensions be adjusted to the cost of living starting in April 1990. Unless there is an increase of 8 to 11 percentage points in contributions, the deficit is expected to escalate (Diéguez and Giral-Bosca, 1988; DGEC, 1989a; BPS, 1988–1989; Mesa-Lago, 1990).

Up to 1981, the sickness insurance program generated a surplus, but in 1982–1987 it ended in a deficit, increasing from 5% to 32% of revenues (5% to 25% of expenditures); data for 1988 indicate a slowdown in the proportion of the deficit. The growing deficit in 1982–1984 was due to the overall economic crisis that provoked a decline in real wages, an increase of evasion, etc. And yet, the deficit continued to grow in 1986–1987, despite the economic recovery, because BPS coverage was expanded to lower income groups that pay proportionally less and possibly use services more given their higher sickness incidence.

In 1987, the combined deficit of sickness and maternity programs was equivalent to 20% of the total BPS deficit, compared with 12% in 1983. Although the pension program continues to be the major generator of the deficit, the deficit share of sickness-maternity is growing. In 1982, 83% of sickness insurance expenditures went to reimburse IAMC services to the insured, and the proportion increased to 86% in 1988 (another 12% of expenditures went to paid leave). Increasing costs of health care at IAMCs (see below) are partly responsible for BPS's sickness-maternity growing deficit.

About one-third of the deficit is financed by the central government out of general revenue. The latter mainly comes from the sales tax, which is regressive: only 16% of the population is insured (and the large majority probably has medium income); consequently the bulk of the population helps finance the coverage of a minority through price transfers and taxes. Such regressivity should have declined since 1984 with the incorporation of lower-income groups, including some poor, into the BPS and the elimination of salary ceilings for contributions (DGEC, 1989a; Banco de Previsión Social, 1988–1989; Saldaín, 1988).

In summary, the BPS sickness-maternity program is increasingly deficitary and takes a growing proportion of the BPS total deficit. The major causes for the deficit are, in terms of income, the twofold increase in population coverage in 1984–1988 that mainly incorporated low income groups that contribute less, and, in terms of expenditures, the growing health care costs at the IAMCs. The expanding disequilibrium of the sickness and maternity programs, combined with the huge imbalance of the pension program, indicates the inability of the sickness-maternity program to maintain current services without a significant state subsidy, much less to expand coverage to include the uninsured poor. Although BPS regressivity has been reduced since 1984 with the incorporation of lower income groups, it is probably still considerable.

Since 1977, the IAMCs have faced increasing financial difficulties. We have seen that in 1979–1984, IAMC premiums and user fees were frozen by the government; due to inflation, their real value deteriorated in that period. This was beneficial for the IAMC affiliates but harmful to its finances; however, due to the economic crisis, the number of IAMC affiliates declined by 3% in 1981–1984 (19% in Montevideo). Towards the end of 1984, premiums again were allowed to be fixed by the market, and rapidly increased. In 1983–1985, the real value of premiums in Montevideo increased 28%, and 14% in the rest of the country. This increase brought on a 6% decline in individual affiliation to IAMCs in 1985, but it was more than compensated by the growing number of BPS affiliates that resulted from the expansion of sickness insurance coverage in 1985–1988. Individual affiliation rose again with the economic recovery, but in 1987 it was still below the 1984 level.

In 1981–1987, the number of IAMCs declined 38% (from 81 to 50) due to bankruptcy; this reduction actually was positive, as the remaining IAMCs competed for the expanded number of BPS affiliates. The number of affiliates in Montevideo decreased by 3% in the same period, but it increased by 64% in the rest of the country, because most of the BPS coverage expansion took place outside of the capital city. Some of the surviving IAMCs are afflicted with large deficits and increasing indebtedness; in 1986, four-fifths of the IAMCs in Montevideo suffered major financial difficulties.

We have seen that the increase in IAMC premiums has contributed to the growing deficit of the BPS sickness and maternity programs. Access of the low-income uninsured to IAMCs has been significantly reduced as well; a comparison of IAMC affiliates by income bracket in 1981 and 1988 indicates that the percentage of those with lowest income declined from 16.5% to 4.4%. A household survey on health care conducted in 1982 showed that the higher the income of health care users, the greater the coverage by private providers, IAMCs, and armed forces institutions, while the lower the income, the greater the coverage by the Ministry of Public Health. However, the lowest-income household spent the highest share (72%) of its total health budget on IAMC premiums. Obviously, the IAMCs are not a feasible vehicle for covering the poor (Arán, 1986; DGEC, 1983, 1989; Mesa-Lago, 1989c; Márquez, 1989).

Public Sector Viability

The public hospital system (Ministry of Public Health and University Hospital) suffers from several deficiencies—facilities are more than 40 years old, the infrastructure has deteriorated due to lack of adequate maintenance, equipment is outdated, and overall services are considered to be of poor quality and regarded as inferior to those in other sectors. The main reason for this situation is the cut in the Ministry's real budget in the late 1970s and the first half of the 1980s, but there are managerial causes as well. The Ministry's network developed without an apparent plan and the distribution and complexity of services have not always been set according to population needs; there is excessive centralization combined with lack of leadership and coordination, as well as gross inefficiencies at the micro level in the use of available resources and the control of costs and utilization; and despite the government's commitment to primary health care, most Ministry resources still are allocated to secondary and tertiary services (Márquez, 1989).

At first glance, the Ministry's resources would seem to be adequate to serve the population legally assigned to that institution (mostly the poor). Table 33, segment A, shows that in the mid-1980s, the Ministry covered 28% of the population, received 27% of total health expenditures, hired 26% of the physicians, and operated 67% of hospital beds. Excluding the health budget, Ministry resources only were surpassed proportionally by those of the IAMCs on its share of physicians and by those of the private sector on its share of hospital beds. The Ministry's per capita expenditures were rather high by regional standards ($US107) and only slightly lower than the national average, although they were much lower than those of the IAMC and, particularly, than the private per capita expenditures. Therefore, on quantitative terms, Uruguay's public health resources compare quite favorably with the rest of Latin America; furthermore, since 1986 the Ministry's budget has been increased.

The Ministry's existing capacity is more than sufficient to expand coverage to any poor potentially left unprotected. Segment B of Table 33 indicates that, although the percentage of national hospital occupancy increased from 50% to 61% in 1980–1987, in the last year there was still substantial unutilized capacity. Furthermore, the table shows that the increase in utilization took place in Montevideo (from 52% to 78%), while in the rest of the country, half of the hospital beds went unused. Data on 1987 for hospitals and health centers indicate that half of the facilities in Montevideo have utilization rates below the average (ranging from 29% to 63%), while in the interior, more than one-third have utilization rates below the average (ranging from 36% to 46%).

Note that the national average of days of stay at the Ministry (chronic hospitals excluded) is high and increasing; in 1987, it was more than twice that of the IAMCs, while the Ministry average in Montevideo was three times higher than the IAMC average. Although these differences are partly explained by the fact that most Ministry hospitals and the University Hospital are specialized and require a longer period of stay, the gap is still so wide that it would also be due to the more intensive use of IAMC facilities. A reduction in the Ministry's average days of stay would exacerbate its unutilized capacity. Finally, although consultations per capita at the Ministry are less than half those at the IAMCs,

Table 33. Comparison of health care facilities, resources, and efficiency by health care providers in Uruguay, 1985–1987.

	A. FACILITIES AND RESOURCES (1985–1986)					
	Percentage distributions				Per capita	
	Population	Health expenditures	Hospital beds	Physicians[a]	Expenditures $US	Hospital beds
MSP[b]	28.2	27.0[d]	67.3	25.7	107.05	10.7
IAMC[c]	42.8	55.2	17.2	54.8	131.45	1.8
Armed forces	10.6	6.2	3.1	5.8	65.60	1.3
Private	2.3	3.9	10.2	0.8	185.71	19.8
Others	16.1	7.7	5.3	12.9	53.72	0.6
	100.0	100.0	100.0	100.0	111.88	4.5

	B. EFFICIENCY				
	Hospital occupancy		Average days of stay		Consultations per person
	1980	1987	1980	1987	(1987)
MSP[f]	50.0	60.9	9.7	10.1	2.4[e]
Montevideo	52.2	78.1	13.2	15.0	n.a.
Interior	49.0	51.9	8.4	8.1	n.a.
IAMC	n.a.	n.a.	5.7	4.8	5.8
Montevideo	n.a.	n.a.	5.4	5.2	5.8
Interior	n.a.	n.a.	6.0	4.1	6.1

Sources: Author's calculations based on Acuña et al, 1987; DGEC, 1981–1989; Márquez, 1989.
[a]1980.
[b]Includes University Hospital.
[c]Includes BPS affiliates.
[d]Another source gives 18.8%.
[e]1985.
[f]Excludes hospitals for chronic diseases.

they remain higher than the PAHO recommended rate of two annual consultations per capita (Márquez, 1989).

If indeed there are poor without access to health care in Uruguay, the reason is certainly not a lack of Ministry facilities. Transportation difficulties do not seem to be an important obstacle, either, and Ministry services are free to the poor. Quality on the other hand, is a serious problem—although there are differences among Ministry services, in general, their quality is poorer than those of IAMCs and, particularly, than those of the private sector. We have already noted the age and deterioration of the Ministry physical plant and the obsolescence of its equipment. In 1982, only 2% of the hospitals had been built after 1963, and 37% had been built prior to 1930. Since the mid-1980s, there has been some improvement: two new hospitals have been built, one has been re-equipped, and a few are under construction. In addition, users prefer IAMCs because they have the right to request proper care and are offered more privacy and better lodgings and meals (Arán, 1989; Mesa-Lago, 1989c). Some of these problems require attention, but with proper maintenance and increased efficiency, the Ministry would seem to be quite capable to cover all the poor population, if it does not already.

EVALUATION OF COVERAGE OF THE POOR AND ITS IMPACT ON HEALTH STANDARDS

This section evaluates real access of the poor to health care, and the potential impact of universalization of coverage on overall health standards and income distribution.

Real Access of the Poor to Health Care Services

As mentioned in Chapter 2, legal and statistical coverages don't necessarily imply real access to health services. In Uruguay, Costa Rica, and the Dominican Republic, real access of the poor can be evaluated on the basis of household surveys. In 1982, a National Household Health Survey conducted in Uruguay gathered information on health care access by income level, location, age, and providers; results of this survey are summarized in Table 34.

According to the survey, 79.6% of the sample population reported having "institutional coverage" on health care by either the Ministry of

Table 34. Real access of the poor to health care in Uruguay, 1982 (percentage distributions).

A. HEALTH CARE COVERAGE										
		By income (thirds)				By area			By age	
	Total	Lowest	Middle	Highest	Montevideo	Other cities[a]	Rest	0–14	15–59	60+
Covered	79.6	73.1	79.9	86.2	83.5	78.2	70.7	75.7	81.1	83.7
Not covered	19.9	26.4	19.7	13.3	14.2	21.4	28.9	23.7	18.4	16.0
Unknown	0.5	0.5	0.4	0.5	0.5	0.4	0.4	0.6	0.5	0.3
Total	100.0	100.0	100.0	100.0	100.0	100.0	100.0	100.0	100.0	100.0

B. COVERAGE BY PROVIDER[b]									
		By income (thirds)			By area		By age		
	Total	Lowest	Middle	Highest	Montevideo	Rest	0–14	15–59	60+
MSP	30.5	55.4	28.7	11.0	15.8	46.8	37.2	25.3	32.4
Armed forces	10.2	5.9	12.2	11.7	9.3	11.1	12.2	9.7	5.6
BPS[c]	1.8	1.7	2.5	1.1	2.1	1.4	10.0	0.4	0.2
Other public	1.3	1.3	1.4	1.3	1.5	1.1	0.9	1.7	1.3
IAMCs	53.8	33.9	53.0	71.8	67.8	38.4	38.6	60.2	55.2
Other private	2.4	1.8	2.2	3.1	3.5	1.2	1.1	2.7	5.3
Total	100.0	100.0	100.0	100.0	100.0	100.0	100.0	100.0	100.0

Source: Apezechea et al, 1984.
[a]Cities with more than 10,000 inhabitants.
[b]Percentage distribution of those with institutional coverage.
[c]Infant-maternity program; those insured in sickness are reported under IAMC.

Public Health, the armed forces, the BPS maternity program, other public institutions, IAMCs (including BPS insured on sickness), or the private sector. ''Institutional coverage'' was not clearly defined, but apparently meant the ''right'' to protection and possible past use of services. The uncovered population (people who reported that either they did not have the ''right'' or had had no access to services in the past or both) was 19.9%. Given that a large percentage of the population declared that it was covered by the Ministry of Public Health, which technically is in charge of all those not protected by other institutions, a team of experts concluded that the ''uncovered'' sector faced some type of inaccessibility to Ministry services, be it cultural, social, administrative (e.g., inadequate hours for outpatient consultation), or related to transportation (Apezechea, Prates, and Franco, 1984). Note that, in Table 29, the statistically estimated uncovered group was 14% in 1981 and 16% in 1984; the 1982 survey suggested that lack of real access was greater.

According to segment A of Table 34, the proportion of the covered population increased with income, degree of urbanization, and age. In the lowest third income bracket of the population (which included indigent, poor, and low-income people above the poverty line), the proportion of uncovered increased to 26.4% (compared with 13% among those in the third highest income bracket); among those living in towns with fewer than 10,000 inhabitants or in rural areas, it rose to 29% (compared to 14% in Montevideo). While only 16% to 18% of the productive-age and retired populations were uncovered, almost 24% of children under the age of 14 lacked coverage.

The overall distribution of the covered population by provider (segment B of Table 34, adjusted based on percentage of total instead of those covered) presents similarities and differences with the 1981 statistics in Table 29: the combined BPS and IAMC coverage is almost identical (45% in the survey versus 44% in Table 29), but the Ministry coverage is smaller (24% versus 28%) and coverage by others is also smaller (11% versus 14%).

The percentage of those covered by the Ministry of Public Health decreases with income and urbanization, whereas the opposite is true of those covered by the IAMCs and the private sector. In the lowest-income bracket, 55% were covered by the Ministry (compared with 11% in the highest bracket), and in the country's interior, the proportion was 47%, contrasting with 16% in Montevideo. Conversely, IAMC coverage was 34% in the lowest-income bracket, versus 72% in the highest, and 68% in Montevideo, versus 38% in the rest of the country. In the same manner, only 1.8% of the lowest-income group used private services versus 3.3%

in the highest-income group; 1.2% did in the interior, versus 3.5% in Montevideo. Because of the lack of or low coverage of children by the IAMCs, except with supplemental coverage, 39% of children below the age of 14 were covered by IAMC, versus 60% of the productive age group; conversely, the percentage of the population covered by the Ministry of Public Health was the highest among children (37% compared with 25% of the productive-age group). The BPS maternity-infant program concentrated its coverage among children, particularly among those younger than six years old. Due to the lack of coverage of many pensioners by BPS sickness insurance, the proportion of this group covered by the Ministry was higher (32%) than the productive-age group (25%).

The results of the 1982 survey confirm many of the previous analyses and suggest that the low estimate of Ministry coverage selected for inclusion in Table 29 is more realistic than the higher estimates we rejected. Unfortunately, the 1982 survey was conducted in the first year of the economic crisis, and there is no recent survey that can shed light on the improvement in health care coverage, both overall and of the poor, that has taken place since the mid-1980s.

Impact on Overall Health Standards

As a pioneer welfare state in the Region, Uruguay rapidly achieved unique health standards in the Region by the mid-20th century, but stagnation of both its economy and of public health expenditures led to a slowdown in the improvement of health standards. In the meantime, other Latin American and Caribbean countries accelerated their health improvements and left Uruguay behind (Apezechea, Prates, and Franco, 1984). For instance, in 1950–1960, Uruguay had the lowest infant mortality rate among 25 countries in the Region, but by 1980–1990, ten countries had lower rates (ECLAC-CEPAL, 1989a).

Therefore, to properly assess the impact of universalization on health standards, we would need accurate statistical series going back to the 1900s, which is impossible. Available series, such as those in Table 35, go back to the mid-1960s or the 1970s, when the improvement of health standards had already slowed down. According to segment A of the table, the rate of physicians per 10,000 inhabitants increased twofold in 1965–1987; actually, the country has a surplus of physicians and the third highest rate

in the Region. The rate of hospital beds per 1,000 inhabitants peaked in 1980 (the second highest in the Region at that time) and declined in 1987 to 5.0, returning to the 1965 level; it has been shown that there is excess capacity here, too (see Table 12). Rather than being affected by physical plant and personnel problems, budgetary allocations have been buffeted by deficiencies, particularly, managerial inefficiency.

Uruguay has the oldest population in Latin America and the Caribbean, and, consequently, the general mortality rate has slowly increased, from 9.6 to 10.2. Life expectancy increased rapidly in 1908–1956, but gains slowed significantly in 1957–1963, and life expectancy became almost stagnant until the mid-1970s; some gains have occurred since then (Apezechea, Prates, and Franco, 1984). In 1960–1970, Uruguay had the highest life expectancy in the Region, but increased less than three years in 1970–1990; in other countries, life expectancy rose much faster, and by the end of the 1980s, six countries had higher life expectancies than Uruguay. Infant mortality rates declined sharply in 1930–1955, almost stagnated until 1971, and declined thereafter (Apezechea, Prates, and Franco, 1984). Recent data on infant mortality rates are inconsistent. Table 35 offers three different series that show a drop in the rate, from 11 to 26 points in 1970–1988. The acceleration in the annual rate of decline in the infant mortality rate since the late 1970s (or 1980s) has been largely the result of the use of oral dehydration salts throughout the country, combined with immunization (Márquez, 1989).

Uruguay's change in causes-of-death and morbidity profiles took place much earlier than in the rest of the Region. By the end of the 1970s, 62% of all deaths were caused by "diseases typical of development" such as cardiovascular diseases and malignancies, while only 8% were the result of "diseases typical of underdevelopment" such as intestinal, parasitic, perinatal, and respiratory diseases. The previous trend continued in the 1980s, so that by 1987 the proportions were 63% and 6.6%, respectively (see Table 35, segment B). Widespread vaccination in the last decade eradicated polio and diphtheria and dramatically reduced the incidence of tuberculosis, whooping cough, measles, and tetanus.

Among infants, the proportion of intestinal infections as a cause of death sharply declined from 17% to 1.8% in 1978–1987 (mainly as a result of the rehydration campaign). As the proportion of these diseases (and of respiratory dis-

Table 35. Health care facilities and standards in Uruguay, 1965–1988.

A. FACILITIES AND STANDARDS								
				Mortality rate				
					Infant[a]			
	Hospital beds per 1,000	Physicians per 10,000	General	(1)[b]	(2)	(3)	Life expectancy[b]	
1965	5.1	11.4	9.6	47.9	49	n.a.	68.4	
1970	5.9	10.9	9.6	47.1	48	50.2	68.6	
1975	n.a.	14.1	10.0	46.3	41	48.6	68.8	
1980	6.0	17.5	10.3	41.7	38	38.2	69.6	
1987–88	5.0	22.1	10.2	35.8	28	23.8	71.0	

B. CAUSES OF DEATH (%)		
	1978–1979	1987
All the population		
Cardiovascular	40.9	41.1
Tumors	21.0	22.1
Accidents	5.6	4.8
Infectious and parasitic	2.7	2.0
Perinatal	3.8	2.1
Respiratory	1.9	2.5
Children below 1 year		
Perinatal	42.9	47.3
Congenital abnormalities	8.2	15.3
Intestinal infections	16.9	1.8
Nutritional deficiencies	5.2	6.1
Respiratory	6.4	5.6

Sources: MSP, 1987; ECLAC, 1989; Mesa-Lago, 1989c: DGEC, 1981–1989; Márquez, 1989; World Bank, 1989.
[a]The three series are from ECLAC, Mesa-Lago, and Márquez.
[b]Values for five-year periods.

eases) decreased, the percentage of perinatal diseases and congenital causes of infant death increased. Malnutrition as a cause of infant death is relatively small, but appeared to be growing in the 1980s. Massive immunization of children has cut down morbidity and mortality; in 1983, 95% of children below one year of age were vaccinated against tuberculosis, 73% against polio, 70% against DPT, and 62% against measles (Márquez, 1989).

Finally, access to potable water and sewage services also expanded. In 1960, 73.7% of the urban population and only 2.4% of the rural population had access to potable water (piped and well), but the proportions increased to 96.5% and 69.2%, respectively, in 1985, for a national average of 83%. In 1985, 96% of the total population had toilets, 97.5% in urban areas and 86.5% in rural areas (ECLAC-CEPAL, 1989a; DGEC/ECLAC, 1989).

As noted, however, there are departments (the poorest) in Uruguay where health and sanitary standards are considerably below the national average. For instance, the national infant mortality rate in 1986 was reported as 27.9 but there were three departments with rates rang-

ing from 38.8 to 44.8 (Ministerio de Salud Pública, 1987).

Effect on Income Distribution

A 1982 household survey on social public expenditures evaluated the impact on income distribution of state subsidies to health care, social security (pensions), water and sewage, education, and housing. In health care, the survey included the Ministry of Public Health, the University Hospital, BPS sickness insurance and maternity-infant program, armed forces hospitals, and other public institutions; the IAMCs were excluded. The distribution effect was disaggregated by providers and zones as follows: Montevideo, capitals of departments, other cities, and rural areas. Table 36 summarizes the survey's main results.

Among social public expenditures, those on health care had the highest progressiveness, contributing most to an egalitarian income distribution. The state transfer to all health services was 2.5% of GDP and averaged 2.8% of household income. Because of the high priority as-

Table 36. Impact of state health subsidies on family income distribution by income levels in Uruguay, 1982 (in percentages).

| Household quintiles | Income distribution | | Distribution of subsidy by provider | | | | Distribution of subsidy by area | | |
	Before subsidy	After subsidy	Total	MSP	BPS Infant-maternity	BPS Sickness insurance	Montevideo	Other cities[a]	Rural
Poorest 20%	7.2	8.1	34.0	47.9	49.3	11.4	48.2	25.6	44.5
Second 20%	11.8	12.4	29.7	28.9	33.1	23.5	19.0	8.4	21.2
Third 20%	14.8	14.9	16.1	8.5	10.0	22.5	6.1	52.9	18.6
Fourth 20%	19.9	19.5	8.4	7.0	7.6	26.0	6.7	9.3	10.3
Fifth 20%	46.3	45.2	11.8	7.7	0.0	16.6	20.0	3.8	5.4
Total	100.0	100.0	100.0	100.0	100.0	100.0	100.0	100.0	100.0

Sources: Davrieux, 1987; Petrei, 1987.

[a]Excludes capitals of departments.

signed to health care by the poor families, they spent proportionally more on it than on other social services; as household income increased, a lower proportion of the budget was spent on health care. However, the relative impact of the health subsidy on income distribution was lower than that of other subsidies (e.g., pensions), because fewer resources were assigned to the health sector vis-a-vis the rest. A reallocation of the state subsidy that increased the relative share of health would, therefore, augment the subsidy's progressiveness and its redistributive impact. Consequently, the reduction in the Ministry of Public Health's budget in the early 1980s should have reduced the progressiveness of the state subsidy, while the budget increase in the second half of the 1980s should have augmented it (Davrieux, 1987).

Table 36 shows that the poorest population quintile received only 7.2% of income but 34% of the health subsidy, which increased its income by about one percentage point. The poorest 40% of the population received 64% of the subsidy, which raised its income share by 1.5 percentage points. As household income rose, the share of the subsidy decreased. The Ministry channeled 60% of the subsidy received by the poorest families (54% of the households covered by it fell in the lowest quintile) and next in importance was the BPS maternity-infant program; the poorest quintile received 48% to 49% of the total subsidy allocated to each provider. Conversely, the distribution of the subsidy to the BPS sickness insurance was considerably less progressive, because few within the poorest quintile were covered by that program and, hence, received only 11.4% of the subsidy (see the section on ''Social Insurance (BPS) and IAMC Viability,'' beginning on p. 73). However, with the expansion of BPS coverage since 1985 to incorporate lower income groups, the pro-

gressiveness of this program may have improved. Subsidies to the military and other public agencies were the least progressive (Davrieux, 1987; Mesa-Lago, 1989).

In terms of areas, the most progressive impact of the total health subsidy was registered in rural areas (a reduction of −0.36 in the Gini coefficient), followed by Montevideo (−0.27), other capitals (−0.23), and other cities (−0.17). The poorest quintile of the rural population received 44.5% of the rural subsidy and the poorest quintile in Montevideo received 48% of the subsidy allocated to that capital (Table 36). The distribution of the total health subsidy by areas was proportionate to the population living in them, but the Ministry's distribution clearly targetted the rural areas as a priority: these received 23.4% of the subsidy vis-a-vis a share of population of 13.3%. In contrast, all other providers except one allocated 3% to 4% of the subsidy to rural areas where poverty incidence is higher (Davrieux, 1987). Potable water and sewage subsidies were third in progressiveness (subsidies to education ranked second), followed by housing and social security (pensions).

Although we were unable to fully evaluate real access of the poor to health care, this section indicates that universalization of coverage in Uruguay has had a positive impact in raising health standards (although the impact was stronger earlier and slowed down in the last two decades), as well as on improving income distribution and helping the poor. The Ministry emerges as the key vehicle, both for coverage of the poor and progressiveness in income distribution; a higher allocation of the state subsidy to the Ministry (combined with the proper policies to improve quality and efficiency) would therefore have significant beneficial consequences for the poor.

Private Alternatives to Expand Coverage and Improve the Quality of Health Care for the Poor

General Review

The poor who are not covered by BPS are entitled to free Ministry of Public Health health care, but if they do not have real access to the latter's services or the quality of available services is inferior, few of them could offset this by joining IAMCs or buying private services. Furthermore, the families of the poor who are insured at BPS are not covered in most health services, such as children older than three months for curative medicine, those above 6 years of age for preventive medicine, and those over 9 years old for dental care; also uncovered are spouses for any health care except maternity. The insured poor cannot afford IAMC supplementary coverage for their family on those services not provided by sickness insurance (in 1989, supplementary coverage for a wife and two children cost $US45 monthly); hence, their only option is free but poor quality Ministry services. Furthermore, many low-income (not poor) families of BPS insured or IAMC affiliates cannot afford supplementary coverage either and, unlike the poor, they have to pay for Ministry services according to their income.

The private health sector (outside of the IAMCs) in Uruguay is small, covering only 2.3% of the population and spending 3.9% of total health expenditures. There are some NGOs which help poor and low-income people to get more comprehensive and better quality health care. In addition, there are some groups of low-income workers that have organized into unions, associations, or cooperatives that have been able to obtain supplementary services. In Montevideo, the Association of Municipal Workers has an outpatient clinic and an agreement with an IAMC, the Housing Cooperative operates a small clinic, and a sandal factory has a dental clinic; in the interior, the Omnibus Cooperative of Paysandu manages an outpatient clinic. As a case study of these supplementary services for the poor and low-income families, we have selected the clinic of the Cooperative of Thermos Bottles Production (COTER) of Montevideo (Inter-American Foundation, 1987; Roura et al, 1989).

The COTER Clinic and Health Package

History

This cooperative of artisans manufactures thermos bottles and other glass goods using a traditional glassblowing method. In 1966, the private enterprise that preceded the cooperative went bankrupt, and 26 of its workers decided to purchase the factory. In its 25 years of existence, COTER has had its ups and downs: in the 1970s, when there was much demand for its products, output expanded rapidly, but the crisis of the 1980s brought the coop to the brink of bankruptcy. Yet, the workers managed, with modest outside help, to overcome the crisis and make the factory profitable again; output has tripled since 1982. The number of members increased from 26 in 1966 to 80 in 1982, and to more than 200 in 1989. Each member contributes a minimum capital of $US50 at the start; all workers are guaranteed a minimum salary and members are entitled to a share of the profits.

Not only is COTER a healthy self-managed enterprise, but it is one of the few urban industrial cooperatives in Uruguay that has a broad social program that includes medical and dental care through its own clinic. In 1985, coop members voted virtually unanimously to forfeit a wage increase in order to create a clinic. COTER rented a house across the street from the factory and hired a few medical professionals; in the same year, IAF provided a $US5,700 grant to purchase dental equipment for the clinic. COTER also signed an agreement with one IAMC, MIDU, to provide supplementary curative services to the workers' families, 90% of whom joined the program. In consideration of the clinic's services and the number of people in the group, MIDU reduced the monthly fee for supplementary coverage. In 1987, IAF awarded the cooperative a second grant for $US28,000 to buy the house where the clinic operates; in exchange, COTER agreed to pay $US10,000 in five years, into a development fund to finance coverage extension of clinical primary health care services to workers at six other factories located in the neighborhood, as well as to poor residents of an urban slum adjacent to the cooperative.

The Population Served by the COTER Clinic

By the end of 1989, there were 620 persons (180 cooperative members and 440 relatives) covered by the clinic and IAMC supplementary services. By 1992, the clinic is expected to have the development fund in place and to incorporate 200 additional people, many of them poor, raising the total to more than 800 users. COTER members' average ages run between 25 and 30, the average household has 3.5 members, and most of them live near the factory and clinic, which is the only in the area.

COTER members are not poor, but most of them have low incomes. According to COTER officials, the household monthly average income in 1989 was $US121, about 2.4 times higher than the poverty line estimated by ECLAC for Montevideo in 1988, but about one-fourth the average monthly household income of that city in 1989. If the capital's population were divided into three income brackets, coop officials placed the cooperative members in the upper level of the lowest income bracket.

Before the clinic was established and the agreement with MIDU signed, most of the COTER workers did not have health care coverage for their families, and all lacked dental care. They either went to Ministry of Public Health facilities and paid user fees or to the private sector and paid even more; when the required health service was too expensive for them, the cooperative had to help them financially. The workers also complained about the low quality of Ministry services. According to the president of COTER, coop members were in a worse situation than the poor, because they had to pay for Ministry services and occasionally went without medical treatment.

Facilities, Services, and Financing

The clinic has a reception room, a dental cabinet with all the needed equipment, a gynecological room, a well-stocked pharmacy, and a bathroom. Its personnel consists of five physicians, two dentists, one dental assistant, and one secretary; except for four physicians supplied by MIDU, the remaining personnel is paid for by COTER. Members and their families have access to all clinical services: outpatient consultation on general medicine, pediatrics, and gynecology every weekday; minor surgery and emergencies; dental care (including orthodontics) three times weekly; laboratory tests and medicine; and preventive services such as immunization, maternity care, health education, and control of tuberculosis, diabetes, and high blood pressure. Low user fees are charged for various services: $US1 to $US2 per dental filling and extraction (these fees are about one-fifth of those charged elsewhere), $US162 for complete orthodontic treatment (payable in 12 monthly installments), $US0.35 for laboratory tests, and $US0.10 for each prescription; all other services are free.

MIDU facilities provide all services that are unavailable at the clinic, such as hospitalization, major surgery, complex curative care, rehabilitation, ambulance transportation, and home visits by physicians; MIDU services also are available when the clinic is closed. Cooperative members are entitled to freely select from MIDU facilities and personnel; they also can change from MIDU to another IAMC if they choose to, but by doing so they would lose many of the current advantages they enjoy under the COTER plan.

COTER pays half the supplementary family coverage at MIDU and workers pay the other half. Total annual costs of all the health services to COTER are $US30,000 (this comes out of profits), and it is estimated that with all the health packages, the workers save approximately 90% of average costs of similar services elsewhere. The only financial aid received by COTER for its health services has been the two IAF grants totalling $US33,700, a sum similar to the annual costs of the services paid by COTER.

Evaluation

The average annual cost per person for the entire health package, including the COTER fee to MIDU but excluding depreciation of the clinic's building and equipment and the workers fee to MIDU, was $US48 in 1989; when those other costs are added, the per capita cost increases to $US90. Although this figure is not strictly comparable to per capita health expenditures for 1986 as shown in Table 33, the COTER per capita cost is 16% lower than that of the Ministry's and about one-half that of the IAMC average.

Users of clinic services pinpointed other nonfinancial advantages of the clinic such as proximity, a personal relationship with the medical personnel, fewer clients and no waiting lines, and better quality of services. Some users said that even if a MIDU clinic was closer than COTER's, they would keep using the latter. A few problems noted by clinic personnel and users were insufficient nursing help and lack of some medicine in the pharmacy; there were no complaints regarding the low user fees.

Whether the COTER clinic will extend its primary health care coverage to workers in six other factories and poor people in the nearby slum is yet unknown. The IAF-COTER agreement on the second grant is not clear on when the extension of services ought to begin; one interpretation holds that it should be in 1992, when the development fund is completed. My feeling is that unless IAF puts pressure on COTER, the expected extension of services will not materialize.

A final important question is whether the COTER health care package can be duplicated elsewhere. There certainly seems to be a need for it, because, as this evaluation shows, it tackled some key deficiencies facing health care in Uruguay, such as poor quality and inefficiencies of public services and overall financial difficulties. Furthermore, the COTER health plan has reached a segment of the population that, although not poor, has a low income, is not insured by the BPS, and would have been unable to join an IAMC with its own means. The catalyst here undoubtedly was this unusual cooperative that has been successful both economically and socially. COTER officials, although aware that their institution had unique characteristics, have optimistically stated that its model could be replicated if workers in unions and cooperatives were educated and some external support became available. The modest investment in this project has paid high dividends and should be expanded.

COSTA RICA

POVERTY: SIZE, TRENDS, AND CHARACTERISTICS

According to ECLAC, in 1988 Costa Rica had the third lowest poverty incidence (population) among ten Latin American countries (only Argentina and Uruguay had lower rates): 25% national, 21% urban, and 28% rural (Table 2). In 1961–1981, the national poverty incidence (households) in Costa Rica declined from 51% to 22%, but increased to 25% in 1988. Data on the total population show a rise in national poverty incidence from 24% in 1981 to 27% in 1988; the number of poor increased by 35% in 1981–1988 (ECLAC, 1990).

Costa Rica's economy grew at a very good rate in the 1960s and 1970s; open unemployment and inflation were low and real salaries steadily grew. The 1981–1982 economic crisis interrupted that process of development: real GDP declined almost 10% in those two years, inflation reached peaks of 65% and 82%, open unemployment set a record of 9.4% in 1982 (while underemployment rose to 14.4%), and real wages fell by almost 30% in 1981–1982. During the rest of the 1980s the economy recovered: real GDP grew at an annual average of 4% (for a cumulative rate of 21% in 1981–1989), inflation declined to an average of 16%, open unemployment decreased to 5.5% in 1989, and real wages recovered somewhat, but by 1988 remained at

12% below the 1980 level (Vedova, 1986; ECLAC, 1989, 1989a).

Altimir's (1984) estimates for 1979 indicate that the national poverty incidence (households) actually had declined that year to 17% (as compared with the 24% figure given by ECLAC for 1970). He also estimated that in 1982, in the midst of the crisis, poverty incidence rose to 29% (considerably higher than ECLAC's figure of 22% for 1981). The ECLAC survey followed Altimir's methodology, so we assume that both series are comparable and conclude that poverty incidence had reached a peak in 1982 and had declined to 25% by 1988.

In 1965–1988, the urban population of Costa Rica rose modestly, from 38% to 45%. In 1988, Costa Rica ranked as the fifth least urbanized country in the Region (the fifth most rural) and had a very low annual rate of increase in urbanization, which was actually lower in the 1980s than in 1965–1970 (World Bank, 1990). Urban poverty incidence (households) was almost stagnant between 1970 and 1981 (15% and 16%), but jumped to 21% by 1988. Rural poverty incidence declined from 30% to 28% in 1970–1981, and remained at 28% in 1988 (Table 2). The bulk of the poor is still concentrated in rural areas: in 1988, there were twice as many indigents in rural areas as in urban areas. In the same year, there were 726,300 poor in Costa Rica (35% of them indigents); 62% lived in rural areas and 38%, in urban areas (ECLAC, 1990).

The Urban (Informal) Sector

As a percentage of the EAP, the informal sector was basically stagnant from 1950 until at least 1980, when it was estimated at 12.4%. That percentage was the lowest registered by PREALC (1981) among 14 Latin American countries; excluded from the PREALC study were the least developed countries that probably have higher informal sector percentages (except for Cuba, which has a tiny informal sector). Other estimates of the informal sector are higher: about 27% in 1979 and increasing to 29% or 32% in 1982, at the peak of the crisis (Fields, 1985; Pollack and Ulhoff, 1985). The ILO office in San José roughly estimated this sector from 18% to 22% in 1988. There is consensus that the 1981–1982 crisis induced an increase in the informal sector, but there is no solid data on what has happened in the recovery period. A study on the informal sector began in 1988, but I have not been able to obtain the results.

The quarterly National Survey of Households, Employment, and Unemployment provides data for a comparison of occupational categories of the labor force in 1980, 1982 (the worst year of the crisis), and 1986. The combined percentage of urban self-employed and unpaid family workers increased from 13% of the EAP in 1980 to 15% in 1986; probably all unpaid family workers and most of the self-employed work in the informal sector. In addition, there were 5.3% domestic workers (considered informal) in 1980; no data are available for 1986 (Ministerio de Trabajo y Seguridad Social, 1980 to 1986). Some salaried workers and employers also should have been within the informal sector. In 1987, half of industrial employment was in 15,000 micro- and small enterprises with an average of five employees each, most of them unpaid family workers. Interviews with leaders of three associations which embrace about 7,000 micro- and small enterprises, including cooperatives, indicated that each employs from one to two workers, mostly unpaid relatives, and both owners and employees earn very low incomes. Given the above information, the informal sector should have been somewhat higher than 20% in 1986 (Mesa-Lago, 1990a).

The informal sector income as a percentage of formal sector salary increased from 42% to 46% in 1979–1982, but declined to 34% in 1983. In 1980, 16% of the EAP in the lowest income strata were self-employed and unpaid family workers; 85% of these two groups were in the lowest income bracket. In 1979, 15% of all urban manual workers and workers providing services (categories where informal workers are concentrated) were poor, and this proportion had increased to almost 27% by 1982. Income distribution data indicate that the percentage of income of the poorest 10% of the urban households declined from 2.1% to 1.5% in 1971–1983, but increased to 2.3% in 1988 (Altimir, 1984; Fields, 1985; Vedova, 1986; Rovira, 1988; ECLAC,

1990). There is no information on other characteristics of informal workers.

The Rural Sector

The rural population in 1988 was 1.5 million (55% of the total population), of which 447,100 were poor (30% of the rural population); 173,100 of the latter were indigents (11.6% of the rural population). The poorest 20% of the rural population received 5.5% of total rural income in 1988, and the average income of that rural quintile was about half the average income of the poorest urban quintile (ECLAC, 1990). Poverty incidence (households) among agricultural workers rose from 34% to 53% in 1979–1982; about 60% of the increase in national poverty incidence during the crisis was concentrated in that group (Altimir, 1984). Combined open unemployment and underemployment in rural areas grew from 11.6% in 1977 to 25% in 1982, but sharply declined in 1983–1988 (Vedova, 1986; ECLAC, 1989).

A study of the rural areas conducted for the 1971–1980 National Health Plan found that 51% of the national population lived in villages with fewer than 2,000 inhabitants and 35% lived in settlements with fewer than 500 inhabitants. The most dispersed rural population was also the most geographically isolated and the poorest (with the lowest income per capita); it was severely afflicted by underemployment, illiteracy, precarious and crowded housing, water contamination, lack of adequate services for excreta disposal, and high rates of malnutrition and infant mortality (Saenz, 1985). Because of its dispersion, isolation, and low living standards, this segment of the population had little or no access to health care. The cost of providing health services to that population was estimated to be high, because of the absence of infrastructure, problems in construction and transportation, and difficulties in attracting qualified medical personnel (Beirute, 1988).

The most rural, least developed counties (*cantones*) in the regions of Brunca (southeast, bordering Panama), Chorotega (west, bordering with Nicaragua in the north), and Huetar Atlántica (northeast, bordering the Atlantic) are those with the lowest health standards, such as the highest infant mortality rates and malnutrition among children (see the section on ''Evaluation of Coverage of the Poor and Impact on Health Standards,'' beginning on p. 95). Although there have been impressive health improvements all over the nation, serious health problems persist in a few counties and among some vulnerable groups, especially in remote rural areas (Overholt, 1986).

HEALTH CARE COVERAGE OF THE URBAN (INFORMAL) AND RURAL POOR

Administrative Structure and Legal Coverage

The Costa Rican Social Security Fund (CCSS) was established in 1941, and began operating in 1943 to provide sickness-maternity coverage and pensions for urban salaried workers. It was introduced late by Latin American standards, and initially was limited to the capital city and the provincial capitals. Coverage includes general and specialist care, maternity care, surgery, hospitalization, laboratory services, dental care, limited optometry services, and medicine for the insured (and pensioners) and their dependent spouses and children; the insured also are entitled to paid leave for sickness and maternity.

In 1961, a law mandated that the government expand social insurance coverage to all the population within a ten-year period; the law's implementation was delayed almost a decade because of a lack of needed infrastructure. In 1971, a new law ordered CCSS to proceed with the "universalization" of coverage; to that end, a 1973 law transferred all Ministry of Health hospitals to CCSS. In exchange, the latter took on the provision of free health care for the poor (indigents), with the state paying the bill. The 1973 law also established that CCSS would concentrate on curative medicine, while the Ministry would focus on preventive medicine.

As part of the thrust for health care expansion in the 1970s, CCSS granted mandatory coverage to domestic servants and employees of microenterprises and their dependent relatives, as well as voluntary insurance coverage to the self-employed, unpaid family workers and employers, and their dependent families. In addition, welfare (noncontributory) coverage became mandatory for health care and pensions to indigents and their dependent families. An indigent household is defined as one that cannot satisfy the basic food, clothing, housing, and health care needs; the dispossessed or those who earn below 75% of the minimum agricultural salary are eligible for welfare programs. The condition of indigence is checked twice a year by CCSS, but the record does not show whether the person is insured or an indigent, legally assuring equal health care treatment for all users. The state is legally bound to reimburse CCSS for the cost of indigent health care, while the program of Social Development and Family Allowances (DESAF), begun in 1974, finances welfare pensions awarded by CCSS.

The 1971–1980 National Health Plan entrusted the Ministry of Health (established in 1927) with the task of expanding primary health care to the most remote, dispersed rural population, as well as to the urban marginal population. The rural health program, which began in 1973, first targeted settlements with fewer than 500 inhabitants and, later, those with fewer than 2,000 inhabitants, where poverty was concentrated. A group of villages and settlements constitutes a "health area" of 150 km^2 with some 3,000 inhabitants; a rural health post serves such an area, and paramedical personnel visit the population in their homes; services are provided according to local needs; several health posts depend on a Ministry health center.

The Ministry's urban community program began in 1976, and was geared to the urban population in shantytowns, which basically consisted of rural migrants. An infrastructure similar to that of the rural program was developed, consisting of Ministry "work areas," health posts, and health centers. The Ministry also operates mobile units for general medicine and dental care that provide services to people who live too far from population centers and who lack access to health care.

Furthermore, the Ministry provides general services to the entire population, such as epidemiological control, environmental sanitation, immunization, nutrition, health education, and family planning. Finally, the Ministry operates education-and-nutrition centers (CEN) that provide milk and nutritional supplements and education to children and pregnant women and manages integral-care centers (CINAI), which are day-care centers that supply three daily meals to children under the age of 6, as well as other services. The Ministry of Education dispenses school meals to children between the ages of 6 and 12.

DESAF finances part of the Ministry's health care for the rural and urban poor, some of its general prevention programs (potable water, latrines), and its education-and-nutrition and integral-care centers.

Other public institutions that provide some health care services are the Costa Rican Institute of Water Supply and Sewage (ICAA); the National Institute of Insurances (INS) in charge of employment injury, which basically excludes the poor from coverage; and the Institute of Social Aid (IMAS) which helps poor or low-income people (many of them in the informal sector) with monetary support, training, and credit, but not health care—those in need of it are transferred by IMAS to Ministry and CCSS facilities.

In 1979, the concept of a national health system was legally introduced and, with it, functions for all health care institutions were determined more clearly. The 1982–1986 National Development Plan and the 1983 National Health Plan launched advances in integration, primarily between CCSS and the Ministry, that included the following: a National Health Council was established under the direction of the Ministry of Health and charged with the development of the National Health System; functions were separated and coordination was enhanced, as was uniformity in terms of health regions; if only one institution served a given location, it was determined that it would assume full responsibility for health care; and, in newly built facilities, all programs were integrated and housed together. And yet, less than half of the health facilities have been integrated; both institutions basically continue to function with their own top authorities, bureaucracies, and budgets; and most services are not functionally unified. Integration has been partly achieved at the local level, but not at the top, and problems of overlapping, inefficient use of resources, inadequate coordination, and flaws in the quality of services persist.

As we have said, the Ministry is responsible for preventive medicine, while CCSS is devoted to curative medicine, with functions and levels of care coordinated between the two institutions in a pyramidal structure. The first level of attention is provided by the Ministry's prevention and primary health care services to the overall population and targeted groups through the following facilities: health posts (control of contagious diseases, vaccinations, infant-maternal health care, home visits); mobile units (complete medical teams, including dentists, for diagnosis and first aid); dental clinics; and nutrition and education centers. The second level combines prevention and curative services through facilities of both institutions: the Ministry health centers (prevention, outpatient consultation, emergency, obstetrics, pediatrics, and general medicine) and rural assistance centers (with similar functions, including hospitalization, particularly for child delivery), and the

CCSS clinics (outpatient consultation and similar functions as the Ministry's health centers) and outpatient consultation and minor surgery services at hospitals. The third and fourth levels are the curative services provided by CCSS peripheric, regional, and national (specialized) hospitals.

In summary, the Costa Rican health system is one of the few in the Region that is more typical of social security than social insurance, and that offers one of the most complete legal coverages of the poor. Urban and rural indigents and their families are entitled to free and full Ministry preventive and primary care and all curative services (but not monetary benefits). Coverage of the poor is not limited to the working-age population and their dependent families, but extends to welfare pensioners (noninsured who receive noncontributory pensions from CCSS) and their families.

The law extends mandatory full coverage (health care and monetary benefits) to all salaried workers (urban or rural), including domestic servants and employees of microenterprises, even those with a single employee and regardless of the enterprise's capital and income. However, owners of clandestine enterprises often request their employees to join CCSS as self-employed, in order to save the employer's contribution. The self-employed (and employers) can join CCSS voluntarily (with full sickness-maternity benefits), either individually or through a collective agreement if they are members of an association, union, cooperative, or self-managed enterprise. Unpaid family workers, if not already covered by CCSS as dependents of the insured, can also join voluntarily. All dependent family of these groups of workers also are entitled to health care coverage in CCSS. Finally, those insured who become unemployed and indigent are entitled to free health care coverage (Saenz, 1985; Rodríguez V., 1986; Overholt, 1986; Beirute, 1988; Miranda, 1990; Mesa-Lago, 1990).

Statistical Coverage

Statistics on CCSS population coverage are among the most comprehensive and reliable in Latin America and the Caribbean, and include historical series that go back three decades. Coverage increased from 15.4% of the total population in 1960 to 38.4% in 1970, and, with the rapid expansion during the 1970s, it reached a historical peak of 84.4% in 1979 (Mesa-Lago, 1990, Table 37). Because of the economic crisis,

CCSS coverage declined to 77% in 1981, but rose again in 1984–1987, almost recuperating its 1979 level. Table 37 shows that the number of insured (contributory program) declined in 1979–1981 and, due to the increase in population, the proportion of insured covered decreased from 77.3% to 69.7%. Conversely, the number of indigents covered augmented during the crisis, surpassing the increase in population and sustaining the rate of coverage above 7%. If we assume that the top 15% to 20% of Costa Rica's population ranked in the top income quintile buys its own health care, we conclude that the whole population (and hence the poor) are protected by curative care.

The CCSS annual report gave a total population coverage of 89.3%, in 1987, because it used lower population estimates than those in Table 37; if the official figure is taken, the percentage of the uncovered population in 1987 was only 10.7% (CCSS, 1988). The report asserts that this group has enough income to pay for its own care, either at the CCSS (which charges fees according to users' income) or from the private sector. The latter, however, is very small in Costa Rica and, hence, most of the highest income group depends on CCSS services.

Even if some of the poor (mainly rural in remote, isolated areas) are not covered by CCSS curative medicine, almost all of them are reached by the Ministry's preventive and primary health care services. Table 37 shows that the combined coverage of Ministry programs for the urban and rural poor reached almost 61% in 1979, declined to 50% in 1981 due to the economic crisis, and increased again to 53% in 1987. During this last year, the combined CCSS and Ministry health services coverage was 136%, the overlap being a result of the different services provided by each institution.

In addition to focusing on the poor, health care services in Costa Rica target other vulnerable segments of the population such as pregnant women and infants. In 1983, 81% of all pregnant women were insured by CCSS, plus another 7% who qualified as indigents; the remaining 12% either were financially able to pay for care or were protected by the Ministry. In 1987, 90.7% of all births in the country (including those in indigent families) were taken care of in CCSS facilities. A survey of consultations given at CCSS/Ministry facilities in 1983 revealed that infants had an annual average of 8.7 consultations per capita, 3.5 times the total population average of 2.5; furthermore, from 81% to 85% of all children were immunized against the most common contagious diseases.

Table 37. Official data on population covered on health care in Costa Rica, 1979–1987 (in thousands and percentages).

	Population[a]			Coverage social insurances (CCSS)			% of population covered			Coverage Ministry Health			% of population covered		
	Total (1)	Urban (2)	Rural (3)	Insured[b] (4)	Indigents[c] (5)	Total (6)	Insured (4/1)	Indigents (5/1)	Total (6/1)	Urban (7)	Rural (8)	Total (9)	Urban (7/2)	Rural (8/3)	Total[d] (9/1)
1979	2,170	927	1,243	1,678	155	1,833	77.3	7.1	84.4	600	718	1,318	64.7	57.7	60.7
1981	2,342	1,016	1,326	1,631	170	1,801	69.7	7.2	76.9	527	641	1,168	51.8	48.3	49.8
1984	2,534	1,128	1,406	1,878	206	2,084	74.1	8.1	82.2	486	812	1,298	43.1	57.7	51.2
1987	2,774	1,265	1,509	2,082	223	2,305	75.1	8.0	83.1	602	859	1,461	47.6	56.9	52.7

Sources: Author's calculations based on CCSS, 1984, 1988, 1988a; Beirute, 1988.
[a] The CCSS and the Ministry of Health give lower total population estimates for the entire period; we chose the higher estimates according to data from international agencies. Urban and rural populations are the author's estimates based on population census data for 1973 and 1984, and projections.
[b] Insured by CCSS includes active, pensioners, and dependent family (a small number of those covered by independent pension funds are also included).
[c] Noncontributory coverage of indigents by CCSS; includes both active and pensioners.
[d] The overlap in coverage results from different services: CCSS provides curative medicine while the Ministry of Health is predominantly involved in prevention, sanitation, and primary health care in dispersed rural and urban marginal areas.

Finally, from 400,000 to 500,000 children (54% to 68% of the population below 10 years of age) received daily meals through the Ministry of Health and the Ministry of Education in 1988; however, DESAF officials reported that the most isolated, needy rural areas did not benefit from this program (Overholt, 1986; CCSS, 1988, 1988a; Rodríguez Cubero, 1988; Fernández Campos, 1988).

Urban Poor

The Ministry's program for the urban marginal population steadily increased its coverage from 10% of the total urban population in 1976 to a peak of 65% in 1979, but, due to the economic crisis, coverage dipped to a trough of 43% in 1984. During the 1981–1982 crisis, services were reduced; for example, 44% in child care and 11% in home visits. With the economic recovery, most of these services were restored, and by 1987, Ministry facilities covered 281 marginal urban areas with 146,094 homes. Coverage increased again to more than 47% in 1987, but remained below the 1979 peak. Despite this decline, in 1987 the percentage of urban coverage by the Ministry (47%) was twice as high as the urban poverty incidence (24%). Furthermore, the Ministry's program is targeted to the urban marginal (poor) population, hence, its degree of coverage is higher than that of the total urban population. However, it has been reported that 20% of the urban poor who are visited by Ministry medical or paramedic personnel do not utilize Ministry or CCSS facilities to which they are referred (Secretaría Ejecutiva de Planificación Sectorial de Salud, 1984; Overholt, 1986; Beirute, 1988).

Population coverage by the CCSS cannot be disaggregated by urban-rural residence, but we can roughly evaluate the protection of some informal groups. In 1980–1986, the number of self-employed covered by the CCSS sickness-maternity program increased 69%, from 93,941 to 158,488. As a percentage of the total self-employed in the labor force, those insured increased from 81% to 109%, while the percentage of coverage of salaried workers declined from 79% to 74% (see Table 38). The explanation for the 1986 overcoverage of the self-employed is that 45% of those registered as self-employed are actually salaried workers employed in small enterprises (71,320) who pretend to be self-employed because of either owners' pressure (to save the employer's contribution) or incentives offered by group agreements signed with CCSS. (Therefore, the actual number of self-employed insured in 1986 was approximately

87,168, and their coverage was 60%.) In 1987, there were 70 group agreements in effect, covering 39,871 self-employed with membership in some type of association, who benefitted from a lower percentage contribution than the one paid by salaried workers and individual self-employed (see the section on "Social Security Policy," beginning on p. 91). In any case, the percentage of coverage of the self-employed in Costa Rica seems to be the highest in Latin America and the Caribbean (see Table 9).

According to Table 38, the average earnings of all the insured self-employed in 1987 were about one-third of the average earnings of all the insured in the CCSS. However, the average of the individually insured self-employed was less than one-tenth of the overall average earnings; since 76% of all the self-employed insured are in this category, we can assume that most of them are poor or have very low incomes (but, see the section on "Social Security Policy," beginning on p. 91). Conversely, 24% of the self-employed who are insured through group agreements have average earnings 7% above the overall average (Table 38).

We have data on the number of domestic servants covered by the CCSS, but not on the total number of these informal workers; a rough estimate for 1980 is 40,800, with 9,772, or only one-fourth, insured that year. The average earnings of insured domestic servants in 1987 were the lowest of all insured groups, 30% of the overall average; hence, they can be considered poor or with a very low income. The number of domestic servants insured by CCSS reached a peak of 9,885 in 1982, but steadily declined to 6,065 in 1987 (Table 38; CCSS, 1988a). This was probably the result of a decline in this type of employment, but could also be the result of evasion in an occupation which is very difficult for CCSS to control.

There is practically no information on the number of small employers or owners of microenterprises who are insured by CCSS. The leader of one employer association reported to me that only 20% of its members were insured, another that the majority was not insured, and still another that very few of its members were insured (Mesa-Lago, 1990).

The combined number of self-employed (including those who are actually salaried informal workers or employers) and domestic servants insured in the CCSS sickness-maternity program steadily increased from 18% of the total insured in 1979 to 26% in 1987 (Table 38; CCSS, 1988a). This is an impressive figure, even considering the relatively small size of the informal

Table 38. Number of insured, average earnings, and degree of coverage by social insurance (CCSS) sickness-maternity program, by occupational groups, Costa Rica, 1987.

Occupational groups	Number of insured (thousands)	Distribution (%)	Average monthly earnings (colones)	Ratio to all insured	% of group coverage[a]
Salaried workers	493.5	74.8	15,733	1.22	74
Private[b]	322.7	48.9	13,230	1.03	n.a.
Autonomous agencies	96.1	14.6	23,867	1.86	n.a.
Government	68.7	10.4	17,153	1.33	n.a.
Domestic servants	6.0	0.9	3,943	0.30	25
Agricultural[c]	72.6	11.0	11,377	0.88	48.8
Self-employed	166.2	25.2	4,158	0.32	109[d]
Individuals	126.3	19.2	1,115	0.08	n.a.
Group agreements	39.9	6.0	13,800	1.07	n.a.
All insured	659.7	100.0	12,816	1.00	66.9

Sources: Author's calculations based on CCSS, 1988, 1988a; ILO, 1988; Mesa-Lago, 1990.
[a]Percentage of EAP insured, total and by specific groups, 1986 data.
[b]Excludes domestic servants.
[c]Included in total salaried workers.
[d]Some 71,000 informal salaried workers are registered as self-employed; when they are excluded, insurance coverage of the self-employed declines to 60%.

sector in Costa Rica. Furthermore, informal workers who are indigents are entitled to free health care from CCSS.

Unfortunately, we only have data on the self-employed indigents, and they are not disaggregated by urban-rural residence, hence we subsequently refer to the total (including the rural self-employed). In 1987, there were 57,870 self-employed workers receiving health care as indigents in CCSS, or 32% of the total indigent population covered and about 40% of the total number of self-employed. When one adds the number of self-employed covered as both indigents (57,870) and insured (87,168), the resulting total (145,000) equals the total number of self-employed in 1986, indicating that all of them were covered in one way or another.

Rural Poor

The Ministry program for the rural poor steadily expanded its coverage from 12% of the rural population in 1973 to a peak of 58% in 1979. The economic crisis brought on cuts in practically all services (16% in settlements served, 23% in home visits, 20% in prenatal care) and population coverage declined to 48% in 1981. With the economic recovery, services were restored, and by 1984, coverage had returned to the 1979 peak level, indicating that priority was given to rural over urban areas. Even in the midst of the crisis (1982), 53% of curative health expenditures and 61% of preventive medicine expenditures were assigned to rural areas (Pfefferman, 1989). In 1987, the program provided services through 393 rural health posts to 236,840 homes in 4,966 locations. It should be noted that although 58%

of the total rural population was protected, the targeted population (settlements with fewer than 2,000 inhabitants) was estimated to be covered by 95% in 1983. Finally, rural poverty incidence in 1988 was smaller (30%) than the Ministry's rural coverage, which was 57% (Secretaría Ejecutiva de Planificación Sectorial de Salud, 1984; Overholt, 1986; Beirute, 1988).

In 1987, the average earnings of agricultural workers insured by the CCSS equalled 88% of the average earnings for all the insured, so, they can hardly be considered as poor. Close to half of all agricultural salaried workers were insured (Table 38). However, most self-employed are rural, CCSS coverage of the self-employed is practically universal, and the insured self-employed (particularly individuals) have very low income. We can, consequently, conclude that a high percentage of the rural self-employed poor is insured by CCSS.

Unfortunately, we lack information on the number of indigents in rural areas covered by CCSS. It is safe to assume, however, that CCSS curative services do not reach the most remote areas as do the Ministry of Health services. Although it is true that those in need of more complex treatment should be referred by Ministry personnel to CCSS hospitals, transportation difficulties and other economic and cultural barriers probably preclude some of the neediest rural poor from using such services. If 20% of the urban poor who are transferred fail to use hospitalization services, the percentage is probably higher among the rural poor.

Table 39 gives an overview of the distribution of Ministry and CCSS health facilities in the five

Table 39.   Percentage distribution of health resources by region in Costa Rica, 1984.

Health regions	Population	CCSS			Ministry of Health	
		Hospital beds[a]	Physicians	Nurses	Physicians	Nurses
Central[b]	52	80	79	81	61	37
Huetar North	18	2	2	2	15	24
Huetar Atlantic	7	4	5	3	8	15
Chorotega	14	8	9	9	10	14
Brunca	10	6	5	5	6	10
Total	100	100	100	100	100	100

Sources: Author's calculations based on Saenz, 1985; Overholt, 1986; CCSS, 1988a.
[a] 1987.
[b] Merges North and South regions.

health regions. As we pointed out, the most rural and isolated regions, Brunca and Chorotega, include most of the counties with the lowest health standards in the nation. Although we have to expect some concentration of CCSS facilities and resources in the Central region (where the capital city is located), the table shows excessive disparities between the central and the other regions: with 52% of the nation's population, the Central region has between 79% and 81% of CCSS hospital beds, physicians, and nurses. Conversely, Ministry facilities are more evenly distributed; in fact, the proportion of nurses in the Central region is lower than its proportion of the population. For instance, Chorotega has 14% of the population but only receives 9% of CCSS physicians and nurses, but it receives 10% of Ministry physicians and 14% of its nurses. Once again, the nature of Ministry and CCSS services partly justifies the more even distribution of the former, but does not entirely clear the question of access to hospital services in remote areas.

REASONS FOR THE HIGH COVERAGE OF THE POOR

The previous section showed that practically all the urban and rural poor are covered by health care in Costa Rica through the combination of CCSS and Ministry of Health services. How is this possible, particularly in a country with fewer natural resources and lower per capita income than others, such as Venezuela and Mexico, that have been unable to reach such a goal? Compared with Uruguay, which also has higher income per capita and a much older social security system than Costa Rica, the latter has achieved a wider health care coverage of the poor. General factors and social security policy can explain this phenomenon.

General Factors

Costa Rica is the fourth smallest country in Latin America, it has no significant topographical barriers, and its population is highly homogenous ethnically; there is only one language spoken, and cultural differences among its people (who enjoy the fourth highest literacy rate in the Region) are unimportant. Finally, there is a good communication system and very few areas are completely isolated. For more than three decades, the country has been blessed with political stability and democracy; there are no extreme differences between the two major political parties which have alternated power. The National Liberation Party (PLN) has been the major political force since the 1960s, and quickly implemented a social policy (with emphasis on education, health care, and social security) that has been basically endorsed by the executive and legislative branches regardless of the party in power. Although CCSS was created in 1941 (by a visionary president who was ahead of his time), its coverage expansion in the 1960s and, particularly, in the 1970s, was the result of the PLN political commitment and continuous push. Because Costa Rica has no armed forces, defense expenditures have been available for social programs.

Costa Rica has the third lowest poverty incidence among the ten countries surveyed by ECLAC. It also has the fifth smallest degree of urbanization in Latin America and the Caribbean and probably the smallest informal sector in the Region, with the exception of Cuba. Furthermore, it has the second highest percentage of salaried workers in the labor force (even higher than Uruguay and Argentina), which has facilitated the expansion of population coverage by social insurances. Conversely, occupational groups that are difficult to cover (the self-employed, unpaid family workers, and domestic servants) are the smallest in the Region.

Although the rural sector in Costa Rica is proportionally one of the five largest in the Region, it has traditionally been relatively prosperous. In the late 1980s, rural income inequality in Costa Rica (measured by the Gini coefficient) was the second lowest among seven countries in Latin America (urban income inequality also was the second lowest among nine countries). Even more important, the gap in income inequality between urban and rural areas in Costa Rica was the smallest (0.005 in the Gini) among seven countries (ECLAC-CEPAL, 1990). There are no significant differences in literacy and other social indicators between urban and rural areas, contrary to other Latin American and Caribbean countries.

Social Security Policy

Political commitment undoubtedly has played a key role in Costa Rican social security policy since the 1970s, but health care has advanced the most. Ministry of Health programs for dispersed rural and marginal urban populations and CCSS programs for indigents, self-employed, and domestic servants have allowed health care to become universal. Conversely, insurance coverage on pensions, particularly among the self-employed, is considerably lower: in 1987, the CCSS pension insurance program covered 45% of the EAP, versus 67% by the sickness-maternity insurance program (coverage of the self-employed was 3.4% and 100%, respectively). Even though there is a program of welfare pensions for indigents, it has to fill the enormous vacuum left by social insurance.

The difference in coverage between the two social insurance programs is explicable by the priorities of the population (health care is an immediate need, while pensions are a long-term concern) and also by the two programs' different financing structure.

Table 40 shows that the total percentage contribution for CCSS sickness-maternity for salaried workers is 16%, but the insured only contributes 5.5% (including domestic servants). Usually, the self-employed must pay the total percentage contribution as he/she does not have an employer, and the burden of such contribution has been a deterrent to their affiliation in many countries. In Costa Rica, however, the self-employed pay from 5% to 12.5% according to a scale based on income; as most of them declare a low income, they pay the lowest percentage on the scale. In 1988, the individually insured self-employed contributed an average of 5.8%, while those insured through collective agreements paid 6.8%, and the contribution average was 6% (versus 5.5% paid by the salaried workers).

Conversely, the percentage contribution paid by salaried workers to pensions is 2.5% while that paid by the self-employed is 7.25%, three times higher. This largely explains why the affiliation of the self-employed in the pension program is so low, whereas it is very high in sickness-maternity. As we mentioned earlier, some of those registered as self-employed are actually salaried workers in informal enterprises, whose owners save 26% of employer contributions through that ruse—the owner saves money even if he "generously" reimburses his employees for the insured's contribution.

The minimum base for applying the sickness-maternity scale of contribution to the self-employed is 75% of the minimum agricultural wage. This wage has gradually risen, but the salary base for the scale of contribution has remained unchanged; hence, the percentage of self-employed paying the lowest contribution has increased with time. Furthermore, the CCSS claims that the income declared for con-

Table 40. Contributions of salaried and self-employed workers to CCSS, Costa Rica, 1988 (percentage of salary or income).

Programs	Salaried[a]				Self-employed
	Insured	Employer	State	Total	
Sickness-maternity	5.50	9.25	1.25[c]	16.00	5.0–12.25[d]
Pensions	2.50	4.75	0.25	7.50	7.25
Others[b]	1.00	11.66	0	12.66	0
Total	9.00	25.66	1.50	36.16	12.25–19.50

Source: Legislation.
[a]Includes domestic servants.
[b]Employment injury, family allowances, training, IMAS, etc.
[c]It is not clear if the current state contribution is 1.25% or 0.75%.
[d]The scale is based on income; the average for all insured is 6%; the minimum base is 75% of the minimum agricultural wage.

tribution purposes by the individually insured self-employed is lower than the actual income and, because it is impossible to control such fraud, they pay less than they should and are subsidized by the rest. However, this subsidy probably has a progressive effect on distribution, due to the very low income of the self-employed. Moreover, CCSS contends that the percentage contribution paid by the self-employed in group agreements, although higher than that paid by individuals, is low for these groups, which have an average income 7.6% higher than that of the salaried worker; in this case, the subsidy should have a regressive effect (López Vargas, 1988).

Group agreements have been a mechanism to accelerate the incorporation of the self-employed, because it is difficult and costly to collect from each of them individually. The association, union, or cooperative is responsible for the collection of contributions and is liable for any debts; but there are disadvantages. Frequently, these associations cover middle-income groups (such as taxi drivers, small manufacturers, mid-size farmers, professionals) who reportedly declare lower incomes than their actual ones. Although the contribution can be adjusted annually, it has been nearly impossible to raise it because of the power of some of these associations. Because their contributions are lower, group agreements further encourage salaried workers to pass themselves off as self-employed and promote the shift from the formal to the informal sector. Theoretically, the associations should prevent this simulation (if fraud is found, CCSS can cancel the agreement), but in practice there is no effective control (Quirós, 1987; Acuña, 1988).

Finally, a self-employed or informal salaried worker who requires medical care and is neither indigent nor insured at CCSS, can register, pay the first contribution, and stop paying after receiving care. Legally, the CCSS cannot refuse to deliver medical services, but can only check into the financial record of the user. Consequently, a self-employed person in debt can receive medical attention again and the worst that could happen is that he/she can be forced to sign a debt-payment agreement, which is difficult for CCSS to execute afterwards (Mesa-Lago, 1990).

The above discussion shows how easy and inexpensive it is for the self-employed and informal salaried workers to be insured by the CCSS sickness-maternity program. Obviously, there are financial costs to the institution and some abuses must be eliminated (to be discussed in the next section), but this flexibility

has been a key factor in the universalization of coverage, particularly in the urban sector.

FINANCIAL VIABILITY OF SOCIAL INSURANCES AND THE PUBLIC SECTOR TO MAINTAIN COVERAGE OF THE POOR

The few poor who are left unprotected by Costa Rica's nearly universal coverage, particularly those without hospitalization, are in the least developed, most isolated rural counties. They probably could be incorporated with the existing infrastructure and resources, along with a better referral system and education of the population in the poorest counties. The question is whether the current health care system is financially viable to maintain both universal coverage and the quality of services in the long run. Because of the relative integration of CCSS and the Ministry of Health, we will discuss the viability of both institutions together, while noting the important differences that exist between them.

Health expenditures per capita (in constant colones) jumped twofold between 1970 and 1979, but dropped by more than one-half in the midst of the crisis; although they have grown since 1983, by 1987 they remained below their 1973 level. As a percentage of GDP, total health expenditures increased from 4.9% in 1973 to a peak of 7.4% in 1979, declined to 5.6% in 1982 (in the midst of the crisis), and grew to 6.9% in 1985 (see Table 41). Despite the decline, this percentage is still among the highest in the Region, and Costa Rica has been one of the few countries to rapidly emerge from the regional trough in health care. After the decline in population coverage in both CCSS and the Ministry during the crisis, previous levels of coverage had been recovered by 1987, except for the Ministry's urban program. But some experts claim that the quality of services has deteriorated (see the section on "Evaluation of Coverage of the Poor and Impact on Health Standards," beginning on p. 95).

The CCSS, which covers 83% of the population on curative medicine, receives 80.4% of total nonprivate health revenue and spends about 81% of the corresponding expenditures. It also has between 90% and 93% of all hospital beds, physicians, and nurses. Conversely, the Ministry, which covers 52% of the population on pre-

Table 41. Health care facilities, resources and efficiency in Costa Rica, 1965–1987.

	1965	1973	1979	1982	1987
Facilities					
Hospitals (CCSS)	33	33	32	32	29
Clinics (CCSS)	n.a.	69	94	107	129
Health posts (Ministry of Health)	0	61	360	367	444
Mobile units (Ministry of Health)	0	6	63	44	88[c]
Health centers (Ministry of Health)	22[b]	65	83	84	84[c]
Hospitals					
Beds x 1,000	4.3	3.9	3.5	3.2	2.7
Hospital occupancy (%)	n.a.	71.5	72.0	75.3	77.6
Average days of stay	11.2	9.4	7.2	7.2	6.4
Physicians x 10,000	4.5	6.1[b]	8.9	9.8[c]	10.4
Consultations per capita	1.5	2.7	3.5	3.4	3.1[a]
Childbirth in hospitals	n.a.	n.a.	n.a.	85.7	90.7
Health expenditures					
% of GDP	n.a.	4.9	7.4	5.6	6.9[c]
Colones (1978) p/c	545[b]	703	1,022	457	693[c]

Sources: Saenz, 1985; Overholt, 1986; Rodríguez V., 1986; DETEC, 1987; Beirute, 1988; CCSS, 1988a; ECLAC, 1989a.
[a]CCSS only.
[b]1970.
[c]1985.

ventive medicine and primary health care, receives 19% of total revenue and spends a similar proportion of total expenditures; the Ministry manages between 7% and 10% of all health resources (see Table 42, segment A).

The disparity in the allocations of health resources between the two institutions can be partly explained by the different nature of the services provided by each of them—CCSS curative services are capital intensive and require more expensive installations, equipment, and personnel than the Ministry's preventive services. The proportion of health expenditures going to preventive medicine in Costa Rica is less than one-tenth of that going to curative medicine (it should be noted that some Ministry services are curative). Per capita health care costs (in 1978 colones) for the two institutions and their respective clients are presented in segment B of Table 42: CCSS spends six times more per capita than the Ministry. Furthermore, Ministry programs for the urban and rural poor have per capita expenditures which are 24% and 3% of the Ministry's overall average expenditures per capita, and negligible when compared with CCSS per capita expenditures. Interestingly, per capita expenditures of the insured and indigents in CCSS are fairly close, particularly considering that the latter are not eligible for monetary benefits; this is an indication that there is no discrimination between them. However, the disparity in resources and costs between the CCSS and the Ministry is not fully explained by the stated reason. To a large extent, the problem is related to the shift in the pathological and morbidity profiles toward dis-

Table 42. Comparison of health care facilities/resources and expenditures per capita among providers in Costa Rica, 1985.

A. PERCENTAGE DISTRIBUTION			
	CCSS	Ministry of Health	Total
Population coverage[a]	83.1	52.7	135.8[b]
Income	80.4	19.5	100.0
Expenditures	80.9	19.1	100.0
Hospital beds[a]	93.4	6.6	100.0
Physicians	90.4	9.6	100.0
Nurses	90.5	9.1	100.0

B. HEALTH EXPENDITURES PER CAPITA		
	1978 colones	Ratio over total
CCSS	707[c]	1.02
Insured	765[c]	1.10
Indigent	549	0.79
Ministry of Health	116	0.16
Urban poor	28	0.04
Rural poor	4	0.006
Total	693	1.00

Sources: Author's calculations based on Saenz, 1985; Overholt, 1986; DETEC, 1988.
[a]1987.
[b]Overcoverage due to different services offered by CCSS and Ministry of Health.
[c]Includes transfers; if eliminated, figures are 587 for CCSS and 634 for insured.

eases which are more complex and costlier to treat. Higher costs in the CCSS have been also the result of an excess of personnel and other inefficiencies (Mesa-Lago, 1989c).

Table 41 summarized health facilities and their efficiency in 1965–1987. Although the number of hospitals slightly declined, the number of CCSS clinics and Ministry health posts increased sevenfold during that period, while the number of Ministry health centers augmented almost fourfold; Ministry mobile units increased 15 times in 1973–1987. Therefore, the expansion of the physical plant in the last two decades has been truly impressive, particularly in facilities at the first and second levels of care.

Efficiency also has improved. Hospital occupancy increased from 71.5% to 77.6% in 1973–1987, while the average length of stay declined from 11.2 to 6.4 days in 1965–1987. These changes, combined with the reorganization of infant medical care and the decline in the birthrate, allowed for a small reduction in the number of hospitals and in the ratio of hospital beds per 1,000 inhabitants, which declined from 4.3 to 2.7. Practically all hospital beds belong to CCSS, but Ministry health centers have some beds for delivery, minor surgery, and emergencies. Although the average hospital occupancy for CCSS hospitals was 79% in 1987, there were three hospitals with very low rates of 57% to 59% (two of them in the Brunca Region), and four hospitals with rates of 65% to 68%; there is, therefore, room for improvement here. The average length of stay was 6.1 days in 1987, but this figure included hospitals for chronic diseases; when these were excluded, most of the remaining hospital averages ranged from 3 to 5 days. Occupancy rates in the Ministry were considerably lower than in the CCSS, and declined from 59.9% in 1982 to 50.9% in 1987 (CCSS, 1988a).

The ratio of CCSS employees per 1,000 insured reached 12.6 in 1981, one of the highest in the Region. The 1983 emergency plan brought down the ratio to 10.4 in 1987, but it still was excessively high. The percentage of expenditures in the sickness-maternity program going to personnel salaries and fringe benefits declined from 54% in 1983 to 50% in 1987, but the CCSS average monthly salary in 1987 was twice the average salary of all the insured and 5% higher than the average salary in autonomous institutions (the highest in Costa Rica). Among the fringe benefits received by CCSS employees, the exemption from paying insured's contributions, which are paid by CCSS, is particularly offensive (Mesa-Lago, 1989a; CCSS, 1988a).

The number of total physicians per 10,000 inhabitants doubled in Costa Rica in 1965–1987, increasing from 4.5 to 10.4. Consultations per capita increased more than twofold in 1965–1979, from 1.5 to 3.5, but seemed to have stabilized thereafter. Deliveries in hospitals increased from 85.7% to 90.7% of total births in

1982–1987 (Table 41). Finally, in 1981–1982, from 81% to 85% of children were immunized against DPT, polio, and tuberculosis; in 1984–1987, 81% of children under one year old were immunized against measles (Overholt, 1986; Beirute, 1988; Pfefferman, 1989).

The CCSS sickness-maternity program took up 74% of current CCSS expenditures in 1987; it ended in a financial deficit in six years in 1975–1982. Reasons for the deficit, in terms of revenue, were: insufficient percentage of wage contribution; the state's failure to fulfill part of its financial obligations to CCSS, mostly its contribution as a third party and the reimbursement of the cost for treating indigents (the total cumulative state debt in 1987 was $US61 million, 86% of which was in the sickness-maternity program); and evasion, payment delays, and loss of income because of underdeclaration of income by the self-employed and registration of informal salaried workers as self-employed. In terms of expenditures, the reasons for the deficit were overgenerous benefits such as partial cost of orthodontics and contact lenses; excessive personnel and overly high salaries and fringe benefits; and some hospital inefficiencies.

The 1983 emergency plan corrected some of these problems. For example, the percentage of contribution was raised from 14% to 16% (by far the highest in Latin America and the Caribbean and four percentage points above the next highest); agreements were signed with the state, so it could pay its debt with bonds; and controls over evasion and *mora* were improved. In addition, some generous benefits were eliminated; by 1984, 852 employees were dismissed or retired (still, the number of employees in 1987 was 5.4% higher than in 1982, prior to the emergency plan); and hospital efficiency continued to be improved. As a result of these measures, since 1983 there has been a surplus in the sickness-maternity program. An actuarial study conducted in 1988 recommended a transfer of 1% from the percentage contribution of the sickness-maternity program to the pension program, leaving 15% in the former. The study assured that, notwithstanding the transfer, the sickness-maternity program would generate a surplus for ten years, or until 1998 (Durán, 1988; DETEC, 1988; Beirute, 1988).

Even if the actuarial projections on the sickness-maternity program are accurate, the financial stability of the entire CCSS is in jeopardy because of a disequilibrium in the pension program. Four actuarial studies and/or revisions of this program conducted in 1980–1988 concluded that it will end in a deficit between 1990 and 1996, hence forcing the use of reserves to pay pensions. In 1990, the Chief Actuary acknowledged that there were no savings for the reserves in that year, and that the program would be in serious financial trouble in 1996 and bankrupt by the year 2000.

Some causes for the pension program disequilibrium are similar to those responsible for problems in the sickness-maternity program, but there are specific causes as well. In terms of revenue, the percentage of wage contribution has remained unchanged for 40 years, and real investment yields have been negative, partly because much of the reserves was lent to the sickness-maternity programs, loans were not indexed, and interest rates were lower than inflation rates. Regarding expenditures, the age for early retirement was gradually reduced, while life expectancy rapidly increased and pensions were adjusted above the increase of the cost of living. As a result of these policies, benefits increased far more than actuarially calculated, not all due revenues materialized, and contributions were not increased; to make matters worse, the pension program began to mature, and the number of pensioners rapidly rose. It is not surprising, therefore, that the actuarial deficit rapidly expanded.

In 1983, loans from the pension program to the sickness-maternity program ceased and the emergency program reduced expenditures; however, most of the major problems that caused the pension program's disequilibrium remained unsolved. In order to restore equilibrium, two or more of the following measures must be undertaken: raise the age of retirement, increase the percentage contribution by 1.5% (the transfer of 1% from sickness-maternity would help but would be insufficient), augment real investment yields, reduce pensions, and force the state to fulfill its financial obligations. Most of these measures are politically or economically difficult to implement, and none had been fulfilled by early 1990.

Since the sickness-maternity program is now generating a financial surplus, the temptation to use such funds to compensate for eventual financial deficits in the pension program will increase (the recommended transfer of 1% of the contribution is an indication of this). If the pension program indeed falls into a serious crisis, it could drag the sickness-maternity program with it. Clearly, these are two powerful reasons to stabilize the pension program (Dávila, 1988; Mesa-Lago, 1988b; CCSS, 1990; Carvajal, 1990).

At the beginning of this section, it was mentioned that the group of poor that needs to be covered by hospitalization care probably lives in the most isolated rural counties. And yet, recent CCSS efforts to expand coverage target the self-employed, who, as we have shown, enjoy practically universal coverage either as insured or as indigents. According to the CCSS actuarial office, in 1987 there were 58,586 self-employed who needed to be incorporated, basically the same number that already received health care as indigents (although this group desperately needs pensions coverage). The projects modified the scales of contribution for the self-employed, making them more uniform; the scales would be periodically adjusted according to minimum and top salaries in the private sector, as well as to the self-employed's real ability to pay. Group agreements would be cancelled and substituted by new ones with uniform rules: the associations would collect the insured's contributions and, in addition, would pay their own contribution. Part of the state contribution would be used to subsidize the affiliation of individual self-employed persons who are not associated, and, hence, would lack the association's contribution. Finally, the self-employed would be entitled to sickness-maternity paid leave.

Although these projects encompassed standardization and financing improvements, they also ignored the low income of those self-employed who are incorporated as indigents, overestimated CCSS's ability to exercise control and assess the real income of associated self-employed who have the ability to contribute more to CCSS, stretched even more the state contribution (normally paid late and devaluated) as a means to subsidize individual low income, and added new benefits (paid leave) that are difficult to finance and are not essential. Although these projects were approved by CCSS in 1988, they were not yet implemented by the end of 1989, probably due to the above-mentioned difficulties (Acuña, 1988; López Vargas, 1988; CCSS, 1988b; Mesa-Lago, 1990a).

EVALUATION OF COVERAGE OF THE POOR AND IMPACT ON HEALTH STANDARDS

This section evaluates the combined CCSS-Ministry of Health coverage of the poor in three areas—real access of the poor to health care, impact of the CCSS-Ministry programs on overall health standards, and the effect of such programs on income distribution.

Real Access of the Poor to Health Care Services

In 1984, a household survey on public social expenditure gathered information on health care access by income and poverty level of the population; the results of this survey have been analyzed in a thorough study by Rodríguez V. (1986). The survey characterized absolute indigence by a lack of sufficient household income to buy a minimum food basket, and absolute poverty by an income insufficient to acquire nonfood basic needs, including health care; the rest of the population was considered nonpoor. The survey distinguished between urban and rural zones among the three groups. The average income of an indigent household was found to be 22% of the national average income, while the poor household income was 44% of the national average. A summary of the principal survey results appears in Table 43.

The survey asked the population that had been sick or had had health problems or an accident three months prior to administering the questionnaire if they had sought medical attention. Nationally, 64% answered positively and 36% negatively, but 45% of the indigents did not seek medical help, compared with 36% among the poor and 34% among the nonpoor. Although there was a difference of 11 percentage points between the two extreme groups, the survey indicated that most of the poor sought medical help.

Out of the 64% who sought medical help nationally, 81.4% did so in CCSS, 3.9% in the Ministry, and 14.6% in the private sector. Disaggregation of users by poverty levels showed that the CCSS was the major provider regardless of income level, but the degree of use was

highest among the poor (89%), followed by the indigents (83%), and lowest among the nonpoor (79.5%). It appears that the survey used the term "insured" (at CCSS) in the questionnaire, thus excluding welfare care of indigents paid for by the state; if the latter had been included, the percentage of indigents using CCSS services would have been even higher. Use of Ministry consultations was highest among indigents (almost 10%) and lowest among the nonpoor (2.6%). Conversely, private consultation was highest among the nonpoor (18%) and about the same among indigents and the nonpoor (7%). Average annual per capita consultations were different among providers: 1.95 in the Ministry, 2.61 in CCSS, and 3.19 in the private sector; if the number of consultations, instead of users, had been employed in the calculations in Table 43, the share of the CCSS and the private sector would have been even higher, and the Ministry's would have been lower.

The survey also asked the users why they had gone to a given provider for outpatient consultation. Those who went to CCSS did so, first, because they had institutional coverage and, second, because CCSS facilities were close to their homes (this was found to be more important in rural than urban areas); quality of service was also mentioned but did not appear to be relevant. Ministry of Health users first cited closeness as the most important reason and low cost as the second (particularly among the poor, and even more so among the rural poor). Finally, those who paid for private consultation did so either to receive better care or because they could choose the physician (Rodríguez V., 1986).

The reasons given for not seeking medical care by 36% of the population were: 61% either cured themselves or resorted to a nonphysician friend (60% among indigents, 58% among the poor, and 62% among the nonpoor); 20% felt that medical care was not necessary because the illness was not serious (24% among the poor

Table 43. Members of the population who were ill and did or did not seek medical consultation (providers and reasons), by poverty levels, in Costa Rica, 1983 (percentage distribution).

Poverty levels	Did or did not seek medical consultation[a]		Providers of medical consultation			Reasons for not seeking medical consultation					
	Did	Did not	CCSS	Ministry of Health	Private	Self-cured or cured by friend	Not necessary	Lack of close facility	Long wait, bad quality	High cost	Others
Indigents	54.8	45.2	83.3	9.7	7.0	59.8	19.8	9.6	4.8	3.4	3.5
Poor	64.0	36.0	89.1	4.2	6.7	57.5	24.5	5.7	5.6	5.2	1.5
Nonpoor	66.0	34.0	79.5	2.6	17.9	62.4	19.1	5.4	7.3	1.4	4.4
Total	63.8	36.2	81.4	3.9	14.6	61.1	20.0	6.3	6.3	2.4	3.8

Sources: Rodríguez V., 1986; and author's calculations.
[a]Persons who felt ill or had health problems or an accident three months prior to the survey and either had medical consultation or not.

and about 19% among both indigents and the nonpoor); 6% gave a lack of services close to their residences as a reason (9% among indigents); 6% blamed long lines or poor quality of services (ranging from 4.8% among indigents to 7% among the nonpoor); and 2.4% said that the high cost of the service was the culprit (3.4% among indigents).

In summary, save for a few exceptions, the survey did not detect dramatic differences among the three groups in terms of health access, use of providers and reasons for using them or for causes for not seeking medical attention when ill. Furthermore, the survey underestimated the number of indigents with access to CCSS services. The survey found the following minor differences: the use of CCSS facilities was higher among the poor than among indigents, but higher among the latter than among the nonpoor; indigents resorted to the Ministry of Health as a second provider, but the second choice of the poor were private services (although with a small difference between Ministry and private care), and a significant proportion of the nonpoor used private services; closeness of the facilities to their places of residence, institutional coverage, and low cost of service were the most important reasons for selecting providers for indigents and the poor (closeness for the rural poor and costs for the urban poor), while quality of the service was irrelevant to them but crucial to the nonpoor (Rodríguez V., 1986).

Impact on Overall Health Standards

Costa Rica is one of the Latin American and Caribbean countries that has improved health standards most rapidly. Table 44 shows that in the 1970s, the annual average rate of reduction in the mortality rate was twice as high as in the 1960s, while the decline in the infant mortality rate was six time higher. There was a significant slowdown in the rate of decline in the 1980s, probably due in part to the economic crisis, but also due to the fact that as mortality rates reach low levels, it becomes increasingly difficult to reduce them; in the case of general mortality rates, the aging of the Costa Rican population would eventually induce an increase. In any event, the table shows that in 1960–1987, general mortality rates were cut in half, infant mortality rates were reduced by three-fourths, and life expectancy was increased by 14.5 years.

There has been a dramatic change in the country's epidemiological profile as well. In 1965, 49% of the major causes of death were "diseases of underdevelopment" such as contagious diseases, digestive tract problems, parasites, respiratory diseases, and prenatal conditions, whereas only 22.7% were "diseases of

Table 44.   Health standards in Costa Rica, 1960–1987.

	1960[a]	1970[b]	1980	1987	Change 1987/1960
Mortality rates					
General	8.0	6.7	4.1	3.9	−4.1
Infant	68.6	61.5	19.1	17.8	−50.8
Life expectancy (years)	60.2	65.6	70.8	74.7	14.5
Causes of death (%)					
Contagious, intestinal, parasitical	27.0	19.0	8.4	8.1	−18.9
Respiratory	11.5	10.4	10.2	8.9	−2.6
Prenatal	10.7	6.2	5.9	6.9	−3.8
Cardiovascular	9.1	22.0	25.3	27.9	18.8
Tumors	9.5	12.6	16.7	19.2	9.7
Accidents	4.1	8.8	13.3	10.6	6.5
Others	28.1	21.0	20.2	18.4	−9.7
Total	100.0	100.0	100.0	100.0	0.0
Children malnutrition (%)					
General	57.4	53.2	34.2[c]	n.a.	−23.2
2nd and 3rd degree	13.7	12.7	3.6[c]	n.a.	−10.1
Sanitation; % pop. with:					
Potable water	57	73	84	93[d]	36
Sewage	n.a.	48	87	95[d]	47

Sources: Saenz, 1985; Overholt, 1986; Rodríguez V., 1986; Beirute, 1988; ECLAC, 1989a; Mesa-Lago, 1990; World Bank, 1990.
[a]1965 for causes of death, malnutrition, and sanitation.
[b]1973 for causes of death; 1975 for malnutrition.
[c]1982.
[d]1985.

development," such as cardiovascular diseases, tumors, and accidents. By 1980, the proportions had reversed to 24.5% and 55%, respectively; in the 1980s, although the trend continued, there was a significant slowdown and proportions were 24% and 58%, respectively. Among children below one year of age, 23.4% of the deaths in 1970 were caused by gastroenteritis, infectious diseases, and parasites, but by 1980, the proportion had declined to 10.8%; in addition, 10.3% of deaths in 1970 were caused by bronchitis, tetanus, and measles, but ten years later there were no reported deaths due to such diseases. Among children from 1 to 4 years of age, gastroenteritis was the principal cause of death in 1970 (23.4%), while measles, tetanus, whooping cough, and bronchitis caused 19% of deaths; by 1980 there were no deaths reported due to any of those diseases. There were parallel declines in morbidity rates in the 1970s for diseases preventable by immunization; polio, diphtheria, and measles are practically nonexistent now, while the rates of malaria, whooping cough, and tetanus are extremely low (Overholt, 1986).

Overall malnutrition among children below five years of age declined from 57.4% in 1965 to 34.2% in 1982; second and third degree malnutrition dropped even more dramatically, from 13.7% to 3.6%, respectively, for those same years; the annual rate of decline of the latter in 1970–1982 was almost four times greater than in 1965–1970. Finally, the percentage of the population with access to potable water (aqueduct or easy access) increased from 57% in 1965 to 93% in 1985, while the proportion of the population served by sewage or other means of excreta disposal increased from 48% to 95%. Urban areas have 100% access to both services, while rural areas have 82% and 88% access, respectively (Beirute, 1988). Diseases related to the lack of these services have been dramatically reduced.

Several international and domestic experts on health care and/or development agree that, although the Costa Rican health improvements mentioned above cannot be solely or completely attributed to the 1970s health policies, the two are clearly correlated—the creation of the Ministry of Health programs for rural and urban areas, the acceleration of CCSS coverage expansion (including indigents), and the establishment of nutrition and other programs for pregnant women and children all took place in that decade. The 1974–1980 National Health Plan set goals that experts considered difficult to achieve at its inception, but that were actually over-

fulfilled. In fact, Costa Rica had practically provided health care to all its citizens before the WHO goal of health for all was established in Alma Ata in 1978 (Saenz, 1985; Overholt, 1986; Rodríguez V., 1986; Beirute, 1988; Pfefferman, 1989).

We are unable to precisely assess the respective impact of the CCSS and the Ministry on Costa Rica's rising health standards, but there are indications that the Ministry's impact (relative to its lower share of resources) has been higher because it has targeted more vulnerable groups such as poor women and children; CCSS expenditures on indigents, pregnant women, and infants probably have had a more beneficial impact on overall health standards than expenditures on higher-income and productive-age groups. A CCSS document states that the Ministry's primary health care, immunization, and infant nutrition programs have done more to reduce mortality and morbidity than CCSS's curative programs that treat cardiovascular diseases and tumors. The Director of the best children's hospital in the country proved that the most important factor in reducing infant mortality was the control of infectious diseases, most of which are preventable through vaccination and sanitation. And the Minister of Health pinpointed the lack of basic equipment and medicine in rural areas as the greatest shortcoming, in contrasting it with the ultramodern equipment and high technology that is prevalent in the capital and that treats a proportionally smaller number of patients.

The impact of the Ministry's programs for the poor has been analyzed (see Table 45). A comparison of the degree of coverage by the Ministry's rural program by county and increases in life expectancy between 1970–1972 and 1974–1976, found a positive correlation between both variables—counties with 25% to 49% coverage experienced an increase of 3.5 years, and the number of years gained steadily rose reaching 5.1 years in counties with more than 75% coverage. Counties with less than 25% coverage by the Ministry's rural program are the most developed and the ones where this program is the least important; this explains the high life expectancy of this group.

A comparison of the degree of coverage by Ministry urban and rural programs and the reduction in infant mortality by counties between 1968–1969 and 1979–1980 shows similar results: as the degree of coverage increases from 25% to more than 75%, infant mortality rates increasingly drop, from 41 to 63 points. Again, coun-

Table 45. Impact on health standards of the Ministry of Health programs for the poor in Costa Rica, 1968–1980.

Grouping of counties by degree of population coverage	Life expectancy[a]		Change (years)	Infant mortality[b]		Change[c]
	1970–72	1974–76		1968–69	1979–80	
Less than 25%[d]	68.7	71.1	2.4	49	20	−29
25% to 49%	63.9	67.4	3.5	64	23	−41
50% to 74%	67.3	71.3	4.0	76	22	−54
More than 75%	67.9	73.0	5.1	80	17	−63
Nation	67.7	71.1	3.4	63	20	−43

Source: Saenz, 1985.
[a]Rural program only.
[b]Rural and urban programs.
[c]Reduction of points in the rate of children below one year who died per 1,000 born alive.
[d]These counties are the most developed and the ones where the Ministry of Health programs for the poor are not important.

ties with less than 25% coverage are the most developed and have the lowest infant mortality. Unfortunately, we lack data on CCSS coverage by county to replicate this type of analysis.

Another comparison divides counties into six groups according to infant mortality rates (from less than 10 to more than 50) and compares the percentage distribution in 1972–1974 and 1986. At the beginning there was no county in the less-than-10 group, and the percentage of counties increased in each of the following groups, reaching 33% in the 50-and-more group. But by 1987, there were 12.7% of the counties in the less-than-10 group and 53% in the 10-to-19.9 group; the percentage then steadily declined, reaching zero in the 50-and-more group. Not only was there an overall reduction of rates throughout the country, but there was considerably less dispersion of the rates among counties, more concentration around the national average rate, and a reduction in the gap among counties (Saenz, 1985; Ministerio de Salud, 1987).

Still, there are a few counties in Costa Rica that have infant mortality rates well above the national average. In 1986, the national rate was 17.6, but the following counties had much higher rates: Turrubares, 47.6%; La Cruz, Carrillo, Aguirre, and Garabito, from 31.6% to 29%; Limón, Tarrazú, San Mateo, and Corredores, from 28.8% to 26.1%; and Tilarán, Talamanca, Oreamuno, Acosta, and Alfaro Ruiz, from 25.9% to 25.1%. The highest concentration in these counties was in the regions of Chorotega and Huetar Atlántica (Ministerio de Salud, 1987). With few exceptions, these counties are the poorest in Costa Rica, an indication that there are still some areas where access to health care should be improved. And yet, with the exception of Turrubares, the remaining counties' rates are well below the national rates of most

Latin American and Caribbean countries (see Table 12).

Effect of Income Distribution

The household survey on public social expenditures evaluated the impact of the 1982 state subsidies to health care services on family income distribution (Rodríguez V., 1986). The health services covered by the survey were curative medicine, basically provided by CCSS, including consultation and hospitalization and preventive medicine, basically provided by the Ministry, including direct services (such as those geared to the rural and urban poor), and general services. The study evaluated the impact of the subsidy on different income strata, poverty levels (indigents, poor, nonpoor), and zones (national, urban—disaggregating the capital city—and rural).

The total health subsidy in 1982 was estimated at $US131 million, or 5.3% of the GDP and 17.9% of central government expenditures. It should be noted, however, that the study did not consider contributions and payments of the users of services. Of the total subsidy, 89.2% went to curative medicine (59% to hospitalization, mainly specialized, and 30.2% to outpatient consultation) and 10.8% to preventive medicine (8.2% to direct services and 2.6% to general services).

The distribution of the subsidy by location systematically favored rural zones over urban zones, but more so for preventive than curative services. According to the survey, the distribution of the population was 51.8% urban (27.4% in the capital and 24.4% elsewhere) and 48.2% rural, while the distribution of the subsidy was 46.5% urban (with no significant difference between the capital and the rest of the urban zone) and 53.5% rural. Of the total subsidy, the rural zone received 46.9% and the urban zone 42.3% in curative medicine; in preventive medicine, the rural zone received 6.6% and the urban zone 4.2%.

The distribution of the subsidies was progressive for all programs and all zones. The highest degree of progressiveness was that of preventive medicine (particularly direct programs) and the least, that of hospitalization (particularly specialized hospitals). However, because of the lower subsidy share assigned to preventive services and the higher share assigned to hospitalization, prevention subsidies had less actual impact on reducing income inequality than did hospitalization subsidies. An inversion of current subsidy shares assigned to those programs would, therefore, dramatically increase the progressive redistribution impact of the subsidies. Put more simply, an increase in the subsidy to prevention services available for the rural and urban poor would reduce income inequality significantly (Rodríguez V., 1986).

Table 46 shows the impact of the health subsidies by income and poverty strata, as well as by areas. Nationally, the subsidy induced an increment of 8.4% in the average family income, more in the rural area (14.2%) than in the urban area (5.7%). The subsidy-induced increment was inversely correlated with income; in other words, it was 61% for the 10% of the population with the lowest income (57% for indigents), and

declined as income increased to 2.4% for the wealthiest 20% of the population. In the rural area, the poorest 10% of the population benefitted from an increment of almost 78%, versus 61% in the urban area. Reduction of income inequality (Gini coefficient) was greater in the rural area than in the urban one. However, urban indigents experienced a greater increment than rural indigents, because prevention services (concentrated in the rural area) received a much lower share of the total subsidy than hospitalization services (concentrated in the urban area, particularly specialized hospital services in the capital).

The evaluation made in this section clearly shows that Costa Rican health programs for the poor have been very successful: there are no dramatic differences in real access between indigents and the poor, and the nonpoor; in the 1970s these programs contributed to one of the most rapid improvements in health standards in the Region (placing Costa Rica among the three countries with the best standards); and state health subsidies have a progressive impact on distribution. These achievements are even more remarkable in a country that in 1987–1988 ranked seventh in per capita income among 20 Latin American and Caribbean countries (World Bank, 1990) and ninth among 23 of the Region's countries (ECLAC, 1989a), but surpassed most of the wealthier countries in health standards and protection of the poor.

Table 46. Impact of state health subsidies on family income distribution by income levels, poverty strata, and areas in Costa Rica, 1982 (in percentages).

Households	Percentage distribution of income before (B) and after (A) subsidy								
	National			Urban			Rural		
	B	A	Ia	B	A	Ia	B	A	Ia
Income quintiles									
Poorest 10%	2.2	3.3	61.1	1.9	2.8	61.1	3.1	4.8	77.5
First 20%	6.1	7.9	41.4	6.1	7.5	29.8	7.8	10.2	49.2
Second 20%	11.2	11.9	14.1	10.4	10.8	9.6	13.4	14.3	22.1
Third 20%	14.9	15.3	11.8	15.1	15.2	6.3	17.7	17.5	12.9
Fourth 20%	21.4	21.1	6.6	21.1	20.9	4.7	21.5	21.4	13.7
Fifth 20%	46.4	43.8	2.4	47.3	45.6	2.0	39.6	36.6	5.5
Total	100.0	100.0	8.4d	100.0	100.0	5.7d	100.0	100.0	14.2d
Poverty strata									
Indigentsb	2.8	4.1	57.2	1.4	2.2	62.7	5.8	7.8	54.3
Poorc	6.0	7.0	25.4	4.1	4.7	21.2	10.2	11.5	29.0
Nonpoor	91.2	89.0	5.8	94.5	93.1	4.2	84.0	80.7	9.7
Total	100.0	100.0	8.4d	100.0	100.0	5.7d	100.0	100.0	14.2d
Gini coefficient	.387	.346	−.041e	.395	.366	−.029e	.299	.249	−.050e

Source: Rodríguez V., 1986.
[a]Percentage increment of average family income when subsidy is added.
[b]Household income is insufficient to buy a minimum food basket.
[c]Household income is sufficient to buy minimum food basket but not to cover other basic needs such as housing, clothing, health, and education.
[d]Average increment among all families.
[e]Absolute difference between Gini coefficients prior to and after subsidy.

PRIVATE ALTERNATIVES TO IMPROVE HEALTH CARE EFFICIENCY

The remarkable development of social security in Costa Rica has left little room for the private sector in health care. It should be noted that CCSS and, to a lesser extent, the Ministry of Health have private patients (neither insured nor indigents) who pay for their services; for example, 2% of CCSS dental consultations in 1986 were for private patients. Hence, although 15% of the population is not covered by CCSS, a portion of it uses its services, paying user fees. In 1982–1985, the private sector only managed 1.9% of the total number of hospital beds, 3% of total hospital discharges, 1.1% of total days of hospital stay, and 0.3% of total outpatient consultations. In 1987, occupancy in the private sector was 45.9% and the average length of stay was 2.7 days, both much lower than the national averages (Rodríguez V., 1986; Overholt, 1986; CCSS, 1988, 1988a).

We have seen that a small proportion of indigents and poor reported in 1983 that they used private consultation services. There is information on only one association of small entrepreneurs and informal workers, ADAPTE, that was considering a collective voluntary insurance with a private hospital for its members. The Federation of Voluntary Organizations embraces 50 NGOs that help low income groups; it manages a house for persons who come from the countryside to receive outpatient health care in the capital city (Mesa-Lago, 1990a).

Perhaps the most important role of the private sector is its collaboration with CCSS. In the 1980s, CCSS developed the following three programs to incorporate the private sector, transfer part of CCSS costs to it, and induce an increase in CCSS efficiency and quality of services: enterprise physicians, mixed medicine, and medical cooperatives. In 1982–1983, CCSS signed an agreement with the private sector introducing the first two programs, both for ambulatory services: in enterprise physicians, 630 private enterprises hire and pay a doctor and provide him with an office and a nurse, while CCSS supplies support services (laboratory and other diagnostic services and medicine); under the mixed medicine program, the insured selects a physician from those enrolled in the program and pays for his services, while CCSS provides support services and medicine.

Table 47 summarizes information on both programs for 1986–1987: combined, they served 7%

Table 47. Resources and services of enterprise physicians and mixed medicine in Costa Rica, 1986–1987.

	Enterprise physicians	Mixed medicine	Total
Population served	111,576	51,773	163,349
% of population covered by CCSS	4.8	2.2	7.0
Total outpatient consultations	502,094	93,191	595,285
% of total CCSS consultations	7.0	1.3	8.3
Consultations per capita	4.5	1.8	3.6
Expenditures (thousand colones)	50,468	19,578	70,046
Expenditures per capita	452	378	428
% of total CCSS services			
Medicines	5.6	1.7	7.3
X rays	2.5	1.5	4.0
Lab tests	2.0	1.3	3.3
Sickness paid leaves approved	6.2	—	6.2

Sources: Author's calculations based on Beirute, 1988; CCSS, 1988, 1988a.

of the population covered by CCSS (two-thirds of those served are in enterprise physicians and one-third in mixed medicine); jointly they provided outpatient consultations equal to 8% of CCSS medical consultations (more than their share of CCSS covered population); per capita annual consultations averaged 3.6 (4.5 in enterprise physicians versus 1.8 in mixed medicine), slightly higher than the CCSS average of 3.1. The combined average per capita expenditure was 428 colones (20% higher in enterprise physicians than in mixed medicine), about one-fourth of the CCSS per capita cost. Jointly they received the following proportions of total CCSS services: 7% of medicines, 4% of X rays, and 3% of laboratory tests; they also approved 6% of all sickness paid leaves. Since these proportions are lower than the enterprise physicians/mixed medicine share of the CCSS covered population, except for medicines, they utilize fewer diagnostic services and are stricter in awarding paid leaves than CCSS.

Practically all these indicators suggest that enterprise physicians and mixed medicine are more efficient than CCSS and/or have helped it to reduce costs. About 92% of the enterprise physicians and 76% of the mixed medicine programs are located in the Central Region, because both enterprises and enrolled physicians are concentrated there (CCSS, 1988a). Although this program may help CCSS financially, it does not help the poor, since they are neither employees in large enterprises nor have resources to pay a private physician; furthermore, most of the poor are concentrated in rural areas, and these two programs are urban.

A new program, which began in 1988, has the potential to reach the urban poor; it is a health cooperative organized in the neighborhood of Pavas in San José, which has 45,000 inhabitants. The cooperative consists of 100 health professionals who are expected to buy coop shares; CCSS has transferred to the cooperative a fully equipped clinic for the period of the contract (the coop pays a symbolic sum as rental), and CCSS also pays a monthly sum per user and the Ministry of Health pays a monthly lump sum. The cooperative provides the following services to users: prevention, nutrition, immunization, and antiparasitical treatment; physicians' visits to homes, schools, and workplaces; curative medicine (consultation, obstetrics, minor surgery, dentistry); diagnostic services (X ray, laboratory tests); medicine; and milk to pregnant women and undernourished children.

The population (insured and indigents) freely selects the physician from the cooperative. The cooperative must maintain the building and equipment and return them to CCSS in good condition at the end of the contract. The cooperative receives some input, such as milk, from the Ministry of Health, but hires and is responsible for all its personnel and buys medicines and other supplies in the open market or from CCSS (Ministerio de Salud/CCSS, 1988). This experiment, if successful, could use the surplus of physicians in Costa Rica to expand services to urban areas with poor coverage and/or services.

MEXICO

POVERTY: SIZE, TRENDS, AND CHARACTERISTICS

According to ECLAC, in 1984 Mexico had the fifth highest poverty incidence (total population) among the ten Latin American countries in the survey: national 37%, urban 30%, and rural 51%. Mexico's poverty incidence was higher than that of Argentina, Uruguay, Costa Rica, and Venezuela, but lower than the regional average and than that of five other countries in the survey, including Peru (see Table 2). In 1950-1970, the country's national poverty incidence (households) declined from 52% to 34%; it further decreased to 32% in 1977 and to 30% in 1984 (ECLAC, 1990). The series on the total population, only available for 1977-1984, indicates a decline in poverty incidence from 40% to 37%. We lack data on poverty, both for 1980-1981, the growth peak prior to the crisis, and for after 1984, when the economy deteriorated further.

In the 1970s, the Mexican economy boomed: GDP per capita grew at an annual rate of 3.5% (5.8% in 1980-1981), annual inflation averaged 16%, and open unemployment was about 3%. The crisis began in 1982, and in the rest of the decade, cumulative GDP per capita declined by 9%, inflation averaged 80% annually, real wages fell by 34%, and unemployment doubled (6.6% in 1983). By the end of the decade, the economy

was still sluggish and, although inflation had been cut to 18% and unemployment was back to 3%, there was no increase in real wages (ECLAC, 1988a, 1989). The number of poor increased 7.8% in 1977-1984, and, due to the crisis, poverty doubtlessly grew at a faster rate in the rest of the decade.

Mexico has one of the highest rates of urbanization in the Region, and by 1988, about 71% of its population was urban, an increase of 16 percentage points since 1965. Rapid urbanization caused the poverty incidence (households) in the urban area to increase from 20% to 23% in 1970-1984; in the rural area, it decreased from 49% to 43%. However, the incidence of indigence in the rural area in 1984 was more than three times that of the urban area. In that year, there were 28 million poor in Mexico (10 million indigents); 52% of them lived in urban areas and 48% in rural areas (ECLAC, 1990).

The Urban (Informal) Sector

In 1970, about 25% of the urban workers in Mexico earned less than the minimum wage and were considered poor; 73% of them worked in the informal sector. As a percentage of the EAP, the informal sector steadily grew from 14% in 1960, to 18% in 1970, and to 22% in 1980. In that last year, Mexico had the sixth largest informal sector in Latin America (Tokman, 1980; PRE-ALC, 1981a, 1982). A national survey of the informal sector conducted in 1976, estimated that 38% of the urban employed EAP were in the informal sector, distributed as follows: 64%, salaried (including almost 14% in domestic service); 26%, self-employed; and 10%, unpaid family workers (the survey did not identify informal employers). The degree of informality within each occupational category was 100% in unpaid family work, 79% in domestic service,

62% in self-employment, and 32% in salaried work. About 55% of the informal workers were in the tertiary sector (services and commerce), and another 31% were in manufacturing and construction. Informal workers were younger than formal workers, and there was a higher proportion of females in the former than in the latter; 94% of them lacked any skills, 96% did not belong to a labor organization, and 71% had no income or earned less than 2,000 pesos per week—the percentage of informal workers in this income bracket was seven times higher than that of formal workers (Secretaría de Salud Pública et al, 1979; Secretaría de Trabajo y Previsión Social, 1985).

According to the survey, 76% of the informal salaried workers did not have access to health care services and 82% were not covered by social insurance, versus 8% in the formal sector. Self-employment was much less protected than salaried work: 86% of informal workers lacked health care services (66% among formal workers). The least protected informal workers were street vendors, providers of personal services, and domestic servants (Montaño, 1985).

Although no survey of informality has been conducted in Mexico since 1976, scattered data indicate a rapid increase of its importance. The nonsalaried EAP (either self-employed, unpaid relatives, employers, or unclassified) increased from 37% in the 1970 census to 56% in the 1980 census. Household surveys conducted in 1982–1985, although reporting smaller percentages of the EAP (employed) in nonsalaried work than in the census, showed it increased from 17% to 24% in that period. Self-employment in the Federal District rapidly expanded in the first half of the 1980s in services, commerce, construction, and manufacturing. Finally, open unemployment peaked in 1983 at 6.6% of the EAP and reportedly declined later to 3% in 1989 but these figures are a subject of discussion (Diéguez, 1986; Samaniego, 1986; ECLAC, 1989).

The Rural Sector

Mexico's rural population falls into two groups: concentrated population, living in settlements from 2,500 to 14,999 inhabitants, and dispersed population, living in settlements of fewer than 2,500 inhabitants; the latter is officially considered the rural population. In 1987, it was estimated—improperly using the same proportions as in 1980—that the former group embraced 11.8 million people (14.5% of the total

population), while the latter covered 27.3 million (33.7% of the total population). Within the dispersed group, which suffers from a higher poverty incidence than the concentrated group, there were 110,000 villages with fewer than 500 inhabitants, for a total of 11.4 million people (14% of the total population). This segment, considered "marginalized" because it is left out of the development process, is where the critical poverty is concentrated. The above figures on the dispersed population should have declined in 1981–1987 based on projections of the proportion of the population in that category. In 1980, almost half of the rural sector was traditional as opposed to modern (PREALC, 1982). According to ECLAC, in 1984 there were 13.4 million poor in rural areas of which 6.4 million were indigents (ECLAC, 1990).

According to a study conducted in 1981, the marginalized rural population is highly dispersed and isolated, inhabiting the least developed states; 77% of them live in largely arid or semi-arid locations above 1,000 meters. Practically all the marginalized rural population works in agriculture, uses rudimentary tools with a very low level of productivity, and is affected by seasonal unemployment and underemployment. About 38% are illiterate and 38% consume a diet of corn and beans and have a high degree of malnutrition; 90% live in houses that lack any type of excreta disposal, 67% in dwellings that do not have piped water, and 50% in homes without any electricity; 32% of the households live in one-room dwellings that house an average of six persons. The ten major causes of death among the marginalized rural population are diseases typical of underdevelopment, such as contagious, intestinal, respiratory, and perinatal diseases. Close to half of the deaths are among children under one year of age. According to the World Bank (1990), infant mortality in all rural areas (not only poor ones) was 79 per 1,000, almost three times the rate of urban areas. About 67% of the rural marginal are not in the cash economy and, out of the 37% who earn some income, half are temporary workers who receive less than the national minimum wage. Some 56 Indian tribes (5.2 million people or 7.7% of the total population) live in the rural marginal zones (IMSS, 1983; IMSS and COPLAMAR, 1988a).

Because of its dispersion, isolation, high altitude home, and lack of communication, the marginalized rural population is highly inaccessible. Providing social services to this group is difficult and extremely costly given such problems as transportation, construction and supply of facilities, and training and incentives for medical personnel.

HEALTH CARE COVERAGE OF THE URBAN (INFORMAL) AND RURAL POOR

Administrative Structure and Legal Coverage

The Mexican Institute of Social Security (IMSS), established in 1943, is the main social insurance agency; its sickness-maternity program is geared to the protection of salaried workers in the private sector, mostly urban residents. Coverage includes general and specialized care, surgery, maternity care, hospitalization, laboratory services, dental care, and medicine for the employee, his spouse, children below the age of 16, and parents. The insured also is entitled to paid sickness and maternity leave. If the insured becomes unemployed, coverage on health care continues for six and one-half months. The second largest social insurance agency, the Institute of Social Security and Services for State Employees (ISSSTE), was created in 1959 and covers federal government employees. There are two other independent social insurance agencies covering the armed forces (ISSSFAM) and petroleum workers (PEMEX). With the exception of IMSS, social insurance agencies do not provide any health care for the poor.

In the mid-1950s, IMSS gradually began to extend its population coverage. Interestingly, this effort coincided with growing agricultural union organization and violent protests in the countryside. First to be incorporated were rural groups in fairly developed areas or economic branches, such as salaried plantation workers (sugar, sisal, tobacco, coffee, palm) and some members of credit associations and communal farms (ejidos). In his inaugural address, then President Echeverría declared that social security could not be a "prerogative of a minority," but should cover marginal groups and the neediest sectors; to delay this action—he said— would be "imprudent" and would "deepen the differences among the inhabitants of the country" (Mesa-Lago, 1989c). In 1973, an IMSS Social Solidarity Program began to offer health care protection to the poor in rural areas and, theoretically, to marginal urban areas. In 1977,

the General Coordination of the National Plan for [Rural] Depressed Zones and Marginal Groups (COPLAMAR) was established and, two years later, it signed an agreement with IMSS for health care coverage. COPLAMAR was abolished in 1983, but IMSS continued to provide and rapidly expand its medical-hospital services to the marginalized rural population. In 1985–1988, some of those services were transferred from IMSS to state governments (see the section on "Evaluation of IMSS-COPLAMAR Health Care Program for Rural Poor," beginning on p. 115).

Coverage of the urban poor by IMSS has been considerably less significant. A 1973 law mandated the compulsory coverage of domestic servants, the self-employed, small entrepreneurs, unpaid family workers, and other non-salaried workers. However, the law was suspended until the Executive Branch's enactment of regulations to specify the financing and benefits of each group, an action that had not occurred by 1989. Nevertheless, all of these groups can voluntarily join IMSS individually or through collective agreements. Owners of microenterprises with two or three employees are required to register them at IMSS, but enforcement is weak (these employers may voluntarily join). Employers of domestic servants are not required to register them.

The requirements for voluntary group agreements with IMSS are complex and, in practice, exclude the poor because the group must have economic resources and an administrative organization to be eligible. IMSS requires that a given association, cooperative, trade union, or corporation be capable of registering its group members, of collecting and sending their contributions to IMSS, and of guaranteeing such payments. IMSS has entered into agreements with lottery vendors, street musicians, and taxi drivers who own their vehicles; salaried taxi drivers should be registered by their employers, but most of them are not because they operate illegally.

The above-mentioned individuals or groups who have joined IMSS usually are entitled to health care protection (medical-hospital benefits), but not to paid sickness or maternity leave. Domestic servants and taxi drivers are entitled to all IMSS benefits.

The urban poor not covered by IMSS could have access to health care services from public sector institutions. The federal Secretariat of Health supervises the 1984 national health system, but in reality provides little coordination. The Secretariat administers preventive medicine and sanitation for the population as a whole, as well as a national network of hospitals and outpatient clinics. Its curative medicine services charge low flat user fees, but we do not know whether such fees are still high for the poor. The Federal District Department manages hospitals and primary health care centers for the resident population that is not covered by social insurance. Users are classified into one of five income brackets, which is noted on the ID card: the lowest level pays only a nominal fee, while the other levels pay an increasing percentage of the costs of services, reaching 100% at the highest (fifth) level; it is said that there is no discrimination in treatment based on payments. There is a special Federal District Department hospital for nonsalaried workers, such as street musicians and shoe shiners, but they must be organized as a group. The National System for Integral Family Development, a federal program, helps particularly the noninsured urban infant-maternal population with nutrition, health care, and other services (Mesa-Lago, 1990a). Finally, states and municipalities also provide services to the poor.

The rural poor outside of the marginalized area—those living in settlements with more than 2,500 inhabitants—may have access to Secretariat of Health and state services. In addition, the National Indian Institute also provides some health services.

To summarize, the rural poor in Mexico can be legally covered by the IMSS-COPLAMAR special program; a few, such as plantation workers and members of cooperatives, may be eligible under other IMSS programs. Those not covered by IMSS are eligible for Secretariat of

Health care by paying small user fees for some health services. Legal coverage of the urban poor is much more limited. IMSS offers voluntary incorporation to domestic servants, the self-employed, small-business employers, and other groups within the informal sector; however, except for a few such as lottery vendors and street musicians, regulations for joining IMSS through associations practically exclude the poor. The urban poor not insured at IMSS are entitled to Secretariat of Health and Federal District services for a nominal user fee.

Statistical Coverage

There are no accurate statistics on the total health care coverage of the Mexican population, so it is difficult to estimate the uncovered population. Each of the many providers produces its own figures on population covered, and there have been only occasional official attempts to combine all these data. Table 48 consolidates all the official statistics available in selected years in 1982–1988, dividing them into two groups of providers: social insurances (IMSS, contributory programs; ISSSTE; PEMEX; ISSSFAM) and programs that offer services to the uninsured: IMSS (COPLAMAR and Social Solidarity) and Secretariat of Health. Excluded from the table are institutions for which there are no systematic data on coverage, such as the Federal District Department, the National Indian Institute, and the National System for Integral Family Development as well as decentralized services that used to belong to IMSS until 1985—which re-

Table 48. Official data on population covered on health care in Mexico, 1982–1988 (in millions and percentages).

| | Population | | Coverage social insurances[b] | Reported coverage of noninsured | | | | | Total coverage | % of population covered | | | |
| | | | | Secretariat of Health[c] | IMSS | | | Total[d] | | Total | Rural | | |
	Total (1)	Rural[a] (2)	(3)	(4)	COPLAMAR (5)	Solidarity (6)	Total (7)	(8)	(9)	(9/1)	(5/2)	$\frac{5+6}{2}$	e
1982	73.1	24.1	33.7	11.5	7.7	1.9	9.6	21.1	54.8	75.0	32.0	39.8	39.8
1984	76.8	24.7	36.6	13.5	9.4	2.4	11.8	25.3	61.9	80.6	38.0	47.8	47.8
1985	77.9	25.1	39.2	14.8	11.6	2.8	14.4	29.2	68.4	87.8	46.2	57.4	57.4
1987	81.2	25.3	43.0	19.0	8.5	1.6	10.1	29.1	72.1	88.8	33.6	40.0	56.1
1988	82.8	25.4	43.8	21.8	8.4	1.5	9.9	31.7	75.5	91.2	33.0	39.0	55.9

Sources: INEGI, 1987; Galván, 1988; Salinas, 1989; Mesa-Lago, 1989c; Wilkie, 1990.

[a]Rural "dispersed" population is based on projections for 1980–1990, of the proportion of 33.7% (population below 2,500 inhabitants) estimated by the 1980 census (INEGI, 1987; Wilkie, 1990). IMSS-COPLAMAR (1988) used the same 1980 proportion to calculate the rural population of 1987.

[b]IMSS, ISSSTE, PEMEX, and ISSSFAM.

[c]In 1987–1988, Secretariat of Health is assumed to include the decentralized IMSS-COPLAMAR services which covered 4.1 million in 1987 and 4.3 million in 1988.

[d]Excludes the Federal District Department, the National Indian Institute, the National System for Integral Family Development, and other services for which no systematic data are available.

[e]After 1985, includes the health care services transferred by IMSS-COPLAMAR.

portedly covered 4.1 million in 1987 (see the section on "Evaluation of IMSS-COPLAMAR Health Care Program for Rural Poor," beginning on p. 115). It is difficult to believe that in 1985–1986, in the midst of the economic crisis when the public sector health budget was drastically cut and after the 1985 earthquake destroyed 30% to 40% of hospital beds in the Federal District (Wilkie, 1990), the Secretariat of Health could expand its population coverage by 41% (from 13.5 to 19 million people) at almost twice the rate of expansion of 1982–1984. However, if the 4.1 million people transferred by IMSS-COPLAMAR between 1985 and 1987 are added to the Secretariat's coverage, then the sudden expansion of the latter can be explained. Moreover, the health care coverage by some of the other institutions is questionable. For instance, in 1987, the population cared for by the National System for Integral Family Development was given as 7.6 million, but only 398 physicians were reported; this institution has many functions such as care of children, old people, nutrition, and vacation/recreation, and health care is not its major concern. The Federal District Department services are important, but there seems to be considerable duplication, such as Federal District people who are covered by both the National System for Integral Family Development and the Secretariat of Health.

According to Table 48, 91% of the total population was covered in 1988, but if we add those institutions excluded from the table (which supposedly covered 12 million people or more), the resulting population covered (87.5 million) would be 5.6% higher than the actual total population, even without considering the population group that uses private health care. Based on this type of data, the 1989 report on the implementation of the 1989–1994 National Development Plan stated that 94.5% of the population was covered, leaving only 4.7 million people without protection (Poder Ejecutivo Federal, 1990). These figures are obviously inflated, particularly the protection of the noninsured. For 1987, Wilkie (1990) estimated that only 65.7 million people were covered (6.4 million fewer than in Table 48); this gives a percentage of coverage of 79%, leaving 21% of the population unprotected (versus 11% in Table 48).

Urban Poor

The very few informal workers that might be insured in Mexico would be covered by IMSS, since the majority of rural poor are insured in IMSS-COPLAMAR; a minority would be covered by the decentralized services. All the insured in ISSSTE, PEMEX, and ISSSFAM are formal workers, basically urban and not poor.

The first question to address is whether there are informal *poor* insured in IMSS. Table 49 shows that in 1987, 93% of the total insured were urban, but few of them might have been informal workers. About half of the employed EAP represented nonsalaried workers (self-employed, unpaid relatives, and employers, where the poor are concentrated) and fewer than 12% (5% of the EAP) were insured. About 96% of the nonsalaried EAP was uninsured. Of the total number of workers insured, only 13.6% were urban temporary workers, which may include some poor. A meager 0.3% of the insured workers were urban nonsalaried, 0.1% each self-employed, employers, and taxi drivers.

Table 50 presents all available data on potential informal workers insured by IMSS. Not all of them are informal; for instance, among employers (almost half of the insured), some have mid-sized enterprises and mid-level income; among the self-employed, there are professionals with relatively high incomes; and practically all taxi drivers own their taxis and must be registered in the municipality and be associated with a union. It should be recalled that, to be voluntarily associated, these groups must have a required level of economic resources and administrative organization.

The table shows that in 1986–1987 the number of some insured declined (e.g., −26% of self-employed, −9% employers, −6% domestic servants); alternative data indicate a much lower number—in decline—of taxi drivers insured. The total number of potential informal insured equals about 0.5% of total (and urban) insured at IMSS, and the actual informal poor insured should be a fraction of that. Among all urban self-employed, between 0.4% and 1.2% were insured, and among domestic servants less than 0.1% were insured (Table 50). Regarding taxi drivers (using IMSS targets, not actual numbers), between 1.6% and 4.5% were covered, as were between 0.6% and 1.5% of street musicians (Mesa-Lago, 1990a).

I roughly estimate that there are from 4 to 6 million informal workers in Mexico (to whom we must add the open unemployed), and fewer than 1% are insured. Wilkie (1990) has combined open unemployed, underemployed, agricultural, and nonagricultural workers and employers to reach a total of 14.4 million people (plus their families) not covered, or about 60% of the EAP; possibly one-half of them are in the

Table 49.   Analysis of social insurance (IMSS) coverage of the population, Mexico, 1987 (in percentages).

1.	**TOTAL POPULATION MEXICO** (% insured)[a]		4.	**WORKERS INSURED**[b]	100.0
	Without COPLAMAR-PSS	42.2		Permanent	84.0
	Urban	57.2		Urban	78.5
	Rural	9.1		Rural	5.1
	With COPLAMAR-PSS	54.6		Temporary	16.0
	Urban	57.2		Urban	13.6
	Rural	49.0		Rural	2.4
2.	**TOTAL INSURED**[a]		5.	**PERMANENT INSURED**[b]	84.0
	Without COPLAMAR-PSS	100.0		Salaried	74.9
	Urban	93.4		Urban	74.4[c]
	Rural	6.6		Rural	.5
	With COPLAMAR-PSS	100.0		Nonsalaried	4.9
	Urban	72.1		Urban	.3
	Rural	27.9		Rural	4.6
				Nonspecified	4.2
3.	**EMPLOYED EAP**[b]	100.0			
			6.	**PERMANENT URBAN**[b]	78.5
	Salaried	47.9			
	Urban	42.6		Salaried	78.2[c]
	Workers insured	37.7			
	Not insured	4.9		Nonsalaried	.3
				Employers	.1
	Rural	5.2		Self-employed	.1
	Workers insured	1.2		Taxi drivers	.1
	Not insured	4.0			
			7.	**PERMANENT RURAL**[b]	5.1
	Nonsalaried	52.1			
	Workers insured	2.1		Salaried	.5
	Not insured	50.0			
				Nonsalaried	4.6
				Sugar	1.6
				Ejidos, credit	1.5
				Small farmers	.2
				Others	.5

Source: Author's calculations based on Galván, 1988; Salinas de Gortari, 1989.
[a]Includes dependents.
[b]Excludes dependents and COPLAMAR/Social Solidarity Program (SSP).
[c]Includes a negligible percentage of domestic servants (.005 of workers insured).

informal sector. Compare these figures with total coverage of the EAP by all social insurance institutions in Mexico: 41.7% in 1983 (Mesa-Lago, 1989c); 48.2% (employed EAP) in 1987; and 40.2% in 1988 (Wilkie, 1990). The uninsured informal can receive health care through the Secretariat of Health, the Federal District Department, and other public charity and NGO's health facilities but there is a total lack of information on this. (ID cards issued by the Secretariat of Health and Federal District Department record employment data on the user—i.e., if self-employed, domestic servant, etc.—but such information is not processed.)

Rural Poor

Coverage of health care for the rural poor (dispersed rural) is shown in Table 48. Until 1985, IMSS-COPLAMAR was the main provider of services, with some health care provided by IMSS Social Solidarity (basically to rural) and by the Secretariat of Health and the National Indian Institute. Coverage by COPLAMAR alone

Table 50. Some potential informal workers voluntarily insured at IMSS, Mexico, 1986–1989.

Insured groups[a]	Dec. 1986	Dec. 1987	% distribution	March 1989	Estimation of coverage % in 1987 based on: 1976 survey[b]	Estimation of coverage % in 1987 based on: 1980 census[c]
Employers	15,080	13,743	41.2	n.a.	n.a.	n.a.
Self-employed	12,146	9,750	29.2	8,995	0.75–1.20	0.39
Taxi drivers	0	5,364[e]	16.1	[e]	n.a.	n.a.
Lottery vendors	3,839	3,791	11.4	n.a.	n.a.	n.a.
Domestic servants	414	399	1.2	391	0.07–0.09	n.a.
Street musicians	0	300[f]	0.9	n.a.	n.a.	n.a.
Total	31,479	33,347	100.0	n.a.	1.06	n.a.
Urban insured	6,463,905	6,912,536				
% informal[d]	0.49	0.48				

Sources: Author's estimates based on IMSS, 1987, 1987a; Galván, 1987; Wilkie, 1990.
[a]Only permanent workers, excludes temporary (urban temporary insured were 13.6% of total insured in 1987).
[b]Employed EAP urban informal.
[c]Self-employed and employers in EAP.
[d]Percentage of informal over total permanent urban insured.
[e]Wilkie gives 1,891 in mid-1988 and 1,430 in mid-1989.
[f]Galván gives 126 in 1987.

increased from 32% to 46% in 1982–1985, and, including Social Solidarity, from almost 40% to 57%. Starting in 1985, IMSS-COPLAMAR services began to be decentralized, and estimates of rural poor coverage became much more difficult to make. Adding scattered data for 1987–1988 on the rural population covered by COPLAMAR-Social Solidarity Program (10 million) and decentralized health care services (about 4 million), the combined coverage seems to have declined to about 56% of the rural population. Note that we are dealing with a rural dispersed population that lives in settlements of fewer than 2,500 inhabitants, but IMSS/decentralized health services target areas with fewer than 500 inhabitants (marginalized rural) where critical poverty is concentrated; hence, coverage of that group should be higher. A rough estimate based on the number of rural poor in 1984 and those covered resulted in an 86% coverage.

The addition of COPLAMAR/Social Solidarity programs to IMSS has had a remarkable impact on IMSS coverage. Table 49 shows that without such programs, IMSS coverage of Mexico's total population in 1987, was 42%; when these programs were added, coverage increased to 54.6% (percentages of Mexico's rural population covered by IMSS increase from 9% to 49% when COPLAMAR/Social Solidarity Program percentages are added). And it should be recalled that in 1987, IMSS had lost about 30% of its COPLAMAR-Social Solidarity population due to decentralization. Without COPLAMAR/Social Solidarity Program, IMSS coverage of the

rural population was minuscule in 1987 (Table 49): 1.2% of the salaried EAP, 6.6% total insured, and 5.1% of permanent insured. Among the latter, almost all are nonsalaried workers engaged in sugar cane plantations, *ejidos*, small farms, etc.

REASONS FOR LOW COVERAGE OF THE URBAN POOR

General Factors

In most of the indicators of Table 28, Mexico ranked in the middle of the five countries. Mexico does not have some of Costa Rica's and Uruguay's advantages: it is the largest of the five countries and its topographical barriers make communication more difficult; a significant percentage of its population does not speak Spanish and has a different culture that isolates them; and the population's illiteracy rate is twice that of the other two countries. Although politically stable (at least until recent years), Mexico has not enjoyed the political competition and openness of the other two countries, and labor and peasant organizations have been much more under the control of the party (PRI) that has dominated political life for many decades. The government, therefore, has been less accountable to the masses and less responsive to pressure from below, although this situation is rapidly changing.

Mexico has abundant resources and enjoyed an enormous economic boom in the 1960s and 1970s, but little of that wealth was invested in improving the living standards of the poor. In 1988, the nation's per capita income was the second highest among the five countries, but there were significant inequalities in income distribution. Social security policy, particularly expansion to the urban poor, has been rhetorical and symbolic, showing little practical progress; COPLAMAR, however, has been a success.

Although population coverage by IMSS-COPLAMAR has been inflated at times—from 75% to 100% over "actual" figures in 1980–1983 (Mesa-Lago, 1989c)—and there is confusion due to the decentralization of services after 1985 and the impact of the 1980s economic crisis, undoubtedly, this program has significantly increased coverage for the rural poor. From practically zero attention in 1973, statistical coverage has increased to more than half of the rural dispersed population, and is even higher among the marginalized rural. The importance of this program, not only in Mexico but in all of Latin America and the Caribbean, caused us to select it for evaluation in the section on "Evaluation of IMSS-COPLAMAR Health Care Program for Rural Poor," beginning on p. 115.

Conversely, about 99% of the informal sector, where the urban poor are concentrated, is not covered by IMSS. Therefore, Mexican social insurance was able to break the Bismarckian barrier through extension of coverage to nonsalaried rural workers, but was not capable of doing the same regarding the urban sector. In the countryside, migration to urban areas, combined with COPLAMAR/Social Solidarity programs, improved the health care of the poor, but in the cities, the flood of rural migrants combined with the growth of the informal sector in the 1980s and the lack of effective IMSS programs to cover this sector left the urban poor largely unprotected. In 1980, Mexico had the third largest informal sector among 13 countries of Latin America (excluding the Dominican Republic and Peru); of the five case studies, only Peru has a larger informal sector than Mexico. The enormous increase in the Federal District population, today the largest metropolitan area in the world, has significantly contributed to the growth of the informal sector. While it is true that the urban poor are legally entitled to use the health care services of the Secretariat of Health and other public programs, these are insufficient to minimally cover the demand of that group (see the section on "Public Sector (Secretariat of Health) Viability," beginning on

p. 114). Reasons given by bureaucrats and experts for the low social insurance coverage of the informal sector are the sector's low income, the high contribution, and other barriers imposed by IMSS.

Social Security Policy

Low Income and High Contributions

As has been seen, Mexican informal workers' income in the mid-1970s was lower than that of formal workers, and specialists agree that, in the 1980s, the former declined as much as the latter, and probably more (Diéguez, 1986; Samaniego, 1986). Because the capacity to contribute is a condition for voluntary affiliation to IMSS, the income of informal workers covered by IMSS should be higher than that of the uninsured. According to Table 51, in 1986 30% of insured informal workers had incomes below the minimum wage (versus 28% of all insured permanent urban workers), 70% of informals earned between one and three minimum wages (versus an urban average of 49%), and only 0.7% earned more than three minimum wages (versus an urban average of 23%). Furthermore, the average income of informal workers has been pushed up by the self-employed, a fair number of whom are professionals earning relatively high incomes, and by employers. Thus, all lottery vendors and 42% of domestic servants earned less than the minimum wage in 1986, compared with only 1% among the self-employed. Employers were the only group with an income higher than three minimum wages (1.3%), while 64% of them earned between one and three minimum wages. Among the potential informal workers insured by IMSS, 41% are self-employed and 29% are employers (see Table 50); most of them are certainly not poor. This leaves less than 30% of insured who could qualify as poor, but 16% are taxi owners who hardly could be considered to be dispossessed. The remaining 14% (lottery vendors, street musicians, and domestic servants) could qualify as poor.

Table 52, Section A, compares the percentage contribution on wage or income paid by salaried workers, including domestic servants, with that paid by informal workers; the latter have to pay the percentage contribution of both the insured and the employer. The percentage contribution paid by informal workers to the sickness-maternity program (7.8%) is 2.6 times higher than that paid by salaried workers (3%), despite the fact that the former are not entitled to cash

Table 51. Percentage distribution of informal workers insured in IMSS according to their income, Mexico, 1986.

Occupational categories	Percentage distribution based on minimum wages			
	Less than the minimum	1 to 3 times the minimum	3 to 10 times the minimum	Total
Informals	29.7	69.6	0.7	100.0
Self-employed	1.3	98.7	0.0	100.0
Employers	34.4	64.3	1.3	100.0
Domestic servants	42.0	58.0	0.0	100.0
Lottery vendors	100.0	0.0	0.0	100.0
Total urban permanent workers	28.0	49.2	22.8	100.0

Sources: Author's calculations based on IMSS, 1986.

benefits. The total percentage contribution paid by informal workers (13.52%) is three times higher than that paid by salaried workers (4.5%), and, in addition to not being entitled to health cash benefits, informal workers are not covered by employment injury—unless they pay an additional 6.5%—and have no access to child day-care centers. Domestic servants and their employers must pay the same percentage contributions as the rest of the salaried sector, but for this employer, the 17.54% contribution is too high. Furthermore, when the domestic servant's salary equals the minimum wage, the employer must pay both his and the employee's contribution. Since employers have the option to register or not register their domestic servants at IMSS, few do. Moreover, each time that a domestic servant changes jobs, the new employer can choose to reregister the employee or not.

The annual average contribution of the self-employed is 30% higher than that of the salaried worker, although this gap narrows because the the salaried worker's contribution is based on actual salary, while the self-employed's contribution is 1.6 times the minimum wage. The employer's average contribution is between 100% and 853% that of the salaried worker (Table 52, segment B). These two groups complain that their contribution is too high (Galván Ulloa, 1988), and yet, their average income is relatively high by informal sector standards. Obviously, this type of contribution is unaffordable for small-business owners and the self-employed who have low incomes.

Other Barriers

It is extremely difficult to detect and register small enterprises in the informal sector and to collect contributions from them, because many

Table 52. Contributions of salaried and informal workers to IMSS, Mexico, 1989.

SECTION A							
Legal contributions by programs (% of income)	Salaried[a]				Informal[b]		
	Insured	Employer	State	Total	Insured	State	Total
Sickness-maternity	3.00	8.40	0.60	12.00	7.82[e]	0.60	8.42
Others[c]	1.50	7.20	0.30	9.00	5.70	0.30	6.00
Total	4.50	15.60	0.90	21.00	13.52	0.90	14.42

SECTION B			
Insured groups	Salary base of contribution (1988)	Annual contribution (thousand pesos)	% increase over salaried contribution
Salaried	Actual salary	488	—
Self-employed[d]	1.6 times minimum salary in the Federal District	632	29.5
Employers	2 to 10 times minimum salary in the Federal District	976 to 4,652	100 to 853
Domestic servants	Average of minimum salary in area	n.a.	n.a.

Sources: Mesa-Lago, 1990; updated by Wilkie, 1990.
[a]Includes domestic servants.
[b]Self-employed, small employers, unpaid family workers, and other nonsalaried workers.
[c]Includes pensions, employment injury, and child day-care for salaried workers, but only pensions for informal workers (optional coverage for employment injured costs 6.5% more).
[d]Includes taxi drivers who own their own vehicles.
[e]Do not provide cash benefits (sickness-maternity paid leave).

operate within the underground economy. In fact, after the 1985 earthquake in Mexico City, hundreds of clandestine enterprises, some of them mid-sized, were uncovered. Moreover, in addition to the above-mentioned financial/administrative requirements for signing agreements, it is difficult to get enough workers willing to join IMSS. For instance, a minimum of 2,000 market vendors is required for affiliation, and in 1988, after two years of effort, this number had yet to be reached. When there are several associations within one group of workers, it can be difficult to choose which association should represent the workers in the agreement. A major problem is that the selected association must accept financial responsibility for payment of its members' contributions by maintaining a bank deposit to cover any payment delays (Mesa-Lago, 1990a).

Financial Viability of Social Insurance and the Public Sector to Cover the Urban Poor

In Mexico, the poor are basically covered by the Secretariat of Health, the Federal District Department, and other public institutions (mostly protecting the urban poor), and IMSS (mostly protecting the rural poor). IMSS-COPLAMAR coverage of the rural poor will be analyzed in the next section; here, we analyze IMSS and Secretariat of Health capacity to extend health care protection to the urban poor.

Social Insurance (IMSS) Viability

The combination of all IMSS programs has traditionally generated an overall surplus, but estimated as a percentage of income, it declined from 17.8% to 4% in 1980–1986. An actuarial analysis conducted in August 1988 had no age population data and its projections were limited to gross income and expenditures; its analysis concluded that IMSS would be sound through the year 2000. It should be noted, however, that the financial system for IMSS pensions apparently changed from scaled premium to pay-as-you-go and that the analysis relied on projected continuation of a young population being incor-

porated into IMSS, but lacked sound demographic data.

In recent years, IMSS has faced a liquidity crisis that has forced it to take out short-term bank loans at high interest rates. Actuarial reserves as a percentage of operating funds declined from 17.9% to 0.4% in 1980–1988; consequently, IMSS has been depleting its cash reserves (the bulk of its investment is in real estate), which appear to be inadequate for meeting long-term obligations (Wilkie, 1990). The main reasons for IMSS's financial deterioration in the 1980s have been, in terms of expenditures, deficits in sickness-maternity and employment-injury programs combined with very high administrative costs and, in terms of revenues, stagnant percentage contributions in the pension program, insufficient contributions in the sickness-maternity program, reductions in state contributions, and a decline in the real investment yield (Mesa-Lago, 1989, 1990).

Since its inception in 1943 until at least 1988, the sickness-maternity program has ended in deficit in all but three years. This program absorbs most of IMSS expenditures, although its proportion declined from 69% to 54% in 1977–1986. The deficit has been covered by transfers (as loans and investments) from the pension and employment-injury programs, contributing to their decapitalization. The total percentage contribution to sickness-maternity increased from 6% in 1943 to 9% in the 1970s, but in 1984, it was actuarially estimated that it had to be raised to 13% in order to bring about equilibrium and for this program to begin to pay its debt to other programs. In 1989, the total percentage contribution to sickness-maternity was increased to 12% (see Table 52), still below the actuarially required premium.

The pension program has been the only one to generate a surplus within IMSS, but it declined from 52% of revenue in 1980 to 14.6% in 1986. As the program matured and the number of pensioners increased, its expenditures gradually increased. The total percentage contribution to this program has remained the same since the program was created in 1943. Due to high inflation rates and inefficiency in investment policies, the average real investment annual yield in 1980–1987 was negative (−21%). The employment-injury program ended in a deficit in 1977–1979 and again in 1983–1986; we lack more recent disaggregated data on this program. As a result, pension surpluses, a major source of financing for the sickness-maternity program, have dramatically dwindled, and the deficit-ridden employment-injury program no longer can provide any subsidies. This situation forced a 33% increase of the legal percentage contribution to sickness-maternity in 1989, which has catapulted Mexico from fourth to second place in the Region (after Costa Rica) in terms of the size of this percentage contribution. We lack information on whether this increase has balanced the sickness-maternity program.

IMSS administrative expenditures are among the highest in Latin America and the Caribbean and show an increasing trend as a proportion of total expenditures—from 13.4% in 1977 to 19.3% in 1983, despite a drop to 17% in 1986. This is mainly due to an excess in personnel, as well as high salaries and overgenerous fringe benefits. The 1982 actuarial study warned that if these expenses were not controlled, they would jeopardize the financial stability of IMSS. And yet, the IMSS ratio of employees per 1,000 insured increased from 6 to 8.9 in 1980–1986, peaking to a historical record in that last year.

Although the federal government has traditionally fulfilled its obligations to social insurance, it cut its overall percentage contribution (as state, not as employer) to IMSS by almost two-thirds, from 1.875% to 0.75%. The sickness-maternity program suffered the biggest cut, but in 1989, the overall state percentage contribution was increased to 0.9% and the difference was assigned to sickness-maternity. It has been reported that in 1987, the state delayed its payments to IMSS-COPLAMAR by as much as three months, forcing IMSS to take funds from other programs. This problem apparently was corrected in 1988.

Even if IMSS has been able to expand health care coverage to only 1% of the informal sector—mostly the relatively high income self-employed and employers—it is doubtful that it would be able to successfully protect the whole sector, including the poor, with such a weak financial base, particularly considering that the informal uninsured workers have low incomes that would require substantial state subsidies. The current contribution to sickness-maternity cannot be increased; in fact, it would have to be reduced if informal workers are going to be effectively incorporated. One possibility for raising revenues would be to eliminate the salary ceiling for contributions, a measure that would also have a progressive effect on distribution. Given that the sickness-maternity program lacks significant reserves, there is no possibility of increasing revenue through a more efficient investment policy. The only logical alternative would be to drastically reduce expenditures, starting with administrative costs. However,

a cheaper benefit program (similar to COPLAMAR's) would have to be designed to permit coverage of the urban poor.

In 1987, IMSS prepared draft legislation to accelerate voluntary coverage of the self-employed and other groups of uninsured and their dependents, mostly in the informal sector. The plan involved introducing a uniform package of health care benefits (without sickness-maternity paid leave, but with a lump-sum payment) to be financed by workers and by the state in equal parts. The total percentage contribution would be 16% (more than twice the current percentage), increasing the state contribution to about 8%. The percentage contribution of the insured would be somewhat smaller, because it would be based on the minimum wage instead of the current 1.6 minimum wages (IMSS, 1987b). Hence, this legal draft acknowledged the need to substantially increase the state subsidy to make up for the lack of employer contributions and to reduce the worker's contribution, although not by enough. In order to make this project feasible, however, a less expensive benefit package would have been required. The need for substantial state funds in the midst of the economic crisis and the adjustment policy sealed the fate of this proposed legislation.

For domestic servants, IMSS proposed a less expensive sickness-maternity program that substituted a lump-sum payment for paid leave. This package would be financed equally by the employer and the worker, instead of 75% and 25%, as it is now. Despite the increase in the workers' percentage contribution, the less expensive package would make the actual payment lower than before. The program would be mandatory—instead of voluntary—but would be limited to high-income urban areas, remaining optional for the rest of the country. It had not been implemented by 1988 (Galván Ulloa, 1988).

If health-maternity coverage is extended to all the self-employed and domestic servants (more than two-thirds of whom are informal sector), IMSS would have to incorporate about 7 million people: 2 million active workers and about 5 million dependents. This would equal 20% of IMSS's current total insured population (15% if COPLAMAR/Social Solidarity Program coverage is included). Although not all of the eligible population would register, IMSS officials consider that its health care services are close to saturation and could not absorb this sizable new group of insured without a substantial expansion of the existing infrastructure, a difficult proposition at this time. Consequently, it has been suggested that the private sector be involved in those locations IMSS or other public health services do not have excess capacity, an idea never considered before (Galván Ulloa, 1988).

The economic crisis of the 1980s has taken a toll on IMSS health care services. In 1982–1987, total revenue in 1980 pesos declined by 32%, while the covered population increased by 27% and expenditures per capita, in 1986 pesos, declined by 42%. Since 1944, there were annual increases in most health services provided by IMSS, but in 1985–1986, there were declines in outside consultations, laboratory tests, pathology, X rays, blood transfusions, surgery, and child delivery (IMSS, 1987; Wilkie, 1990). Under these conditions, it is practically impossible to extend IMSS sickness-maternity protection to the informal sector unless its current model of health care is changed; the COPLAMAR model would be much more viable.

Public Sector (Secretariat of Health) Viability

The 1989–1994 National Development Plan includes important strategies to fight critical poverty and to provide health care for the critically poor. Although it seriously overestimates coverage, the plan acknowledges that full coverage of marginal urban and rural areas has not been achieved, that the quality of care is below a desirable level, and that there are limitations on the supply of equipment, medicines, and other resources. To cope with critical poverty, a National Solidarity Program was launched that involves development agreements between the public sector and marginal urban and rural populations, including Indian communities and arid area dwellers. The health care strategy proposed contemplates four goals: the extension of coverage and improvement of services through increased investment, efficiency, and education, with priority given to the completion of units that will provide primary health care to marginal urban-rural groups; the reduction of inequalities of access and services through the National Solidarity Program and better coordination of welfare health services to the critically poor such as primary care, nutrition, sanitation, water, and housing; a change in the philosophy of health care, giving priority to prevention, immunization, control of contagious and parasitic diseases, and protection of children and mothers, as well as more efficient use of curative medicine; and the reinforcement of

the national health system coordination, eliminating duplication and strengthening decentralization (Secretaría de Planificación y Presupuesto, 1989). It remains to be seen whether these laudable targets will be implemented. The plan's first annual report claims that 2 million Indians and peasants have been covered under the National Solidarity Program through the construction and equipment of 772 rural medical units and health centers. However, the report on the urban sector lacks concrete data to evaluate goal implementation (Poder Ejecutivo Federal, 1990).

Can the public sector provide effective health care to the urban poor? Under the current crisis conditions and without a radical reform of the country's health system, the answer seems to be negative. Compared with social insurance agencies, the Secretariat of Health, by far the largest provider within the public health sector, is obviously underfunded and understaffed (see Table 53). In 1987–1988, while the shares of health care expenditures and physicians were significantly higher than the corresponding share of the population covered in PEMEX, ISSSTE, and IMSS, the Secretariat's share of expenditures was lower than its share of population, and its share of physicians was about the same. Data on the armed forces, not shown in the table, indicate that their health services are on a par with those of PEMEX (Mesa-Lago, 1989). However, if we compare Secretariat of Health resources with those of COPLAMAR, it is obvious that the former is in a much better situation: twice the population of COPLAMAR but twelve times its expenditures and almost seven times its physicians.

The economic crisis of the 1980s has harmed the Secretariat even more than IMSS. In 1982–1987, while IMSS health expenditures (in 1976 pesos) declined by 35%, the Secretariat's

Table 53. Comparison of health care resources and expenditures per capita, among providers[a] in Mexico, 1987–1988 (percentage distributions).

Provider	Population covered	Health care expenditures	Physicians
PEMEX	1.1	4.2	2.8
ISSSTE	10.3	11.6	15.2
IMSS	47.9	61.1	51.1
Secretariat of Health	26.5	21.4	27.3
COPLAMAR/PSS	14.1	1.7	3.6
Total	100.0	100.0	100.0

Sources: Author's calculations based on Salinas de Gortari, 1989; Wilkie, 1990.

[a]Excludes armed forces, Federal District Department, and other public sector and private providers.

dropped by 67%; in the same period, IMSS population coverage increased by 27%, while the Secretariat's coverage jumped by 65% (Salinas de Gortari, 1989; Wilkie, 1990). Table 54 shows that, except for outpatient consultations, all Secretariat of Health facilities and services either peaked in 1986 and sharply declined by 1989 or steadily deteriorated after the crisis began in 1982. Furthermore, out of the ten rates listed in the table, six were lower in 1989 than in 1982. Physicians surveyed in 1989 ranked the Secretariat's primary and secondary level services as the worst in both service and prestige (behind those of IMSS and ISSSTE); these two levels are the ones most used by the lowest income groups of the population (Wilkie, 1990). Although the Secretariat's approach to and costs for health care can more adequately provide effective coverage of the urban poor than those of IMSS, the former lacks the needed facilities and resources to tackle this task.

EVALUATION OF IMSS-COPLAMAR HEALTH CARE PROGRAM FOR RURAL POOR[1]

History

The Program of Social Solidarity that IMSS launched in 1973, was the first to significantly depart from the conventional model of social insurance, but it also changed the Secretariat's historical role as the basic provider of health services to the uninsured low income population. IMSS programs previously had required contributions by both insured and employers, but the Social Solidarity Program was financed 60% by the federal government and 40% by IMSS's own funds. Although the program initially targeted both marginal urban and rural populations, it focused on the latter. Those covered were provided health care, not cash benefits, and, in turn, were expected to contribute 10 days a year in community work. By 1979, IMSS had constructed 310 primary-level clinics and 30 small secondary-level rural hospitals.

---

[1]This section is based on Margaret S. Sherraden's field report, "Primary Health Care for the Rural Poor in Mexico: The Case of IMSS-COPLAMAR (1979–1988)," St. Louis, Washington University, April 1989, supplemented by her June 20, 1989, letter. Technically, she is the author of this section, but I summarized her report and added some materials and calculations, hence I take full responsibility for what is said in it.

Table 54. The impact of the economic crisis on the Ministry of Health (Secretariat of Health) facilities and services in Mexico, 1982–1989.

Facilities/services	1982	1986	1989
Physicians (per 10,000 covered)[a]	5.6	8.4	6.0
Dentists (per 10,000)	1.3	1.7	1.2
Hospital beds (per 1,000)	2.5	2.7	1.9
Outpatient consultation (per person)	1.8	1.9	1.9
Child delivery (per 1,000)	17.3	15.7	12.9
Surgery (per 1,000)	17.0	15.2[b]	13.4
X rays (per 1,000)	67.0	67.2	53.3
Immunization (per 100,000)			
DPT	215	193[b]	169
Typhoid	18	45[b]	34
Measles	67	148	97

Sources: Author's calculations based on Salinas de Gortari, 1989.
[a]Excludes *pasantes*, new graduates who perform mandatory services for one year.
[b]1985.

In 1976, at the height of the oil boom, COPLAMAR was established as an umbrella agency to coordinate an array of programs geared to develop marginal areas. Three years later, COPLAMAR signed an agreement with IMSS to provide the same type of health services that the Social Solidarity Program did. An official document explained: "Despite their good work, social insurances contributed to the creation of a minority covered against all social risks, alongside a majority excluded from all protection. There is a need to enforce the redistributive function of social security beyond the classic scope of social insurance" (IMSS, 1983:15). The decision to give this responsibility to IMSS rather than to the Secretariat reportedly responded to the former's administrative and technical skills, its accumulated experience with the Social Solidarity Program, and its bold initiative, compared to the Secretariat's lack of effective leadership. Furthermore, if that program had been turned over to the Secretariat, it would have become a welfare program—"a palliative rather than a means for getting to the roots of poverty." Blessed with oil resources, the plan was expected to accelerate economic and social protection of the rural poor and to narrow the urban-rural gap, rather than wait for a gradual process of development (IMSS, 1983; Centro Interamericano de Estudios de Seguridad Social, 1987). IMSS was given two years to tackle the health care component of the plan; Table 55 shows that it basically accomplished it.

By the end of 1979, IMSS had built 1,796 rural clinics that provided services to more than 1 million peasant families (3.7 million if combined

Table 55. Evolution of health care facilities and coverage in marginal rural areas of Mexico, 1979–1988.

| | IMSS | | | | |
	Social Solidarity Program	COPLAMAR	Total	Decentralized	Total
1979					
Clinics	310	1,796	2,106	—	2,104
Hospitals	30	0	30	—	30
Population (millions)	2.6	1.1	3.7	—	3.7
1981					
Clinics	310	2,714[b]	3,024	—	2,484
Hospitals	31	10	41	—	41
Population	2.1	6.5	8.6	—	8.6
1983					
Clinics	310	2,720	3,030	—	3,030
Hospitals	31	29	60[c]	—	53
Population	2.2	8.5	10.7	—	10.7
1985					
Clinics	310	2,936	3,246	—	3,243
Hospitals	31	34	65	—	65
Population	2.8	11.7	14.5	—	14.5
1988[a]					
Clinics	187	2,136	2,323	920	3,243
Hospitals	20	31	51	14[d]	65
Population	1.6	8.4	10.0	4.1	14.1

Sources: Author's compilation based on IMSS, 1983; IMSS and COPLAMAR, 1988a; Sherraden, 1989; Salinas de Gortari, 1989; Velázquez Díaz, 1989.
[a]Transfer from IMSS to decentralized state services, from June 1985 to February 1988.
[b]Another source gives 2,174 COPLAMAR clinics.
[c]Another source gives 53 hospitals.
[d]Another source gives 21 hospitals.

with Social Solidarity Program resources). In 1981, there were 2,714 clinics and 10 small rural hospitals covering 6.5 million people (8.6 million with Social Solidarity Program added) and, two years later, 19 additional hospitals increased COPLAMAR protection to 8.5 million (10.7 with Social Solidarity Program added). At the peak of this program in 1985, the IMSS combined health resources to care for the rural poor were 3,246 clinics and 65 hospitals, which covered about 14.5 million people in the country's 31 states. A survey conducted in 1981 and a follow-up study in 1986 provided crucial data on the population served and helped to tailor the program to user needs (Velázquez Díaz, 1989).

When Miguel de la Madrid was inaugurated as President, the situation had changed dramatically. The 1982 economic crisis had imposed a painful adjustment—priority was given to the service of the external debt; the federal deficit had to be cut and social programs became the first target. Decentralized services, which had helped to reduce the burden on the federal government, were partly rationalized with the idea that local needs could be more efficiently and cheaply met through states and municipalities; it also has been argued that the new president was not interested in perpetuating a "monument" to his predecessor (Wilkie, 1990).

In 1983, COPLAMAR was disbanded, al-though IMSS remained temporarily in control of the health program, and in 1984, the concept of a National Health System was introduced and the Secretariat of Health was put in charge of its coordination. From 22% to 29% of IMSS-COPLAMAR facilities and covered population were transferred to the health ministries in the states between June 1985 to February 1988; this undertaking was briefly stopped in 1986 after protests that decentralized services had significantly deteriorated. By the end of 1988, IMSS retained 2,323 clinics, 51 hospitals, and 10 million people in 17 states, while 920 clinics, at least 14 hospitals, and 4 million people were transferred to 14 states (Table 55). Save for one exception, the State of Guerrero, the poorest, most rural states that had most of the clinics, hospitals, and population covered were kept under IMSS; authorities in the poorest states were reluctant to take over the program because they lacked resources and the infrastructure to support it. In 1989, President Salinas de Gortari renewed the appointment of IMSS's Director General, an unusual action in that institution's history. At that point, IMSS-COPLAMAR services in the most developed states had been transferred already, and the politically-strong Director was probably able to halt the decentralization process.

Although some aspects of the decentralization process have been positive, splitting the COPLAMAR health services between IMSS and the states has caused several problems. First of all, the transfer was too fast, sparking administrative complications and a decline in the quality of services. An IMSS official claims that the states had difficulty retaining physicians and other staff abandoning their posts, and supplies and medicines were not delivered; as a result, hospital occupancy declined by 15 percentage points. Further, once the transfer was completed, IMSS stopped providing part of the funding and support services that would thereafter have to be provided by the states (see the section on "Financing and Costs," beginning on p. 120). The states found it difficult to raise taxes, and some resorted to cutting some services; others introduced user fees that reportedly exclude the poorest segment of the population and elicit resistance from the population. Under the IMSS centralized services, the population of one state could receive care in COPLAMAR's hospitals in another state, but under the decentralized system, agreements are required among states. For instance, 60% of the users of a transferred COPLAMAR hospital in Aguas Calientes were from Zacatecas, and the same situation occurred in the states of Tabasco and Chiapas (Velázquez, 1988). Although there is no official position on this, it appears that the above-mentioned problems may have helped stop the decentralization.

Population Coverage and Benefits

Theoretically, the rural areas chosen for COPLAMAR health services were selected according to 19 indicators of marginality that included poverty incidence, concentration of Indian population, and high proportion of uninsured population. In addition, political considerations such as the appeasement of rural areas afflicted by social unrest or guerrilla rebellion and a response to pressure from municipal authorities who wanted to have a clinic also played a role. In practice, it seems that the National Indian Institute staff chose most locations, because they were the most knowledgeable about local conditions. Finally, logistic criteria also were used to establish the clinics and hospitals. These included a lack of similar health services in order to avoid duplication—despite the fact that from 5% to 10% of clinics are located in communities with a Secretariat of Health installation—existence of minimum facil-

ities (such as electricity and potable water), and population size—between 500 and 2,500 inhabitants for clinics (with a sphere of influence from 2,500 to 8,000) and distance among places to be served no higher than one hour; and 5,000 to 10,000 inhabitants for hospitals, as well as existence of 40 clinics in a ratio of influence of 200,000 inhabitants, and access to roads.

As we have said, the program covered more than 14 million people at its peak in 1985; the IMSS-covered population declined to 10 million in 1988, but increased to 11 million in 1989, and the number of clinics also rose by 12% that year (Salinas de Gortari, 1989). By the mid-1980s, about 85% of the target population was reportedly covered. No information is available after 1988 on coverage by decentralized services, but apparently it has declined. In 1988–1989, IMSS-COPLAMAR-Social Solidarity Program covered about 56% of the rural population (see Table 48; the official figure is 65%), 69% of the subsistence agricultural population, and 87% of all Indian groups (from 30% to 40% of the population covered is Indian). Almost 97% of the 20,295 locations incorporated have fewer than 2,500 inhabitants (Velázquez, 1989). About half of those covered are females and about half are less than 15 years old, a larger proportion than in the covered population as a whole (IMSS, 1983); interviews and observations indicate that mothers and children are primary users of clinic services.

Table 56 shows that in 1982–1983, about half of the covered population and half of the clinics and hospitals, were in the nine southern and central states with the lowest IMSS insurance coverage—from 7% to 28%, well below the national coverage of 44%. Oaxaca, Chiapas, and Guerrero concentrated a significant proportion of Mexico's Indian population; Yucatan, the fourth state with a very high concentration of Indians, had a high IMSS insurance coverage at that time (55%). (The remaining half of the population and facilities covered by IMSS-COPLAMAR are in relatively wealthier states in the north and northwest.) In 1981, Chiapas and Oaxaca had the highest infant mortality; Chiapas and Guerrero had the highest illiteracy; Guerrero and S. L. Potosí ranked lowest in terms of lack of piped water; Chiapas had the highest mortality from contagious and parasitic diseases; Guerrero was among the states with the least facilities for excreta disposal; and Oaxaca, Chiapas, Hidalgo, and Puebla were the most affected by diseases preventable by immunization (IMSS, 1983). All available data indicate, therefore, that the poorest and neediest rural sector is being serviced by COPLAMAR.

Table 56. COPLAMAR coverage of the population in the poorest states in Mexico, 1982–1983.

	Indian population	IMSS insurance coverage	Percentage distribution of COPLAMAR's		
			Population coverage	Clinics	Hospitals
Oaxaca	Very high	17.2	10.5	10.6	8.3
Chiapas	Very high	19.9	10.0	10.7	8.3
Guerrero	Very high	23.4	5.1	5.9	4.2
Hidalgo		23.9	5.4	5.3	5.6
Michoacán		19.8	5.6	4.5	5.6
Puebla		28.0	7.4	6.9	5.6
San Luis Potosí		29.0	4.8	5.0	5.6
Zacatecas		18.2	3.0	3.3	2.8
Tlaxcala		6.9	1.2	0.9	1.4
Subtotal[a]			53.0	53.1	47.4

Sources: Author's estimates based on IMSS, 1983; Sherraden, 1989; Mesa-Lago, 1989c.
[a]Percentage of population, clinics, and hospitals in the nine states listed in the table in relation to COPLAMAR's totals.

Coverage includes the head of household, his or her spouse or companion, and dependent children and parents. They are entitled to health care services (but not to cash benefits) at the first level in the IMSS-COPLAMAR clinics, at the second level in the program services, and at the third level in Secretariat of Health specialized hospitals: the percentage distribution of the attended population by level is 85%, 12%, and 3%, respectively. Free-of-charge services provided are detection and control of chronic diseases; prevention and immunization of contagious diseases; curative medical-hospital care at the three levels; medicines; family planning; health education; and promotion/guidance on environmental health, sanitation, nutrition, and housing improvement. Services are free in COPLAMAR, although beneficiaries are expected to contribute community work (see the section on "Financing and Costs," beginning on p. 120); service is rarely denied to those who refuse to do that, although some communities explicitly threaten service denial. The population covered by the decentralized services often has to pay user fees. The Secretariat of Health has used the "integrated health model" of IMSS-COPLAMAR since 1985 to extend coverage to the uninsured population.

Organization and Personnel

Although COPLAMAR is part of IMSS, its administration and financing are separate (see the section on "Financing and Costs," beginning on p. 120) and the model it uses for service delivery and personnel policies is different. IMSS headquarters is directly responsible for program planning, supervision, and evaluation. The two basic units for service delivery are the clinic and the hospital.

The clinics are the same throughout Mexico, because IMSS architects and planners in collaboration with the National Indian Institute developed a "model" clinic for marginalized rural areas. Each clinic has a waiting room, an office and examination room, a two-bed infirmary, and a room for the physician, and provides primary health care, outpatient consultation, maternal-infant care, minor interventions, medicines from a basic list prepared according to local pathology, and community services.

Hospitals serve 40 clinics and provide primary health care to the inhabitants of the immediate area and secondary health care for patients referred from a catchment area of approximately 200,000 inhabitants. They offer emergency services, outpatient consultations, diagnostic services, dental care, medicines, and hospitalization. A surgeon heads a staff of residents in family medicine, pediatrics, obstetrics and gynecology, general surgery, internal medicine, and anesthesiology. When patients require more specialized care, they are referred to Secretariat of Health hospitals; except for isolated cases, COPLAMAR beneficiaries are not entitled to services in IMSS hospitals.

Clinics are staffed by a *pasante*, an advanced medical student who is performing one year of social service, or a recently graduated doctor, also hired for one year, and two clinic assistants. Early on, the program basically relied on *pasantes*, but by 1986, 72% were contract doctors. The clinic assistants are mostly young women recruited from the community who have completed primary school and are bilingual in Spanish and the local Indian language. The main assistant works weekdays, and the other substitutes on weekends. In addition, rural health technicians are placed in inaccessible clinics where there is difficulty to retain a doctor.

Heavy demands are placed on a doctor's time and skills, as he or she must provide curative and preventive health care to a population of 2,500 to 5,000, be a catalyst for the organization of community health groups and projects, and administer the clinic and supervise the assistants. Doctors participate in the program for three reasons: fulfilling the one-year social-service requirement for graduation (*pasantía*), a high rate of unemployment combined with a potential medical career at IMSS (although this possibility was severely reduced in the 1980s), and altruism. Doctors normally try to avoid posts in small communities that are physically and culturally isolated and lack all types of public services and amenities; those who must serve there, usually do not establish real contact with the population, let alone learn about their culture (Centro Interamericano de Estudios de Seguridad Social, 1987).

The clinic assistant is often the doctor's "eyes and ears," but, most of the time she has little autonomy beyond dispensing medications, sterilizing instruments, performing minor medical interventions, and cleaning the clinic and doing some paperwork. The clinic assistant's role has been limited by a combination of factors. Doctors, trained in hierarchical urban medical institutions, tend to view the assistant as a secondary figure; also, the formal training and supervision an assistant receives is geared towards nursing. Moreover, most clinic assistants are young and have little formal education, and in some communities, the clinic assistant job has been given to relatives of local authorities, rather than to the most qualified applicant.

A clinic supervisor, who is always a physician, is responsible for supervising 15 to 20 clinics through monthly visits of one to two days, accompanied by a driver and maintenance technician. A community action promoter visits each community twice a year for up to a week, to consult with clinic staff, local authorities, health committees, and villagers.

Community Participation and Ethnicity

In exchange for free health services, COPLAMAR beneficiaries are urged to participate in family health activities such as prevention, home improvement, excreta and garbage disposal, and adoption of certain health practices or in community health projects such as construction of water and drainage systems and pest control.

The current structure encourages beneficiary involvement at the local level, but not at the state or federal levels. In fact, villagers were not brought into the process until the sites were selected and construction plans were finalized by IMSS authorities. At the local level, there are health volunteers, assistants, and a committee. Volunteers oversee the health needs of ten families, but spend more time helping in the clinic and learning basic nursing skills. Assistants receive a token salary to provide rudimentary health service in outreach communities; insufficient monetary incentives and integration into the program contribute to a high dropout rate among assistants. The health committee maintains the clinic, transports supplies, assesses community needs, and helps to deliver services. Village representatives, along with other authorities, make up a health council at the municipal level.

A state council regulates and evaluates COPLAMAR activities at the state level, but the beneficiaries—peasants and ethnic groups—are represented at the council only through their official organizations. IMSS-COPLAMAR health committees are not represented at the state council. COPLAMAR beneficiaries lack any type of representation on the policy-making national board of IMSS.

There are at least 56 Indian groups in COPLAMAR's catchment area, and their culture and traditional medicine is supposed to be considered. The clinic assistants must be fluent in the predominant Indian language and the clinic doctor is supposed to work with traditional medicine practitioners and midwives. Clinic personnel are encouraged to exchange information and patients with traditional practitioners, to plant medicinal gardens at the clinic, to involve traditional health practitioners in the health committee and volunteer groups, and to train them.

However, doctors' efforts to learn Indian languages, understand Indian traditions and customs, and develop close working relations with traditional practitioners are jeopardized by the short doctor appointments and their conventional medical training. Furthermore, clinic personnel often compete with traditional health practitioners. The former complain that patients go to traditional practitioners first, waiting until "it's too late" to go to the clinic. In turn, traditional practitioners sometime fear that their medicine—and their livelihood—is threatened by the clinic. Relationships with midwives are somewhat better; many communities have come up with an informal division of labor whereby midwives deliver most babies and send high-risk patients to the clinic. IMSS-COPLAMAR train midwives and allocate medical supplies to them to promote family planning and safe births.

Since 1982, COPLAMAR has worked with traditional medicine researchers from IMSS. The most successful, in terms of program personnel, was a project in Chiapas that collected data on traditional medicine while making personnel more sensitive to Indian languages and lifestyles (Lozoya and Zolla, 1983). Unfortunately, the findings from these studies seldom reach clinic personnel.

Financing and Costs

In 1973–1978, the Social Solidarity Program's construction, equipment, and operational costs were financed 60% by the federal government and 40% by IMSS. For COPLAMAR, the federal government agreed to pay all capital and current costs of the new program, while the Social Solidarity Program continued with the same financing. However, indirect support by IMSS to COPLAMAR, for such services as planning and supervision, use of administrative facilities and equipment, training and consultation, and publications, is estimated at up to 50% of total program costs, although this figure may be inflated. In 1983–1986, the average cash share, excluding support services, of IMSS in the COPLAMAR-Social Solidarity Program budget was about 10%. As has been noted, in 1987, the federal contribution to IMSS-COPLAMAR was delayed three months, although this problem was corrected in 1988.

The transfer of COPLAMAR-Social Solidarity Program services to the states meant that the latter lost both the 40% share of the program and IMSS's institutional support. To the best of my knowledge, the federal government continues to pay 60% of transferred Social Solidarity Program services and 100% of transferred COPLAMAR services, but the states must carry a new financial burden (Velázquez Díaz, 1988).

As has been explained, IMSS-COPLAMAR services are free, but the covered population often has contributed with land, structures, and help in building facilities. In addition, they are expected to provide a given amount of commu-

Table 57. Comparison of health care costs in COPLAMAR and other providers, Mexico, 1987.

	Annual per capita expenditures ($US)	Ratio versus COPLAMAR
COPLAMAR	7.52[a]	1.0
National System for Integral Family Development	12.05	1.6
Secretariat of Health	44.00	5.8
ISSSTE	61.66	8.2
IMSS	69.35	9.2
PEMEX	182.00	24.2

Sources: Author's calculations based on IMSS and COPLAMAR, 1988a; Salinas de Gortari, 1989; Wilkie, 1990.

[a]Excludes administrative, training, computing, and other services provided by IMSS.

nity work annually; in 1979–1982, it was estimated by COPLAMAR at 295,890 men years or 17 billion pesos.

IMSS-COPLAMAR stresses low-cost medical services, partly because of the emphasis on prevention and clinic-based services that fulfill 85% of the demand and are much cheaper than hospital services. Program officials claim that IMSS-COPLAMAR expenditures per capita are the lowest of any direct health care program in the nation ($US6.58 per capita in 1986); Table 57 supports this allegation. In 1987, the ratio of COPLAMAR's per capita expenditures in relation to those of other programs was: 5.8 times those of the Secretariat of Health, 8.2 those of ISSSTE, 9.2 those of IMSS, and 24 times those of PEMEX. The gap between IMSS and COPLAMAR costs appears to be narrowing—the ratio was 12.8 in 1981 (IMSS, 1983) versus 9.2 in 1987. Even considering that the cost of IMSS institutional (indirect) support is not included in these calculations, the results are still remarkable. If COPLAMAR has been effective in improving the health status of the poor—a crucial problem that will be analyzed in the next section—its model would be the least expensive and most efficient in Mexico.

COPLAMAR's 1986 budget allocated 45.5% for curative services and 27.9% for prevention. The latter was far above the shares of any other health institution; for instance, the Secretariat of Health spent 17.4% in prevention; IMSS, 2.3%; and the average for the whole sector was 5% (Vázquez Córdova, 1987). Furthermore, prevention has been given increasing attention in recent years (see the following section).

Hospital efficiency shows an increasing trend. The rate of hospital occupancy gradually rose from 42% in 1980, to 67% in 1982, and 83% in 1985–1986; the average length of stay decreased from 4.0 days in 1983 to 3.5 in 1986–1987 (Sherraden, 1989, updated with IMSS and COPLAMAR, 1988a). Although IMSS has not provided data on hospital occupancy since 1981, its average length of stay in 1986 was 4.2 days, 20% higher than COPLAMAR's (IMSS, 1987). However, the poorest states with the highest Indian population are reported to have COPLAMAR's lowest hospital occupancy rates: in 1986, Oaxaca's rate was 61%, largely due to transportation difficulties and cultural barriers for using institutional services.

Evaluation of COPLAMAR's Impact on the Rural Poor's Health Status

Evaluating the potential effect of COPLAMAR on the health standards of the rural population is not an easy task, because the program has been fragmented since 1985 and because other factors such as the economic crisis of the 1980s also have played a role. In addition, program success is influenced by divergent characteristics in the communities.

Fragmentation

Accurate comparisons of data on health services and standards prior to and after 1985 are almost impossible, because there is little information on the decentralized programs. As IMSS-COPLAMAR transferred about 28% of its clinics, hospitals, and personnel to 14 states, data after 1985 should show a decline in IMSS-COPLAMAR services. And, as has been pointed out, IMSS-COPLAMAR retained the poorest states (except Guerrero) with health standards below the national norm; thus, the average health standards of the combined population retained by IMSS-COPLAMAR should be worse than before 1985. To the best of my knowledge, there are no statistical series on all 31 states—the 14 decentralized and the 17 kept by IMSS—that show specific health services such as consultation, child delivery, and surgery and health standards such as mortality and morbidity of the marginalized rural population throughout the 1980s.

Economic Crisis

COPLAMAR's authorities claim that the crisis of the 1980s has not significantly affected this program because its costs are very low and the government would not have dared to cut its services, particularly prior to the 1988 elections.

Thus, it is claimed that IMSS-COPLAMAR has maintained its services in all clinics and hospitals (Velázquez Díaz, 1988). And yet, annual per capita expenditures, in constant 1986 pesos, peaked at 9,071 in 1982, but declined to 4,022 in 1986 (−55.6%) or, converted to constant 1986 $US dollars, the decrease was from $13.90 to $6.58 in the same period (Mesa-Lago based on Sherraden, 1989, and ECLAC-CEPAL, 1988). It is difficult to believe that a reduction of from 56% to 60% in COPLAMAR's per capita expenditures could not have affected its services.

Indeed, in the late 1980s there were indications that IMSS-COPLAMAR had suffered budgetary cuts. Decreases in doctors' salaries, as well as in the number of permanent positions in IMSS, reduced the latter's ability to recruit new doctors and build a rural medicine specialty, and made COPLAMAR less attractive to physicians. There were severe shortages of disposable syringes and materials for repairs in clinics and hospitals; these were particularly serious in the Social Solidarity Program facilities built in 1973. Fewer resources were available from the federal government for joint public health and community projects.

Divergent Local Characteristics

COPLAMAR's success varied significantly from community to community, depending on such factors as geographical accessibility, previous living standards, ethnicity, local authority support, and personnel quality. Geographical isolation, and its concomitant transportation and staffing difficulties, had a negative effect on outcome; furthermore, this factor is positively correlated with the population's low standards of living. In poorer communities, subsistence activities dominate the family's life, leaving little time for community or individual health care activities. High levels of illiteracy are obstacles to the use of institutional medicine, and complicate the work of health personnel; where there is a high proportion of indigenous population, these problems are aggravated by language and cultural barriers. If local authorities do not support the program, encourage participation, and make resources available, the chances for success decrease. Last but not least, if clinic personnel are insensitive to the needs of the community, disrespectful of its lifestyle, and unable to win the confidence of villagers and local authorities, the program's acceptance and the degree of community participation and support drops further. If doctors serve for short periods and if clinic assistants lack the trust of village residents, the probability of fruitful interaction with the community dims significantly. A single standardized health services model and package cannot meet the divergent needs of all communities. Clearly, the most isolated and poor Indian communities require additional resources, special treatment, and services tailored to their needs.

Evaluation of Performance and Policy Recommendations

Even though the above-mentioned factors cannot always be controlled, COPLAMAR results can be tentatively evaluated.

The unprecedented commitment of federal funds and IMSS resources permitted COPLAMAR to rapidly develop a health service infrastructure in most of the country's remote rural areas and to succeed in delivering institutional health care to the rural poor who previously had had virtually no protection—the formidable task of constructing, maintaining, and supplying clinics, even in geographically isolated areas, has been largely successful. The program promotes equal access to clinic and hospital services, ensuring that they are physically accessible and free of charge, and the rights of the community, at least at the local level, are defended. However, although the community's participation has been seriously promoted, two factors have discouraged it. First, as a clinic-based program in an organization dominated by physicians, IMSS-COPLAMAR is geared toward providing curative care and prevention services, rather than community participation. Second, although IMSS-COPLAMAR often successfully involves program beneficiaries in health activities, their involvement more often is defined by IMSS-COPLAMAR planners than by the participants themselves, and sometimes planned priorities do not coincide with community priorities.

Clinic and hospital utilization and services have increased in most communities, at least until the decentralization process began. The 1986–1988 period is difficult to evaluate, but several indicators suggest that population coverage declined somewhat, and that the program apparently did not keep pace with increased needs for health care due to population growth and deteriorating living conditions. Although not enough data are available, it appears that in 1989, IMSS-COPLAMAR increased both population coverage and facilities; the performance of decentralized services cannot be judged due to lack of information.

Table 58 summarizes the most important data on preventive and/or curative services available to the population, in rates per 10,000 people. All rates have been calculated based on the total population reportedly covered by COPLAMAR-Social Solidarity Program, but official statistics (reproduced by Sherraden, 1989) base their estimates on a poorly defined ''beneficiary population'' that is always smaller than the total population (thus resulting in much higher rates) and that changes according to service. Three points in time were selected for the comparison: the beginning of the program (1980 or available year closest to it), the peak before decentralization began (1984), and the most recent year available (1986).

A percentage comparison between 1980–1982 and 1986 shows that prevention and/or sanitation rates have increased dramatically, from 50% to 370%, except for health education; as did the selected treatment of prioritized diseases, 50% to 100%, and all hospital services, 16% to 100%. Conversely, all rates for clinic services have declined, from 7% to 39%. In 1980, there were 2.7 times more clinic assistants than physicians, but by 1986, the gap had narrowed considerably; rates of physicians and other personnel increased from 9% to 16%, while those of nursing personnel declined by 53%; it should be noted that in a few of these services, the peak occurred in the mid-1980s.

Comparable data on IMSS (see Table 53) and COPLAMAR service/personnel rates (Table 58) show that the insured population covered by the former receives many more services per capita than that covered by the latter; in 1986, the IMSS-covered population received 1,357 times more consultations, 3,225 times more child deliveries, 3,350 times more surgery, and 26,650 more X rays than the COPLAMAR population. And yet, immunization rates are similar in both populations, and the rural poor receive other badly needed prevention services and treatment not available to the IMSS urban insured population. Physician rates for COPLAMAR in the 1980s were about one-half those of IMSS, which confirms COPLAMAR's physician-oriented and still curative-oriented services.

Table 59 shows the changes in morbidity rates between 1983 and 1986–1987. These data should be interpreted cautiously, because they are derived from clinic records, not from independent surveys; furthermore, there is no information for 1980, and it cannot be assumed that a decline in disease incidence in 1983–1986 is exclusively due to COPLAMAR. In any event, the table indicates that there has been a significant decline in all diseases, except for scabies, human rabies,

Table 58. Changes in COPLAMAR preventive and curative health services[a] in Mexico, 1980–1986 (rates per 10,000 people covered).

Services	1980–1982	1984	1986	% change 1986/1980–1982
Prevention/sanitation				
Detection of chronic diseases	1.0	2.6	4.7	370
Immunizations	2.7	7.3	8.2	203
Health education	4.0	4.7	4.3	8
Garbage disposal	0.1	0.3	0.4	300
Sewage disposal	0.1	0.1	0.3	200
Water treatment	0.2	0.2	0.3	50
Curative Medicine				
Clinics				
Consultations	6.0	4.2	4.3	−28
Prescriptions	5.7	3.5	3.5	−39
Child delivery	0.02	0.02	0.02	−7
Hospitals				
Consultations	1.2	1.3	1.4	16
Prescriptions	0.7	0.8	0.9	21
Child delivery	0.02	0.03	0.04	100
Surgery	0.02	0.04	0.04	100
X rays	0.1	0.1	0.02	100
Lab tests	0.4	0.6	0.8	100
Selected treatments				
Antiparasitical	n.a.	0.2	0.3	50
Oral rehydration	n.a.	0.2	0.3	50
TB, rheumatic fever, syphilis	n.a.	0.1	0.2	100
Personnel				
Physicians	3.3	4.0	3.6	9
Nursing	8.9	5.0	4.2	−53
Others	3.0	4.2	3.5	16

Sources: Sherraden, 1989; updated with Salinas de Gortari, 1989.
[a]Prevention/sanitation 1980, except detection (1981), curative 1982.

and typhoid fever. In addition, there has been an increase in the incidence of chronic diseases such as malnutrition and rheumatic fever (not shown in the table due to lack of data for 1983), although these increases may be attributable to improved detection. COPLAMAR's emphasis on prevention and/or sanitation should have played a positive role in reducing morbidity in rural areas.

To further improve COPLAMAR's performance, additional federal and IMSS resources should be devoted to that program. Prevention and/or sanitation and local paramedic personnel should be further emphasized over curative medicine and physicians, and, to that end, more public health experts should be brought into the program's planning and organization. The single health model should become more flexible, diversifying sufficiently to take into account significant differences among villages; in those places where the current model is not well accepted, additional effort is needed to involve the community. Health committees and their linkages with the clinic team should be strengthened, and committees should be encouraged to play a more important role in estab-

Table 59. Potential effect of COPLAMAR on morbidity rates among the rural poor, Mexico, 1983 and 1986–1987.

Diseases	% of change 1986/1983
Transmissible	
Influenza	−64.9
Enteritis	−32.6[a]
Acute tonsillitis	−31.9[a]
Amibiasis	−26.8[a]
Ascariasis	−20.0
Pneumonia	−14.3
Oxuiriasis	−12.2
Acute respiratory	−10.8[a]
Scabies	138.1

Diseases	% of change 1986–1987/1983
Preventable by vaccination	
Polio	−83.0
Pertussis	−81.4
Meningitis	−64.0
Tetanus	−58.7
Measles	−30.0
Tuberculosis	−28.6
Diphtheria	0.0
Typhoid fever	20.0
Human rabies	80.0

Sources: Sherraden, 1989; updated with IMSS-COPLAMAR, 1988a.
[a]1987 data indicate a further decline.

lishing program priorities. Qualified clinic assistants must be given increasing responsibility and training in order to perform more important tasks. Doctors should spend at least three years in the community, so as to learn from and become accepted by it; they should receive intensive training before being assigned to a rural post; and they should be given the opportunity for a long-term career. In addition, the number and role of health volunteers need to be expanded and their stipends raised. Community work done in exchange for health care should be specified and tailored to community needs, resources, and interests. Community health projects involving local, state, and federal governments and organizations could be expanded, with increased participation of the community and more outside resources; methods for transmitting grassroots demands and feedback to upper echelons must be improved.

Some experts claim that the health care program for the rural poor should be under one supervisor, and that the current fragmentation between IMSS and state health ministries should end. Some specialists have suggested that the program would be better under the Secretariat of Health, as part of the national health system (Wilkie, 1990), but others stress the need to continue the decentralization process. Before making these important decisions, it is highly advisable to have better data on the performance of both IMSS-COPLAMAR and the decentralized state services since the mid-1980s.

PRIVATE ALTERNATIVES OF HEALTH CARE FOR THE POOR

General Review

In Mexico, private alternatives for health care coverage of the urban poor appear to be limited; those for the rural poor are almost nonexistent. There are solidarity groups in marginal urban areas, financed by domestic and external aid, that offer credit, housing, and food for the poor, but that provide little or no health care. In Reinosa and Tamaulipas, health cooperatives were organized by informal workers who contributed to a common fund to buy a building for a clinic; later on, in negotiations with the Secretariat of Health, members obtained medical equipment and the Secretariat's commitment that major

health care expenditures above fixed user fees in the clinic would be covered.

In Cancún, 1,500 inhabitants of Puerto Juárez, many of whom are informal workers, organized "Common Front," and obtained a house and arranged for a physician to offer daily consultations. Through informal connections with IMSS physicians, the Front was able to arrange for its members to be cared for in the local IMSS hospital.

The Catholic Church also has organized medical consultations in several shantytowns of the Federal District, where a high proportion of its inhabitants are informal workers. Protestant churches persuaded physicians who work for the National System for Integral Family Development, for private clinics, or who are retired to take turns visiting the marginal population in the Federal District without charge. Finally, there are some groups of merchants in the informal sector who have signed agreements with private clinics to receive health care paying a modest monthly fee.

"Tlahuilli," The Mexican Institute of Traditional Medicine

Traditional medicine has strong roots in Mexico, but for many years it was, at best, despised by modern medical institutions. In the first Congress of Traditional Medicine held in 1974, participants criticized modern medicine as an expensive and unaffordable business. Physicians were described as ignorant of Indian languages and culture and as lacking the people's trust, and public health centers were accused of treating the indigenous population badly and ignoring herbal medicine. Although the latter was judged to be good, some participants acknowledged that it could not cure all diseases, and requested training in selected modern medicine techniques to improve their healing abilities. Partly responding to this congress, IMSS-COPLAMAR began, not always successfully, to incorporate traditional medicine into their integral health care model (IMSS, 1983). We have selected for special evaluation a nongovernmental organization that emphasizes traditional medicine, but that has been able to accept modern medicine and provide an alternative for the urban and rural poor.

History

The Tlahuilli Institute was established in Morelos in 1984 by a group of physicians who had individually practiced traditional medicine for more than a decade. Several of them worked in the public health sector and began to experiment with herbal medicine, acupuncture, and indigenous steam baths and other techniques, noting that these had positive results and little side effects, and were inexpensive and well-received by the indigenous population. The group organized a health committee that worked for two or three years in a borrowed house exclusively supported by the community. Responding to demands from small towns, often at the request of their leaders, the group expanded its services to various communities in the State of Morelos; they organized a clinic, established herb gardens, and began to produce medicines from them.

The Institute was given a boost by financial aid from a Dutch foundation, the Interchurch Coordination Committee for Development Projects, to work in four communities. Advised by the Secretariat of Health, they decided to apply communitarian and health promoter approaches to their activities. By mid-1987, Tlahuilli employed several physicians, biologists, and agronomists, and had trained 100 promoters in twelve poor communities; in six of these communities, their work was less than one year old. At that point, the Inter-American Foundation gave a grant to the Institute to expand their activities in those six communities, three of them rural and three urban (Díaz et al, 1989; IAF, 1988).

The Institute's commitment with IAF was to train 120 additional promoters on traditional medicine and to provide new curative services in several clinics. The promoters would learn first-aid skills, natural therapy techniques, and general health information; would identify, collect, and process medicinal plants and establish popular medicine pharmacies; and would research the socioeconomic condition of the communities and their health problems; once their training was completed, they would operate low-cost, self-financing health centers in the 12 communities, half supported by the Dutch foundation and half, by IAF. Institute physicians would visit each of the 12 communities once or twice weekly to offer health training, assist in the preparation of herbal medicines, facilitate the exchange of experiences among communities, and conduct research on health conditions. In addition, physicians would offer curative services in the clinics, to supplement first aid provided by the promoters, and organize local campaigns, in coordination with public health agencies, to fight diseases and epidemics. Finally, Tlahuilli would prepare educational health materials to be distributed to the promoters, and publish an annual bulletin to be disseminated among promoters, public health agencies, and universities (IAF, 1988).

In 1988, the Institute's top leadership changed, and support from the Dutch foundation ended; these events, combined with the conclusion of the Inter-American Foundation's aid in early 1989, brought on a crisis and the need for an overall evaluation of the program, which was conducted in May 1989. In December of that year, I visited several Tlahuilli facilities; interviewed its leaders, staff, and several promoters; and conducted a second informal evaluation.

Population Covered

The Institute serves both urban and suburban communities of blue-collar and informal workers, rural peasants, and indigenous groups. Practically all are poor, and share the following characteristics: unemployment rates over 40%, illiteracy over 30%, alcoholism over 50%, homes without potable water and sewerage services over 30%, annual per capita income under $US160, and high morbidity and mortality rates (IAF, 1988). The ten most common diseases in the communities are those typical of underdevelopment: intestinal diseases (colitis, gastritis, gastroenteritis, parasites); respiratory diseases (bronchitis, tonsillitis); skin conditions; genitourinary diseases; high blood pressure; and nervous system disorders. Most of these communities have no health services, and if they do, they are grossly insufficient. In the State, there is only one secondary-level public health hospital that faces an enormous demand, but about 80% of health needs are at the primary level. According to Tlahuilli's president, its facilities handle one-half of the health demands of the population, while the other half is handled by social insurance and the private sector, but most go unattended. Secretariat of Health facilities are scarce, occasionally one physician twice a month, and physician cooperatives' fees are too high for most of the population (Diaz et al, 1989).

Total population served by Tlahuilli probably exceeds 100,000. This represents about one-tenth of the population of the State of Morelos and one-fifth of the combined health care coverage of IMSS and the decentralized state services formerly under COPLAMAR (IMSS, 1987; IMSS-COPLAMAR, 1988a).

Facilities, Services, and Financing

The headquarters of the Institute, located in Cuernavaca, includes two buildings for offices, classrooms, and one outpatient consultation room. About 12 two-day practical courses are offered annually, with an average attendance of 50 people, between promoters and outsiders. The course is taught by an expert assisted by the most experienced promoters; topics, proposed by promoters, include the ten most common diseases, herbal medicine, acupuncture, and temazcal steam baths. Initially, five physicians worked at the Institute, but when outside funds stopped, only three and one acupuncturist remained; they began visiting the communities twice a week, but after the cut in funds, visits are now decreased to twice a month. Physicians normally do not see patients, but advise promoters and discuss cases with them.

There are between 19 and 21 outpatient consultation posts (consultorios), at least one in each community; these usually have an examination room and a traditional-medicine pharmacy. In addition, there are four clinics that normally consist of a reception room, examination room, bathroom, pharmacy, and a patio and small herb garden. Clinics provide curative services, mostly for respiratory and intestinal diseases, parasites, typhoid, malnutrition, and dehydration, and have a pharmacy stocked with traditional medicines and first-aid modern medicines; they usually offer massages, water treatments, steam baths, acupuncture, and child delivery services. Consultorios and clinics are staffed by two to four health promoters who take turns—initially, working hours were longer than now—to care for the patients. Promoters also identify and harvest medicinal plants or cultivate their own herbal gardens and prepare medicines; other needed herbs are exchanged or purchased in the market. They are expected to collaborate on local vaccination campaigns and to fight diseases such as dengue and parasites and to participate in health education to expand the use of latrines and other sanitation measures.

The Institute has trained 210 health promoters who are now spread throughout the State. Originally, most of them were traditional doctors (curanderos) who were trained by the Institute; all of them are from the community and speak Spanish and some Nahuatl; most are women, and about one-third are illiterate but eager to learn. Currently, most promoters work on their own at home, but some also offer their services at the clinic or consultorio. Each community has a health committee integrated by community members; its number, however, has declined from 20 to 30 to about 4 to 8 now. The committee is expected to manage and support the facilities.

The Institute used the grants from the Dutch foundation (amount unknown) and IAF ($US104,500 for two years) to build one of the headquarters buildings; to buy land and/or a house for some clinics and consultorios; to acquire medical, office, and transportation equipment; to pay salaries for medical and administrative personnel; and to produce educational materials. Tlahuilli personnel contributed from their own savings to construct the first headquarters building; other self-generated revenue included fees for attending training courses ($US4 to promoters and $US20 to outsiders), user fees paid by patients (such as $US1 for consultation or visit, including medicines and $US2 for a steam bath), and profits from the annual medicinal plant festival. Most communities contributed land and a building for the clinic or consultorio and are expected to maintain these facilities.

The annual budget of the Institute in 1987–1988, when outside funding was still available, averaged $US187,000: about 38% came from external aid, 43% was expected to be the community's contribution in kind, and 19% was the Tlahuilli share, also in kind (IAF, 1988). According to its top authorities, Tlahuilli now self-generates about $US12,000 annually, and, even on a shoestring budget, would need an additional $US60,000 a year to operate (Diaz et al, 1989). Therefore, the communities do not seem to be honoring their obligations.

The average maximum expenditure for a person covered by the Institute was $US1.88 in 1987—assuming that the communities' share did materialize, otherwise it would be much lower—that is, one-fourth of COPLAMAR average per capita expenditure, which was by far the lowest in Mexico (see Table 57). Although Tlahuilli charges a user fee for consultation, this is one-tenth to one-twentieth of the fees charged by local private physicians. Furthermore, the fee charged by Institute promoters usually varies according to the patient's economic status and, when a patient cannot pay in cash, he or she can pay in kind, such as empty bottles or produce, or in work (Díaz et al, 1989).

Accomplishments

In mid-1989, the Institute's performance was evaluated by an independent professional financed by IAF. Unfortunately, only promoters from three out of the twelve communities were represented in the collective self-evaluation—a total of nine promoters—and about half of the group left before the exercise ended (Barreiro, 1989).

Surprisingly, the evaluation did not provide information on key issues such as the population's satisfaction with the health services offered by Tlahuilli in terms of cost and quality and in comparison with other potential alternatives. Furthermore, there was no evidence that the beneficiary population was consulted, since the information appears to have been collected exclusively from a very small sample of promoters. And yet, this evaluation is the only document that we have on the Institute's assessment, and its recommendations appear to be wise.

The previous section clearly indicates that the cost of Tlahuilli services is extremely low, and that the amount and the way patients pay for such services are flexible. Moreover, personalized attention by promoters, who usually know the patient well, as well as easy and rapid access add to the advantages of these services. Unfortunately, we cannot evaluate the quality and effectiveness of health care provided by the Institute; its performance is easier to assess in terms of other aspects reviewed in the abovementioned evaluation that are summarized below.

Since 1984, some 120 new health promoters were trained, one-half of them in 1987–1989. At the first regional meeting of promoters held in 1988, 150 attended, 71% of the total. About 21 health committees have been organized, most of them in the State of Morelos, and some in Michoacán, Jalisco, and Guanajuato, and a Council on Traditional Medicine has been formed by representatives of these groups and by promoters. In 1989 alone, the Institute offered 20 courses on topics proposed by the promoters and with active participation by them; courses have been offered in other states with a high proportion of poor population such as Hidalgo, Puebla, and Michoacán.

The Institute participated in local and regional campaigns to fight widespread diseases and epidemics. In 1986, in coordination with public health authorities, it launched a campaign against a dengue epidemic that had badly afflicted the served communities. The Institute discovered a natural-medicine cure made from bark peel and willow combined with a steam bath that was much more effective, faster, and less expensive than modern-medicine treatments; endorsed by public health authorities, this treatment successfully controlled the epidemic. An antiparasitical campaign also produced positive results, albeit not as spectacular as the previous one—it began with a family survey to determine the importance of the infection, and was followed up by laboratory tests, elaboration of antiparasitic medicine made up of a combination of local herbs, application to the patients, and follow-up visits to check results. About 15 promoters worked on this campaign, and it is now being duplicated in some public schools. Unfortunately, the campaign's overall results and effectiveness were not evaluated. Tlahuilli leaders claimed that the traditional medicine, although not as effective as modern antiparasitic medicine, was cheaper and hence more accessible to the poor. However, the independent evaluator questioned the Tlahuilli claim about costs, although she did accept the claim that the Tlahuilli product largely avoids modern medicine's harmful side effects (Barreiro, 1989a).

Finally, the Institute has successfully developed its publication and information dissemination efforts. An annual Medicinal Plant Festival has been held since 1985, and attendance has increased almost fivefold between 1985 and 1989, from 198 to 950. Attendees actively participate in activities such as medicinal-plant exhibits accompanied by literature describing the plants and their curative powers, exchanges of prescriptions and experiences in treatment, discussion panels with herbal doctors, and plenary sessions. The festival covers its own costs and generates a profit. Four issues of the annual bulletin, *Medicina Alternativa*, were published by Tlahuilli between 1985 and 1988; unfortunately, as outside funding ended, that publication was suspended in 1989. These issues included articles by physicians, biologists, and botanists on inventory and classification of medicinal plants and their doses for treatment; evaluation, providing rates of success or failure of specific treatment of diseases using local herbs; and reports on courses and the annual festival. Finally, Institute authorities and promoters participated in several TV and radio programs and attended national and foreign congresses on traditional medicine. This discipline seems to be gaining in popularity, particularly among the poor and indigenous people who cannot afford the increasing costs of modern medicine.

Problems and Lessons

Both the 1989 evaluation and my visits and interviews at the end of that year, detected several problems at the Institute; these are summarized below, along with suggestions for the future.

Although outside funding cuts were responsible for some of the Institute's recent performance problems, others resulted from the failures of some of the initial ideas of its leaders. Initially, the plan involved training health promoters to work, mostly on a volunteer basis, at the *consultorios* and clinics, as well as in other Institute activities. Currently, most promoters operate on their own, offering services in their homes and using community supplies or their own (such as popular pharmacies); they also collect user fees for themselves. Health committees have not been very successful, either: their membership has steadily declined and they seem incapable of providing the expected contribution to the program.

Some communal activities, such as the dengue and antiparasitical campaigns, have been successful, but others such as community herb gardens and the building of latrines, have failed to elicit strong support. It should be noted that some communities responded better than others to the communitarian approach, but, in general, the concept has not really taken root. Because promoters work on their own, it is difficult to mobilize them for prevention and environmental activities, unless they can clearly derive a direct benefit from them, such as the elimination of the threat of dengue. Institute authorities first reacted against shifting from free community service to paid individual work, but eventually realized that it was unrealistic to expect hundreds of promoters to work gratis, particularly in a serious economic crisis, and that the important issue was for promoters to provide low-cost services to the poor, regardless where they did it (Barreiro, 1989a; Diaz et al, 1989).

The success of the clinics and, to a lesser extent, of the *consultorios* has been below expectations. In the 1987 agreement with the IAF, the Institute committed itself to extend curative services to all twelve communities, but, although information is not precise, it appears that there are only four clinics in operation. The failure to expand clinics to the other eight communities, or to convert existing *consultorios* into clinics, seems to stem from their low rate of utilization, and this, in turn, is the result of promoters shifting services to their homes. In addition, according to the agreement, physicians were expected to provide supplementary curative care in the clinics, but this is an exception, not the rule.

Data on frequency of weekly consultations are partial and contradictory: the Institute president reported to me rates of 15 to 20 patients per promoter, but in the 1989 evaluation, promoters gave rates of 8 to 17 consultations per clinic and/or *consultorio* (compared with rates of 12 to 40 reported by IAF in 1988), and the promoters in one community gave me rates of 4 to 5 consultations for the clinic. The president's rates probably include private consultations, but, if true, this confirms the underutilization of institutional facilities. Use of institutional treatment unavailable at the promoters' homes, was higher than consultations in general, but it varied from community to community. For example, in two communities the steam baths were used by 20 to 30 patients weekly, primarily because it had long been a tradition in one community and there was a large urban population in the other. However, in a third community it was used only once in two weeks by five or six people who came from outside the village. The promoters attributed this low utilization to the high cost of firewood, but the village's low population and possible lack of tradition in the use of the steam bath may have been responsible. The low utilization of this clinic could explain the discrepancy between the promoters' view that it was "falling apart," versus the Institute vice-president's justification that the decline was due to the termination of external funds; actually, the facility was very well taken care of and its pharmacy well stocked. I asked the Institute's president whether his policies would be different if he had the opportunity to start over. After thinking about it for a while, he candidly told me that he would put the resources into training more promoters.

A third problem is the sometimes strained relationship between traditional and modern medicine. In the case of the Institute, despite some initial conflicts, it developed a good relationship with public health authorities after its success with the dengue treatment. But a more difficult question is whether promoters systematically refer those patients who do not respond to traditional medicine treatment to the hospitals. Referrals are a matter of policy at the Institute, and promoters are expected to be sensitized to this during training. Once again, behavior varies according to the promoters and the communities: in an urban community, young promoters told me that transfers are frequent, but in a rural isolated community, two old promoters assured me that "all their patients were cured." The independent evaluator confirmed that in one community there is "blind faith," while in another, promoters are "more open." When I asked the Tlahuilli president about this problem, he first acknowledged it, but then offered several examples of promoters who had sent patients to relatives and friends who work at the Secretariat of Health hospital.

A potential cause for some of these difficulties was the type of leadership the Institute had from its inception until its crisis in 1988. The founder and first president, Dr. Horacio Rojas, is extremely dynamic, and is responsible for the institution's initial success and rapid expansion. But both the 1989 evaluation and my own interviews reveal that he exercised a strongly centralized leadership and administration that did not allow room for criticism. Tlahuilli members became accustomed to following orders and fulfilling tasks without any questioning. And yet, the communitarian approach obviously needed true participation by the people to be successful. One could argue that not only was the idea of the clinics not discussed, but obvious realities, such as the fact that promoters were starting to work for themselves or that health committees were not functioning properly, were ignored. The new leadership is aware of these flaws, and seems committed to correcting them; this also is true among promoters, who at the collective evaluation asked for a more pluralistic and open organization that allowed different ideas and objectives.

The above evaluation clearly indicates the need for some changes, particularly under severe budgetary constraints: the training of promoters should be improved, increasing their knowledge of basic first-aid techniques of modern medicine and insisting on the proper need for transfers; the need to continue the operation of clinics/*consultorios*, or of some of their facilities, in various communities should be evaluated; successful activities that are self-supporting, such as the annual festival, should be continued; the restricted time that physicians devote to train, supervise, and advise promoters should be more efficiently used; and the community's involvement in the planning and operation of the program must become more effective.

An important suggestion resulting from the 1989 evaluation was that the Institute should reconsider its role, in order to become a regional center for the collection, systematization, and diffusion of knowledge, rather than for the promotion of institutional care. The six years of cumulative experience on herbal and therapeutical medicine and the campaigns to fight disease cry out for systematization of the developed knowledge to treat, at least, the ten most common diseases that afflict the poor population served by the Institute. Some of that knowledge was published in the four issues of the now defunct bulletin, but much more is needed in the production of instructional materials for training future promoters and for retraining the old ones. This important task may require outside professional assistance and financial aid from abroad.

Last but not least, the Institute needs to become financially self-sufficient. The possibility of deriving significant revenue from the clinics and *consultorios* as they are today is practically nil; these facilities should either become efficient and self-supporting in the future or disappear. Currently, the main sources of funding are the courses and the festival; better courses could attract more students and increase income. If the efforts at systematization and dissemination of information indeed become central to the Institute, they could produce additional revenue from the sale of educational and practical materials, even at the national level. The Institute also should consider establishing a center for the wholesale collection and sale of inputs for the preparation of traditional medicines. Finally, international and regional organizations should provide additional funding to Tlahuilli in order to help it more accurately evaluate its activities and to facilitate its transformation into a more effective vehicle for helping the poor. After all, Tlahuilli costs per capita are among the lowest in Mexico, some of its activities have been extremely successful, and the impoverished population it serves has few or no other alternatives for health care.

PERU

POVERTY: SIZE, TRENDS, AND CHARACTERISTICS

According to ECLAC, in 1986 Peru had the second highest poverty incidence rate (total population) among ten Latin American countries: 60% national, 52% urban, and 72% rural (see Table 2). In 1961–1971, the national poverty incidence (households) in Peru declined from 58% to 50% (Piñera, 1978a); it further decreased to 46% in 1979 but increased to 52% in 1982. Data on the total population show a rise in national poverty incidence from 53% in 1979 to 60% in 1986. The number of poor increased by almost 16% in 1979–1986 (ECLAC, 1990).

The economic crisis hit Peru in 1982–1983; in the latter year, GDP per capita declined 14% and real wages by 15%, while unemployment increased to 9% and inflation by 125%. The American Popular Revolutionary Alliance party (APRA) took power in 1985, and launched an expansionist economic policy that generated a vigorous but brief boom in 1986–1987: real per capita GDP increased 11%, open unemployment was cut by one-half, the real average urban salary rose by 30%, and inflation sharply decreased (Ferrari, 1986). However, this bonanza was followed by a deep recession in 1988–1989: real per capita GDP fell 18.6%, open unemployment rapidly increased and under-employment jumped from 58% to 74%, the average urban salary declined by 62%, and inflation reached a record 3,452% (ECLAC, 1989). Given these deteriorating conditions, both the number of poor and the poverty incidence should have increased considerably in 1988–1989.

Between 1965 and 1988, the urban population of Peru rose from 52% to 69%; due to this rapid urbanization, urban poverty incidence (households) jumped from 28% in 1970 to 45% in 1986, while rural poverty incidence decreased slightly, from 68% to 64% in the same period (see Table 2). In 1986, the incidence of indigence in rural areas was more than twice that of urban areas. In the same year, there were 10.2 million poor in Peru, half of them indigents; 54% lived in urban areas and 46%, in rural areas (ECLAC, 1990).

The Urban (Informal) Sector

In 1970, about 86% of the urban poor in Peru—defined as those who earned less than the minimum wage—worked in the informal sector. As a percentage of the EAP, the informal sector grew from 20.7% in 1970 to 24% in 1982, and to 30% in 1985. In 1980, PREALC ranked Peru as the country with the third largest informal sector in Latin America; if domestic servants were excluded, Peru ranked first. In Lima, possibly the city with the largest informal sector in the Western Hemisphere, estimates of the informal sector as a proportion of the labor force range from 48% to 60% (Tokman, 1980; PREALC, 1981a, 1982; Ministerio de Trabajo y Promoción Social, 1986; De Soto, 1986; Annis and Franks, 1989; Mesa-Lago, 1990a).

The proportion of self-employed, unpaid family workers, and domestic servants—mostly informal workers—in the EAP rapidly expanded in the 1980s, while the share of salaried workers—the vast majority being formal-sector workers—declined. Between 1983 and 1986, nonsalaried work increased from 33% to 39% of employed EAP, while salaried work declined from 61% to 55%. It is noteworthy that these changes occurred at the peak of the economic boom that had helped to create formal jobs. In 1983, Lima's informal sector broke down into 49% self-employed, 18% salaried workers, 16% domestic servants, 8% unpaid family workers, and 9% small entrepreneurs and others. Practically all domestic servants worked in the informal sector, as did 91% of the self-employed, 75% of unpaid family workers, and 59% of employers, but only 12% of salaried workers (Instituto Nacional de Estadística, 1988, 1988a; Pinilla, 1986, 1987).

The profile of the informal worker in Lima in the mid-1980s was as follows: the majority were young, more than half were women, most of them employed their relatives in their trade, the vast majority were uneducated, 40% of merchants were street vendors who did not have a permanent stand, 62% lacked machinery or equipment, and 21% bought what they needed to operate on a daily basis. Almost 73% of informal workers worked in the tertiary sector, mainly in commerce and restaurants and, to a lesser extent, in personal services; 20%, in industry; and 7% each, in construction and transportation. About 83% of Lima's markets were operated by informal workers, and 47% of the city's population lived in informal settlements. Although their productivity was estimated to be one-third that of the formal sector, informal workers generated between 25% and 32% of registered GDP (De Soto, 1986; Pinilla, 1986; Instituto de Libertad y Democracia, 1986; Rossini and Thomas et al., 1987; Mesa-Lago, 1990a).

Informal workers' income is considerably lower than that of formal workers. In the mid-1980s, the self-employed received 91% of the average per capita urban income, domestic servants received 38%, and unpaid family workers, 30%. In Lima, 75% of informal workers earned less than $US100 monthly, with domestic servants earning less than $US40, compared to monthly earnings of $US100 to $US450 by formal workers. A survey conducted in an old neighborhood in the center of Lima, mostly made up of informal workers, found that the average income of 20% of families with six members (several of them working) was below the minimum wage. Lower earnings have been recorded in more recently developed neighborhoods (Instituto Nacional de Estadística, 1988, 1988a; Pinilla, 1987; Barrig and Fort, 1987; Grompone, 1988).

The Rural Sector

Peru's rural population in 1986 was 6.5 million: 4.7 million (72%) of them were poor and 3 million were indigents. The poorer half of the rural households received 22% of total rural income, and the average income of that group was roughly one-half that of the corresponding urban income. About 29% of the EAP in 1985, made up of peasant communities and small farmers, received 10% of the national income (ECLAC, 1990; Ferrari, 1986). The bulk of the rural poor lives in the least developed departments of the Andean highlands.

A study based on 1987 data ranked Peru's 25 departments using a composite index of 21 indicators dealing with socioeconomic development, health status, supply/utilization of health resources, and efficiency/adequacy of such resources; in addition, the study developed a health profile for each department. These health profiles were classified into three major groups; the poorest and most health deprived group consisted of eight departments ranked from worst to best as follows: Huancavelica, Apurimac, Puno, Cusco, Ayacucho, Cajamarca, Amazonas, and Huánuco. The study found that this group systematically scored below national averages, expressed in parentheses, in the following indicators: rural population, 58% to 80% of the total population (32%); annual GDP per capita, 28% to 73% (100%); illiteracy, 22% to 46% of the population 10 years and older (14%); infant mortality per 1,000 children below one year, 96 to 138 (88); and life expectancy at birth, 48 to 58 years (61). The eight departments are in the Andean highlands, or most of their populations live there. Their labor force is basically engaged in agriculture, primarily of a subsistence type—in 1980, 60% of the rural sector was traditional—and most of it consists of landless peasants, self-employed or unpaid family workers, or members of peasant communities. Finally, a very high proportion of the inhabitants in these departments are Indian (Mesa-Lago, 1988c).

According to the 1981 census, these eight departments also had the worst housing conditions in the country: 73% to 85% of them lacked water, sewage, and electricity services, compared with a national average of 49%. A 1981 ''health map'' of Peru, as well as the 1988 study cited above, confirmed that these departments had the poorest health standards, the highest deficits of health resources and services, and the lowest coverage by health care programs. Finally, a national health and nutrition survey conducted in 1984, indicated that the rural population of all Andean highland departments, including the poorest eight and more developed ones, had a morbidity incidence of 34%, but only 12% sought medical attention; the last figure contrasts with a national average of 24% and an urban average of 31%. On the other hand, the survey showed that 33% of the poor population afflicted by disease in the slums of Lima did seek medical attention, slightly below the city average but almost three-fold the percentage registered among the rural poor in the Andean highlands (Suárez-Berengela, 1987).

HEALTH CARE COVERAGE OF THE URBAN (INFORMAL) AND RURAL POOR

Administrative Structure and Legal Coverage

The establishment of the Peruvian Institute of Social Security (IPSS) in 1980 capped a ten-year process of unification and standardization of various sickness-maternity insurance programs covering working groups. Basically, IPSS covers salaried urban workers, but, at the turn of the 1960s, social insurance began to incorporate small groups of self-employed taxi drivers who owned their vehicles, and domestic servants. All insured are covered for general and specialized care, surgery, hospitalization, maternity care, laboratory services, dental care, and medicines. The armed forces is the only salaried group outside IPSS that has its own health care public program.

The APRA party came to power in 1985 with overwhelming support from the inhabitants of Lima's slums and from peasants, and President Alan García's radical economic policy primarily addressed these two poor groups. Public investment was reoriented and credit, training, and technical aid were provided for the informal sector and for small farmers; several public agencies and semiautonomous organizations were created or expanded to channel the funds allocated to those two groups. The National Plan

for Development (1986–1990) targeted the urban-rural areas of critical poverty, specifically the infant-maternal population, Andean peasants, informal workers, and the unemployed with priority programs on health, nutrition, environmental sanitation, drinking water supply, and sewage services. As will be seen later, the plan also contemplated extending social insurance to these groups.

In 1988, President Alan García declared: "Informal workers also have a right to social security and health care through their organizations and collective agreements." Initially, APRA policies seemed to work: the economy boomed in 1986–1987, income distribution favored poorer groups, and the informal economy grew at a higher rate than the formal economy. But the boom was short-lived; the recession that began in 1988 and worsened in 1989, had devastating effects on the informal poor and forced the government to stop its plans to extend health care coverage to the poor (Ferrari, 1986; Annis and Franks, 1989).

Before the mid-1980s, IPSS coverage of dependents was limited to the insured's spouse for maternity and to children below 1 year for vaccination and growth monitoring. Legal coverage was expanded in 1985–1986 to include full sickness-maternity benefits to the spouse and children under 18; pensioners are also covered.

Legislation was enacted in 1986–1987 to extend IPSS compulsory coverage to informal and rural workers and to housewives, but 1987 IPSS draft regulations (see the section on "Public Sector Viability," beginning on p. 142) designed to implement the law were never approved. Prior to the 1986–1987 laws, some of these groups, particularly the self-employed, could voluntarily join IPSS, but very few did. For example, a 1985 agreement incorporating Lima's street vendors into IPSS was never implemented. A new law enacted at the end of 1987, stipulated that the self-employed, rural workers, and fishermen, as well as their dependents, and housewives must be mandatorily covered by IPSS, and added practically the rest of the population—unpaid family workers, students, community volunteers, the handicapped, and indigents. The insured who lost their jobs had the legal right to continue receiving health care during a period to be specified. In short, IPSS was ordered to incorporate 7.6 million people, more than doubling its coverage, without receiving additional resources. But the law had a convenient loophole: the actual incorporation of these groups was again conditional upon IPSS enacting *ad hoc* regulations concerning their registration, financing, benefits, and administration. As it confronted the severe financial crisis, IPSS logically chose to ignore the law.

Even before the 1987 law, IPSS faced a sharp demand increase because of the extension of coverage to dependents, which required a rapid expansion of its primary-level clinics. In 1988, IPSS modestly began to voluntarily incorporate Lima's fruit and clothing street vendors and small groups of peasants organized into associations, and also began to enforce the mandatory affiliation of employees of clandestine garment factories. Limitations in IPSS's medical-hospital infrastructure, difficulties in maintaining control, and the deepening economic crisis brought all these modest expansion efforts to a halt (Mesa-Lago, 1988c).

By law, the Ministry of Health is responsible for preventive medicine, including an important childhood immunization program; curative medicine for all the urban and rural population not covered by IPSS; and special health programs targeted to women and children. User fees, which provided 7% of the Ministry's revenue in 1984, are charged, but we lack data on their amount and whether the poor are exempt (Zschock, 1988). The Ministry of Health infrastructure includes national and regional hospitals, municipal health centers, and health and sanitary posts. Legislation enacted in 1986–1988 mandated the functional integration of IPSS and Ministry health services through a national committee presided over by the Minister of Health. However, each institution maintained its autonomy and kept its facilities, personnel, and services separate, defeating any realistic possibilities of integration from the beginning. The goal was that all Ministry hospitals would be transferred to IPSS, while the Ministry would retain the administration of all health centers and posts; in locations where there was only a facility of one institution, it would provide services to the entire population, whether insured or not. By the end of 1987, six Ministry hospitals had been transferred to IPSS; since the beginning of 1988, political, financial, and administrative difficulties have halted the integration process (Mesa-Lago, 1988c).

In addition to the two public health care providers, there are some small social welfare programs. Lima and other municipalities operate a municipal fund for street vendors (FOMA), financed by a sale tax paid by the vendors; at least one-half of FOMA revenues should be devoted to health care. The municipality of Lima has regulations for street vendors that include

the obligation to provide medical care and sanitary services; in 1986, a mobile health care service began to operate in informal markets, but it lasted only a few months.

To summarize, from a legal standpoint, all salaried workers and their dependent spouses and children are to be covered by the IPSS sickness-maternity program and entitled to benefits in kind, while the insured also are entitled to paid maternity and sick leave; domestic servants are entitled to similar benefits. There also are special health programs established through voluntary agreements signed with fishermen, newspaper vendors, and lottery-ticket vendors. Finally, IPSS administers a program of voluntary incorporation of small groups of self-employed and housewives. Except for urban domestic servants and small pockets of self-employed, the poor are not legally covered by IPSS. Their only alternatives are the Ministry's health services and those offered by the municipality of Lima.

Statistical Coverage

According to Table 60, total population coverage by social insurances (mainly IPSS) increased from 15.7% to 31.6% in 1980–1988, but practically none of those covered are poor. The figures in Table 60 represent gross calculations that are inflated due to the reasons detailed below. Estimates of the active insured are rough IPSS projections of the EAP disaggregated by type of occupation and based on the 1981 census; they assume that all salaried workers legally covered are actually registered, which is not true because evasion by employers and workers is quite high. The estimates also do not consider that, given the economic crisis of the 1980s, projections based on 1981 data are erroneous because formal employment has declined while informal employment and unemployment—not covered by IPSS—have increased. Moreover, since 1981, registration data have not been updated to exclude those who have died, left the labor force, or emigrated; and figures on dependents for 1980–1984 are based on an estimated ratio of spouses and children per insured, and since 1985, they are based on the erroneous assumption that the legal extension of coverage to dependents has been fully implemented. Probably the most accurate IPSS data are for covered pensioners; other segments of the population covered by social insurances, particularly the armed forces and police, are rough estimates.

Checks conducted at the end of 1988, using

Table 60. Official data on population covered with health care in Peru, 1980–1988 (in thousands and percentages).

	Population		Reported social insurance coverage (IPSS)					Coverage others[b]	Social insurance, total covered	Coverage Ministry of Health	% of population covered			
			Active insured	Dependents		Pensioners	Total				Social insurance		Ministry of Health	Total
	Total	Urban[a]		Spouses	Children						Total	Urban		
	(1)	(2)	(3)	(4)	(5)	(6)	(7)	(8)	(9)	(10)	(9/1)	(9/2)	(10/1)	(9+10)/1
1980	17,295	11,069	2,003	70	72	128	2,273	450	2,723	n.a.	15.7	24.6	n.a.	n.a.
1984	19,198	12,766	2,408	82	91	203	2,784	500	3,284	5,000	17.1	25.7	26.0	43.1
1985	19,698	13,198	2,505	767	1,760	211	5,243	500	5,743	n.a.	29.2	43.5	n.a.	n.a.
1988	21,256	14,666	2,818	860	2,191	253	6,122[c]	600	6,722[c]	n.a.	31.6[c]	45.8[c]	n.a.	n.a.

Sources: Mesa-Lago, 1988c; Zschock, 1988.

[a]Author's estimates based on 1981 census and World Bank figure for 1988.

[b]Gross estimate of armed forces and police, fishermen and jockeys.

[c]These figures have been roughly estimated to be inflated by two million people, reducing coverage to 22% of the total population and 28% of the urban population.

data on re-registration of the active insured that resulted from block-to-block inspections of employers in major cities, indicate that at the national level, the figures of active insured in Table 60 were overestimated by 32% or 36%—about one million people. Regarding dependents, it is impossible that in a few months, at the end of 1985, the number of spouses actually covered could have increased nine times (from 82,000 to 767,000), and that the number of children would have increased by 19 times (from 91,000 to 1,760,000). Based on IPSS ratios of spouses and children per insured, an overestimation of 1 million insured has been calculated. Therefore, the overestimation of the total IPSS coverage in 1988 (Table 60) could be 2 million people, hence reducing coverage to 22% of the total population (Mesa-Lago, 1988c).

In the mid-1980s, the Ministry of Health reportedly covered 11 million noninsured poor. (According to ECLAC, there were 10.2 million poor in Peru at that time.) But Ministry officials have acknowledged that of the target population, only 5 million live within access to Ministry health care facilities, leaving 6 million without real coverage (Zschock, 1988). Other public health services are provided by charitable institutions (*beneficencias*) and by municipal governments reportedly covering 750,000 poor, a figure that probably is inflated. The sum of the adjusted coverage of social insurances (4.7 million) and the Ministry (5 million), plus the reported coverage by other institutions (750,000, at most), totals about 10.5 million in 1988, leaving 10.7 million without public protection.

The private health sector in Peru includes direct household expenditures, health insurance, employer and provider plans, cooperatives, and private voluntary organizations. Population coverage of this sector in 1984 was estimated as 346,900 by one source (Suárez-Berenguela, 1987) and as 10 million by another (Zschock, 1988). The first source excluded the six million without access to the Ministry, but considered them as covered by the Ministry. The second source included the six million poor without access to the Ministry in the private sector, and reported that they spent an average of $US4.50 per capita buying services from the private sector. And yet, according to ECLAC, in 1986 there were five million indigents in Peru who could not buy the minimum amount of food, much less afford to pay for health care. In my opinion, there are at least five million critically poor in Peru who lack any kind of health care, plus four million poor who can buy a minimal amount of care only occasionally.

The few informal workers that might be insured in Peru are with IPSS, but we do not know whether any poor informal workers are actually insured. Practically all the insured in IPSS, and in the armed forces, live in urban areas; 58% of them live in metropolitan Lima, which takes 64% of health care expenditures. Based on Table 60, we can estimate that in 1988 about 46% of the urban population was covered by social insurance, but the figure is only 28% after correcting for the overestimation. In 1988, 92.4% of the active insured at IPSS were salaried workers, and practically all were employed in the formal sector; 7.6% were self-employed and domestic servants (Mesa-Lago, 1990a).

Data from the 1985–1986 National Household Survey on Living Standards and the 1986 Lima Survey on Employment, combined with IPSS statistics on the insured for the same years, allow us to roughly estimate the percentage of coverage of some groups of informal workers (see Table 61). The percentage of coverage of the self-employed was 4% nationally and 16% in Lima, while that of domestic servants was 77% and 31%, respectively. Note, however, that the total number of domestic servants reported by the national survey was 78,000 for Peru, while the number reported by the employment survey for Lima, where most domestic servants work, was 122,000. Obviously, the first figure is grossly underestimated and, hence, the percentage of national coverage is significantly overestimated; the 31% figure for Lima is, therefore, more reliable. Regarding the self-employed, the lower percentage of coverage at the national level is explained because almost half of the self-employed work in agriculture, and probably none is insured, while those insured by the IPSS in Lima are urban, explaining the higher percentage reported in the capital. No unpaid family workers are covered by IPSS.

There is no statistical information on the coverage of informal small employers and their salaried workers. One study found that in the mid-1980s, these employers did not honor their social security obligations with their employees. Another study concluded that social insurance was designed for workers with a labor contract, and it was not enforceable in microenterprises. In 1988, none of the 5,000 members of the Association of Artisans and Small Industrialists was insured by IPSS. And in the 1985–1986 National Household Survey, 42% of salaried workers reported that they were not insured; it can safely be assumed that most of them were informal workers (De Soto, 1986; Grompone, 1987; Instituto Nacional de Estadística, 1988; Mesa-Lago, 1990a).

How many of the informal workers insured by IPSS are poor? The answer is most of the domestic servants (2% of total insured at IPSS) because of their low income, but not so the self-employed, because many of them are professionals with relatively high incomes. At best, less than 5% of the potential informal workers are covered by IPSS, leaving between 1.7 and 2 million informal workers and their 3.7 to 4 million dependents—a total of 5.4 to 6 million people—without health care coverage.

The APRA government plans to extend coverage to the informal sector did not materialize. In 1985, IPSS set the following targets for coverage of the urban marginal population: 120,000 in 1987, 750,000 in 1988, 1.5 million in 1989, and 1.8 million in 1990; by 1987, the target for 1988 had been cut by one-half. In 1988, IPSS reported that there were 11,216 informal workers in the "process of being incorporated," of which 93% were owners of market stands and street vendors, 6% were self-employed fishermen, and 1% were newspaper vendors. Information was unavailable on whether those workers were finally insured, but, even if all of them were, they would have accounted for less than 0.5% of the self-employed with an occupation. According to the Federation of Street Vendors of Lima, only 3% of its 13,000 members were insured by IPSS in 1988 (IPSS, 1985 and 1987; Mesa-Lago, 1990a).

Concerning Ministry of Health coverage, Zschock (1988) reports that only 2 million in the urban population had real access to Ministry

Table 61. **Estimates of potential informal workers covered by social insurance (IPSS), Peru, 1985–1986 (in thousands and percentages).**

	Peru	Lima
Number employed[a]	3,608	776
Self-employed	2,660	528
Domestic servants	78	122
Unpaid family workers	870	126
Insured at IPSS[b]	168	122
Self-employed	108	84[c]
Domestic servants	60	38[c]
Unpaid family workers	0	0
Percentage of coverage	4.6	15.7
Self-employed	4.1	15.9
Domestic servants	76.9	31.1
Unpaid family workers	0	0

Source: Mesa-Lago, 1990a.
[a]Peru, according to the National Household Survey of 1985–1986; Lima, based on employment survey of 1986.
[b]Average of the insured in 1985–1986.
[c]Re-registration in 1988; there are no separate data for Lima on 1986 registration.

services, excluding about 10 million. An investigation in El Agustino, a Lima neighborhood inhabited mostly by informal workers, found that between 72% and 77% of them went to the Ministry hospital or health center, 8% to 11% went to a private physician, 7% to 10% took care of themselves, and 5% to 8% did not get any care and did not resort to other services (Barrig and Fort, 1987). In Villa El Salvador, a town close to Lima inhabited mostly by informal workers, the Ministry's health center does not offer childbirth services, and most women deliver in their own homes (see the section on "The Example of Villa El Salvador," beginning on p. 146).

Finally, several sources report that despite legal dispositions and agreements, FOMA does not provide health care to street vendors, and revenues of that fund are used by the municipalities for other objectives (Mesa-Lago, 1990).

Rural Poor

In contrast with IMSS-COPLAMAR, IPSS does not cover any rural poor; in fact, IPSS coverage of the rural population as a whole is very small. In 1981, Peru's eight most rural and poorest departments, where most Indians live, had the lowest IPSS population coverage: Apurimac, 2.5%; Ayacucho, 2.7%; Cajamarca, 2.8%; Amazonas, 3.1%; Huancavelica and Puno, 3.7%; and Huánuco and Cusco, 4.7%; compare these figures with a national coverage of 14% and a coverage of 26% in Lima-Callao (Mesa-Lago, 1989c).

In 1966, IPSS developed a pilot project of peasant social insurance in three rural communities in Junín, a state selected for its relatively high socioeconomic development. Those covered were beneficiaries of the agrarian reform in Indian communities and cooperatives; they contributed land, community work to build the health post, and a symbolic cash amount; the state was supposed to contribute but never did. The health post had a sizable staff—one physician and five assistants—and offered infant-maternal care, curative medicine, environmental sanitation, and health education. The project failed due to the absence of state financing, a very expensive model of health care, and lack of support from the communities (Mesa-Lago, 1989c).

Under the APRA government, at the end of 1985, IPSS developed a new project to extend coverage to peasants, emphasizing primary health care, prevention, and outpatient consultation. It was to start in 14 rural communities selected according to a minimum health care infrastructure, where IPSS would coordinate its activities with the Ministry of Health and community leaders. The project would be financed by a state contribution equal to 1% of the national wage bill; the elimination of the wage ceiling to increase the insureds' contribution; contributions in land, manpower, and maintenance from the beneficiaries; a cash contribution from the head of the insured family equal to one-half of the minimum wage; and foreign aid. Population coverage targets set in 1985 were 1.8 million in 1988, 3 million in 1989, and 5.2 million in 1990; two years later, those targets were cut to 1, 2.8, and 4.4 million, respectively. In 1988, IPSS received a USAID grant to bring a group of experts to plan the extension, but the economic crisis put an end to the project (IPSS, 1985, 1987; Mesa-Lago, 1988, 1989c).

According to Zschock's (1988) estimates, in 1984–1985 the population with real access to Ministry of Health services in rural areas was 3 million; assuming that this figure is correct, it still leaves 3.5 million without protection, 54% of the rural population. The latter is similar to ECLAC's estimate of 3 million indigents in the rural sector who did not have access to health care; still, according to ECLAC, there were an additional 1.7 million rural poor. We can roughly estimate that in 1988, from 3.5 to 4.7 million rural poor, between 53% and 68% of the rural population, did not have access to health care. Ministry per capita expenditures in rural areas in 1984 were less than half those in urban areas (Zschock, 1988).

REASONS FOR THE VERY LOW COVERAGE OF THE POOR

As we saw in the previous section, one-half of the salaried workers (mostly in informal-sector enterprises), from 84% to 96% of the self-employed, about 69% of domestic servants, the mass of rural workers, and an unknown percentage of owners of microenterprises, as well as all of their dependent families, are not covered by IPSS. Furthermore, more than half of the poor population supposedly covered by the Ministry does not have real access to its health services, which are obviously insufficient to perform their tasks (see the section on "Public Sector Viability," beginning on p. 142). The reasons for the extremely low health coverage of the poor are both general and policy related.

General Factors

Peru faces significant general disadvantages vis-à-vis Costa Rica and Uruguay, and shares some features with Mexico—its territory and population are much larger, there are significant topographical barriers that make communication more difficult, a very large percentage of its population has a different language and culture and lives relatively isolated, and the rate of illiteracy is much higher than the previous three countries. Peru also has not enjoyed the political stability of the three countries analyzed previously.

In 1986, Peru had the second highest incidence of poverty and indigence (national, urban, and rural) among the ten Latin American countries surveyed by ECLAC: more than one-half of its population was poor and 30% was indigent, and the deepening economic crisis since 1988 must have increased the number of poor and indigents. In 1980, Peru had the second largest informal sector among the 13 countries evaluated by PREALC. And yet, Peru's per capita income in 1988 was ninth in Latin America, only 14% lower than Chile's, whose social insurance population coverage was about three times higher; Bolivia, which had the second lowest per capita income in Latin America, had a population coverage close to that of Peru. Still, Peru's per capita income was half of Uruguay's and three-fourths that of Mexico and Costa Rica. Part of the problem is inequality in income distribution: Peru had the fifth worst in 1986 among the ten countries in the ECLAC study; in addition, until the mid-1980s, social insurance coverage of family dependents was one of the lowest in the Region. Finally, health care resources are concentrated to serve a small portion of the population, and no serious effort has been made to develop special programs to protect the poor (ECLAC, 1990; World Bank, 1990; Tables 2, 7, 8).

Social Security Policy

Policy, related issues, to be discussed below, are low income of the noncovered and high contributions required for social insurance coverage, combined with poor quality of services; isolation of rural areas and difficulties to detect, reg-

ister, and control informal microenterprises; and weak or ineffective mobilization to demand protection.

Low Income and High Contributions

We have already seen that the income of informal workers in Lima averaged less than one-third that of formal workers, while the poorest half of rural households earned 22% of rural income and the average income of that group was half of the corresponding urban income. It is obvious that the indigent population and part of the poor population does not have enough resources to pay for health care.

Table 62, segment A, compares the legal percentage of contribution to IPSS among various insured groups. The percentage paid by the self-employed voluntarily insured (18%) is three times the percentage paid by the salaried worker (6%), because the former must pay the equivalent of the employer's contribution for sickness-maternity and pensions (12%); the self-employed lacks protection against employment injury. Conversely, the domestic servant's percentage is the same as that of the salaried worker (6%) and, as will be seen later, domestic servants also benefit from a lower salary base of contribution. Peasants who join IPSS voluntarily must be members of associated enterprises or communities; if they live in an economically depressed area, they pay a lower percentage than domestic servants (4%, one-fifth that of the self-employed), but if they live outside economically depressed zones, they pay more (9%, still one-half that of the self-employed). Theoretically, if the self-employed is a member of a union or association, the latter should pay the 12% corresponding to the employer, but in practice, the self-employed pay that 12% because associations lack the resources and refuse to sign payment agreements with IPSS. The self-employed often choose to join only the sickness-maternity program, because it is the one they need most and they lack the resources to pay for pensions.

The salary base for contributions to IPSS is the total compensation for salaried workers, the minimum insured compensation for the self-employed and peasants, and one-third of the minimum insured compensation for domestic servants. Unfortunately, we lack data on income and total contributions to IPSS by occupational categories, such as were available for Mexico; hence, segment B of Table 62 approaches the comparison in a different way. Although the salaried worker's contribution base

Table 62. Contributions of salaried and informal workers and peasants to IPSS, Peru, 1988.

A. LEGAL CONTRIBUTIONS BY PROGRAMS (% OF INCOME)					
	Salaried[a]				
	Insured	Employer	Total[b]	Self-employed[c]	Peasants[d]
Sickness-maternity	3	6	9	9	4–9
Pensions	3	6	9	9	0
Employment injury	0	4[e]	4[e]	—	—
Total	6	16	22	18	4–9

B. INSURED			
		Ratio over salaried average (1.00)	
	Salary base of contribution	Monthly contribution	Income per capita[f]
Salaried	Total compensation	1.00[g]	1.00
Self-employed	Minimum insured compensation	3.00	0.83
Peasants	Minimum insured compensation	0.66 or 1.48	n.a.
Domestic servants	1/3 of minimum insured compensation	0.33	0.35

Source: Mesa-Lago, 1990a.

[a]Includes domestic servants.

[b]In the 1970s, the State legally had to contribute 1% but never paid it; in 1987, the law said the State should pay 1% of the total insured compensation of the previous year, but the State did not do so in 1988.

[c]If a member of a union or association, the latter should pay 12% and the insured 6%, but in practice, the worker pays all.

[d]Only if members of associational enterprises or communities that have signed an agreement with IPSS. The 4% is applicable to economically depressed areas; the rest pay 9%.

[e]Average premium.

[f]1985–1986.

[g]To facilitate the comparison, it is assumed that the salaried worker receives the minimum insured compensation.

is his total compensation, we have used the salaried worker who earns the minimum insured compensation, because by using a similar income to the other groups, it allows for comparisons. Taking the contribution paid by the salaried worker as the base (1.00), the self-employed pay 3.00; peasants, 0.66 or 1.48; and domestic servants, 0.33. Table 62, segment B contrasts these ratios with the average per capita income of the salaried worker, and estimates that the self-employed contributes three times more than the salaried worker, but earns only 83% of the latter's income. This largely explains why so few self-employed have joined IPSS voluntarily. Leaders of associations of informal workers and experts claim that the self-employed contribution is too high in view of their income and other more urgent needs they have; hence, the high contribution becomes the main obstacle in joining IPSS (Grompone, 1987).

Conversely, domestic servants pay 33% of the average contribution paid by salaried workers. Thus, the decrease in the percentage of contribution from 18% (self-employed) to 6% (domestic servant), plus the one-third reduction of the minimum insured compensation, makes the contribution of domestic servants more reasonable and facilitates their coverage. However, note that domestic servants per capita income is less than one-half that of the self-employed. The

fact that their employers pay three-fourths of the total contribution gives an added advantage to domestic servants. The compulsory nature of the affiliation has been given as an additional reason for the higher coverage of domestic servants, but studies in other countries suggest that this is not an important factor in practice (Mesa-Lago, 1990a).

The contribution of a peasant living in an economically depressed area is one-third less than that of the salaried worker and one-fifth less than that of the self-employed, but twice that of the domestic servant. Although we lack data on the per capita income of peasants living in economically depressed areas, their income probably is lower than that of domestic servants. Furthermore, only those peasants in associated enterprises or communities are allowed to join IPSS. Finally, peasants who do not live in economically depressed areas, should pay a contribution 48% higher than that of salaried workers. This largely explains IPSS's ongoing failure to extend health care coverage to this group.

On several occasions, IPSS has considered using a state subsidy to facilitate the incorporation of low-income workers. In fact, according to the Peruvian constitution, the state must contribute to IPSS both as an employer and as a third party. The latter contribution was set in the 1970s as 1% of the total wage bill, but the state never paid and the fee was eliminated at the start of the 1980s. In 1985, President García publicly stated that a portion of the resources saved by reducing the foreign debt payments would be used to extend social insurance coverage to low-income groups. However, that promise never was fulfilled, despite demands from associations of informal workers and peasants to the President and to IPSS. A law enacted at the end of 1987, reintroduced the state contribution of 1%, to be used, among other things, to extend coverage. The contribution was calculated based on the previous year's total wage bill, in order to reduce the state contribution; furthermore, it was not paid in 1988.

Those not insured by IPSS who are poor and have access to the Ministry health services do not pay if they lack resources; if they have some income, they pay minimal user fees. Some Ministry services are free regardless of income, such as treatments for tuberculosis and rehydration.

In addition to their high cost, IPSS health care services are widely considered to be of poor quality. Usual complaints among the uninsured that often are given as reasons for not joining IPSS are long waiting lines to receive care despite an overabundance of personnel who show no concern for the users, long distances to health care centers, and very poor service.

Actual users expressed similar complaints about Ministry of Health services, adding the need to have "contacts" (friends among the personnel) to get admitted into specialized hospitals, improper time schedules for consultation, absentee physicians, inadequate treatment, and poor hygiene. In the survey conducted among women in El Agustino, 65% said that they wasted four hours waiting in line to receive service and 19% said they wasted six hours (Barrig and Fort, 1987; Mesa-Lago, 1990a).

Rural Isolation and Difficulties to Incorporate Informal Enterprises

As noted, the lowest IPSS population coverage is found in the eight least developed, most rural, and poorest departments in the Andean highlands, departments that also have the highest concentration of Indians and the highest illiteracy rates. This population is widely dispersed and physically isolated and must surmount cultural obstacles. A Peruvian expert said that the small user fee charged by the Ministry is not a barrier to access because the population in those areas often pays similar or even higher fees to traditional doctors (*curanderos*), and that they only resort to Ministry facilities when it is too

late. And yet, as was seen in the case study of Mexico, COPLAMAR, despite its flaws, proved that it is feasible to provide health care to isolated rural populations.

In the urban sector, evasion of private enterprises to IPSS was estimated to be between 35% and 40% of contributions in 1985. In 1988, the estimated number of salaried workers in Lima was 36% higher than the number re-registered at IPSS, yet another indication of a high rate of evasion. A survey of enterprises conducted in Lima in the same year, found that 33% of the registered enterprises had more than six workers, employed 90% of insured workers, and paid 96% of total contributions. The remaining 66% of enterprises had fewer than six workers, employed 10% of the total insured workers, and their share of contributions was only 4%. The cost of collecting from and inspecting these small enterprises is quite high compared to the corresponding costs for large enterprises; furthermore, costs to detect, register, and control the smaller evading enterprises would be even higher.

At the end of 1985, IPSS started using a computerized system of registration and collection to reduce evasion and payment delays. Teams of trained inspectors combed cities block by block to detect and register clandestine enterprises and their workers or re-register already listed enterprises, checking the number of workers and the wages paid. Although data were not available on the number of evading enterprises found, IPSS officials reported that hundreds of garment enterprises and repair shops were identified. By 1988, the computerized system was in operation in most of Lima and in 15 of the country's 24 departments. But at that point, a new IPSS administration dismissed 800 system workers, mostly inspectors and computer operators, alleging that their cost was too high; in addition, priority was given to collecting the monthly fees from large enterprises, rather than collecting the quarterly fees from small enterprises. The aggravation of the economic crisis has stimulated the labor transfer from the formal to the informal sector at a time when IPSS has cut resources to detect and control the rising number of informal microenterprises, making the protection of informal salaried workers all the more difficult (Mesa-Lago, 1986a, 1988, 1988c, 1990a).

Weak or Ineffective Mobilization to Demand Protection

A study on the historical evolution of social security in Peru demonstrated that the most powerful and best organized pressure groups were the first to be covered, the ones with a higher degree of protection, and the ones that enjoy better benefits at a relatively lower cost (Mesa-Lago, 1978). Despite advances in the late 1960s and throughout the 1970s, peasants remain the least organized group in Peru, and the one that probably has the worst health care in the country.

Within the informal sector, some groups have become organized, but they have not always effectively pressured the state to obtain adequate health care protection. The two most important federations of transportation workers, FED and ANEXOS, relying on their ability to paralyze the country, have succeeded in extracting a significant package of benefits from the state, including the incorporation of taxi drivers into IPSS. Conversely, the associations of shanty-town inhabitants, where informal workers predominate, have not been successful in this area, and, at most, they have obtained a Ministry medical post; apparently, because their main interest is to legalize their land settlement, they tend to lose enthusiasm as soon as their goal is fulfilled.

Among street vendors, there are 22 federations in Lima alone. They have often mobilized efficiently to defend their right to sell in the streets, but they lack a long-term plan and their strength weakens once an emergency disappears. Some of these federations have fought to obtain health care protection: for instance, in 1985 one of the three most powerful federations signed an agreement with IPSS and the Lima municipality to that end. Unfortunately, the fragmentation of street vendors among many associations with conflicting ideologies has prevented them from steadily pressuring the authorities, and the agreement was never implemented.

Street vendors also have failed to force FOMA to invest part of the excise tax revenue to provide them with health care. Depending on their location, in 1985 informal street vendors paid between 98% and 495% more than formal commercial establishments. In several instances, street-vendor federations have threatened to stop paying the excise tax if its revenue is not used for health care, paid maternity leave, etc. However, these protests have not been successful because they have been local and sporadic, and have lacked a nationwide, steady coordinated effort with clear objectives. In addition, many street vendors do pay this tax as a sort of ''license'' that legitimizes their activities, even though they know the municipality will use its revenue for purposes other than protecting the group (De Soto, 1986; Grompone, 1987; Mesa-Lago, 1990a).

FINANCIAL VIABILITY OF SOCIAL INSURANCE AND THE PUBLIC SECTOR TO COVER THE POOR

According to various estimates, between 9 and 11 million poor lack any public health care protection in Peru, or from 43% to 52% of the 1988 total population; roughly 60% of them live in urban areas and 40% in rural areas. In that year, the combined population coverage (actual access) of IPSS, the Ministry of Health, and other public institutions was 10.5 million; hence, universalization of coverage to the poor would require doubling the current coverage. In the following sections, we analyze the capacity of IPSS and the Ministry to undertake that enormous task.

Social Insurance (IPSS) Viability

IPSS's accounting data are seriously flawed, but they show that all programs combined generated a surplus in 1975–1981 and 1985, but operated with a deficit in 1982–1984 and in 1986–1988. The disequilibrium worsened in 1988, forcing IPSS to take loans and launch an emergency plan. In 1987, the sickness-maternity program took 58% of all IPSS expenditures and was the principal cause of the disequilibrium. Since 1977, this program has ended in a deficit in all years except 1985; that year, contributions and the salary ceiling were increased. In 1987–1988, the contingency reserve of the sickness-maternity program had declined by 94%, practically vanishing. This program's persistent deficit was covered by loans from the pension and employment-injury programs until 1983, when such loans were prohibited; however, they were immediately replaced by accounting transfers that are difficult to trace. These loans and transfers have not been amortized, and, if any interest has even been paid, it has been minuscule; consequently, such practices have contributed to the decapitalization of the pension program. The pension program has usually generated a surplus, but this has declined as a proportion of its revenue; in 1988, the pension program also faced financial ruin (it has suffered an actuarial deficit for many years). In conclusion, there are no resources left at IPSS to subsidize the sickness-maternity program (Mesa-Lago, 1988c, 1989c).

In terms of income, the causes of the sickness-maternity program deficit, and the IPSS overall disequilibrium, are: a total percentage contribution that is already high but insufficient to cover expenditures (Argentina, Chile, and Uruguay have lower percentages of contributions than Peru, but higher population coverage); very high evasion and payment delays (35% to 40% of contributions), aggravated by runaway inflation (1,722% in 1988, 2,948% in 1989), which have increased the incentive for *mora* and drastically reduced the employers' debt to IPSS in real terms; a huge state debt to IPSS (only as an employer); and negative real investment yields of reserves due to nonrepayable loans given to the sickness-maternity program and low yields of investment in public bonds, rental buildings, and banking deposits in national currency.

In terms of expenditures, the causes of the deficit are: extremely high administrative costs that rose from 22% to 35% of total expenditures in 1976–1988 due to an excessive bureaucracy, salary indexation to inflation, and an increase in compensation to Ministry employees incorporated into IPSS by the integration process; expansion of the population covered under health-maternity since 1986, mainly due to the incorporation of dependent family; paid sickness leave with 100% salary replacement, one of the highest in the Region, that fosters simulation of disease; a sharp increase in the cost of medicines, most of which are either imported or use foreign-made inputs; hospital inefficiency (average hospital occupancy in 1986 was 73.6% but fluctuated widely among departments, the average length of stay was too high (11.3 days), and physicians only worked 53% of the daily schedule); and an increase in real pensions that were indexed to inflation each quarter during 1984–1988 (Mesa-Lago, 1988c).

In September 1988, IPSS approved an emergency plan to tackle the crisis that proposed the following measures: an increase in the percentage of contribution; enforcement of the collection of the debt owed by private employers and adequate monitoring and collection of the state debt; better control of evasion and improvement in the investment yield; freezing of jobs to gradually reduce personnel; restrictions in pay-

ments of overtime, travel, and fringe benefits to personnel; elimination of or reduction in expenditures for supplies, electricity, phone, and other services; and austerity in investment.

The already mentioned 1987 draft regulations to expand IPSS coverage to informal workers specifically mentioned the following groups: self-employed vendors in public markets who had permanent stands, street vendors without permanent stands, street shoeshiners and car cleaners, small manufacturers, artisans, miners, fishermen, eventual and temporary wage earners who worked for multiple employers, home workers, and workers without an employer but organized in associations or cooperatives. The regulations granted full health care for the insured and dependent relatives, plus paid leave for sickness or accidents; they also reduced the contribution of the self-employed to 4% and, if they were associated, charged 2.5% to the public Regional Development Corporation (CORDES) and only 1.5% to the worker. The resulting reduction in revenue was to be compensated with part of the state's 1% contribution (IPSS, 1987b).

The 1987 draft regulations to incorporate peasants, including those working in agriculture and rural merchants and artisans, distinguished between the self-employed and the associated and between small and mid-sized operations. A self-employed small farmer was defined as one who worked between one to eight hectares or owned one to five head of cattle; a small artisan was defined as someone who worked for himself or with his family and did not have paid employees. A self-employed, mid-sized farmer was one who worked more than four or eight hectares of land or owned more than six head of cattle; a mid-sized artisan was one who hired paid employees. Associated peasants included those organized in cooperatives, communities, or other groups. The worker and his dependent family would be eligible for full health care protection, but was not entitled to paid leave. The program would be financed by a 4% contribution on the minimum insured compensation by the self-employed small operator and a 9% contribution by the self-employed mid-sized operator; if associated, CORDES would make a contribution, and the state also would contribute. Payments could be in cash, in kind, or in work, to be delivered either monthly or twice annually according to the type of work; the self-employed peasant would be directly responsible for payment, but the association would be responsible if peasants were grouped together. The selection of the rural locations to be covered would be done according to the following criteria: size of the population, road access, literacy, percentage of the EAP employed, type of ownership (enterprise or collective preferred over individual), type of production (for local or national markets preferred over self-consumption), incorporation into economic plans and sociopolitical associations, availability of health care infrastructure from IPSS and the Ministry), and percentage of the population already insured at IPSS. A system of 0 to 4 points was given, depending on whether or not the criteria were met; for example, zero points would be given if illiteracy was 100%, versus 3 points if literacy was 60% (IPSS, 1987a). Thus, the Peruvian criteria were opposite those used in Mexico, because the poorest communities were given the lowest rank.

In May 1988, IPSS still considered the extension of coverage feasible through the construction of 73 clinics, a substantial improvement in hospital and medical personnel productivity, more emphasis on primary health care, and the integration of IPSS and Ministry of Health services. The financial crisis that began in September 1988 made it painfully clear that the extension plans were too optimistic: the expansion of clinics was insufficient to absorb even the demand increase caused by including coverage of part of the dependent family; the integration with the Ministry became too costly for IPSS, because the latter had to raise the salaries of transferred Ministry personnel to equalize salaries with those of its own personnel, and it was halted; and the productivity of medical personnel and hospitals did not improve substantially. By the end of 1988, IPSS leaders informed a USAID-financed technical mission hired to facilitate the expansion, that it was not viable because of the crisis (Mesa-Lago et al., 1988c).

Although we lack comprehensive data to evaluate the results of the 1988 emergency plan, scattered information indicates that several of its measures have not been implemented—rather than decreasing, the number of IPSS employees increased by 8% in 1989; the government promised to start paying its debt to IPSS in 1989, but had yet to do so by the spring of 1990; the drastic cuts in personnel of the computerized system of registration and collection made it impossible to reduce evasion by and to collect debts from private employers; and a 3,000% rate of inflation in 1989 further eroded IPSS reserves and aggravated real negative investment yields ("La seguridad. . .," 1990).

IPSS's failure to control its crisis raises serious doubts about that institution's long-term capability to continue delivering adequate health care to its current users, let alone to expand such services to cover the poor.

Public Sector (Ministry of Health) Viability

Traditionally, the Ministry has had to serve a much larger population than IPSS, but has been assigned fewer resources to do that. Table 63 summarizes three comparisons, at different points in time and sometimes without comparable data, of the population covered by and resources of IPSS, the Ministry of Health, the armed forces, and the private sector. In 1981, the armed forces and the private sector had much higher shares of physicians—the private sector had a larger share of hospital beds as well—than both IPSS and the Ministry; IPSS, in turn, had proportionally more physicians and hospital beds in relation to its population than the Ministry. In 1984, the share of health expenditures of IPSS and the armed forces, in relation

Table 63. Comparison of health resources/facilities by provider in Peru, 1981–1987.

Providers	Percentage distributions (1981)			Percentage distributions (1984)		Ratios (1987)		
	Population covered	Hospital beds	Physicians	Population covered	Expenditures	Expenditures per capita (intis)	Physicians x 10,000	Consultations per capita
IPSS	17	16	21	18	41	1,616	7.55	1.12
Ministry of Health[a]	62	57	35	58[b]	34	200	4.33	0.47
Armed forces[a]	7	7	14	3	7	n.a.	n.a.	n.a.
Private	14	20	30	21[b]	18	n.a.	n.a.	n.a.
Total	100	100	100	100	100	n.a.	n.a.	n.a.

Sources: Zschock, 1988; Mesa-Lago, 1988c, 1989a.

[a] In 1981, other public institutions were clustered with the Ministry of Health, while in 1984, they were clustered with the armed forces.

[b] The original distribution assigned 26% to the Ministry of Health (actual population with access) and transferred to the private sector (originally 53%) all the Ministry of Health population without access (32%).

to their respective share of population, was more than 2 to 1, but the Ministry's share of expenditures in relation to its population share was 0.5 to 1. In 1987, expenditures per capita of IPSS were eight times higher than those of the Ministry, while the ratios of physicians and consultations were about twice as high in IPSS as in the Ministry. With such meager resources, the Ministry does not appear capable of extending real access to the poor; and yet, its model of health care is less expensive and more appropriate to the needs of the poor than that of IPSS.

The full impact of the 1980s economic crisis on the health care provided by the Ministry and IPSS cannot be measured because available comparable data are for 1981–1984, and so do not include the aggravation of the crisis in 1988–1989. The existing data suggest, however, that by 1984 the crisis had affected IPSS even more than the Ministry: total health care expenditures declined by 21% in IPSS, compared to a decline of 16% in the Ministry; in per capita terms, the declines were 33% and 17%, respectively. More recent information for IPSS indicates that total expenditures declined by 75% in 1981–1988. A comparison of the composition of expenditures between both institutions in 1981 and 1984 shows that the share of salaries and fringe benefits increased in both (19% in IPSS and 26% in the Ministry) at the expense of reducing the share of supplies such as medicines (mostly in the Ministry, for a decline of 33%) and, particularly, in the share of investment in physical plant (declines of 64% in IPSS and 30% in the Ministry). Investment in physical plant was paralyzed in both institutions after 1988, and the scarcity of medicines and other medical supplies reached a crisis level (Zschock, 1988; Mesa-Lago, 1988c; ''La seguridad. . .,'' 1990).

The USAID-financed study on expanding IPSS population coverage, conducted at the end of 1988, calculated how much it would cost to expand such coverage to various groups of the population with different health care packages. Incorporating informal workers and their dependent family into IPSS with full health care benefits (as mandated in the draft regulations) would cost $US309 million annually, while the estimated cost for incorporating peasants and their dependents was $US437 million annually. The incorporation of the two groups would cost $US746 million annually or twice the cost of the population already covered in 1988. If only IPSS first-level primary health care had been provided to both groups, the cost would have dropped to $US326 million annually, similar to the cost of the population already covered.

Informal workers and peasants have considerably lower incomes than the group currently covered by IPSS, and most of them are self-employed or unpaid family members. The IPSS health-maternity program suffered steady deficits in the 1980s, even with a group covered that has relatively high income and benefits from substantial employer contributions. The state was not able to honor its obligations as employer to IPSS, much less subsidize a massive expansion of the population covered. Therefore, the IPSS model of full health care coverage was judged unsuitable to cover the poor; provision of primary health care only, also through IPSS, would have cut costs by half, but still would have been unfeasible. However, if only medical consultation were provided, based on the much less expensive model of the Ministry's sanitary posts, the cost would have dropped to less than $US3 million annually. Although this service is quite limited, it still would be an improvement for the poor who lack any type of health care, particularly in rural areas. Furthermore, it would be financially viable. The conclusion of the study was that the Ministry of Health model, even with all its flaws, would be more suitable for providing coverage for the poor than the current IPSS model (Mesa-Lago, 1988c).

PRIVATE ALTERNATIVES OF HEALTH CARE FOR THE POOR

In the second half of the 1980s, there were various antagonistic positions in Peru concerning the state's role in the economy, but they coincided in questioning the viability of the current model of social security and health care to accomplish the task of universalization. The poor in the informal and rural sectors cannot finance their coverage under that model, and neither the state nor the formal sector is capable of subsidizing such coverage.

For the market-oriented Institute of Freedom and Democracy, the solution is to deregulate the economy, streamline the state apparatus, decentralize the administration, and eliminate barriers against the informal sector. According to this model, these changes would foster the informal sector's economic progress, which, blessed with increased income, would be able to contribute to social insurance or, even better, buy its health care from the private sector. The latter, in turn, would compete with IPSS, which would lose its monopoly and be forced to improve its efficiency. In short, the Institute maintains that there is no need to protect the poor in the informal and rural sectors, because the market, if allowed to function freely, would solve the problem on its own (De Soto, 1986). This position specifies neither how long it would take for the market to promote development and solve the problem nor what should be done in the meantime to provide health care to the poor.

Conversely, a state-oriented approach proposes to transform the informal and rural sectors through a government long-term plan that would create two million new productive jobs fueled with a state fund for credit and investment; part of the IPSS reserves would be used to that end. Planners estimate that in six years, the informal sector would contribute $US83 million to social insurance, and that in 25 years it would have paid the funds invested to create the jobs. Until the jobs are created, this model recommends changing the financing of social insurance by fixing the insured's and employer's contributions according to the enterprise's productivity. In this way, large and highly productive enterprises that have few workers and contribute little to social insurance would pay more, while small, labor-intensive enterprises with low productivity would contribute less (Vereda, 1988). This position does not explain how the productivity of the enterprise would be effectively measured, nor does it tackle the negative effect that this type of financing could have on productivity.

In 1988, President García, attempting to strike a middle ground, stated that the solution to the problem was to enforce Article 14 of the constitution to allow other institutions to compete with IPSS and for the population to freely select among various social insurance and health care providers; competition, in turn, would force IPSS to improve efficiency. Both public agencies and private corporations, as well as unions and cooperatives, could enter the market under state supervision; such alternative providers must offer additional or better-quality benefits than those already in existence; joining these new agencies would be entirely voluntary. Finally, 10% of the contributions collected by the new agencies would be transferred to IPSS, in order to help it to expand coverage to peasant communities, informal workers, the unemployed, and other groups unable to finance their own protection (García, 1988).

The presidential interpretation of Article 14 of the constitution has been criticized, using the argument that the article establishes the obligation and exclusiveness of the sole institution (IPSS) in charge of social insurance, and, therefore, it is not legally possible for the insured to withdraw their affiliation with IPSS and shift to another insurance agency. According to this interpretation, the article only allows public or private agencies to offer supplementary benefits to those already granted by IPSS (Montes, 1988). This interpretation is correct concerning those mandatorily covered by IPSS, but not for those who may join it voluntarily, such as informal workers and peasants who legally can freely select between IPSS and other providers.

In the political campaign for the 1990 presidential election, IPSS became the focus of heated discussions among contending political parties, although they agreed on the institution's inability to solve the nation's social security problems. There seems to be a consensus developing among contending groups that the state, through different ways, should help the informal sector to become an "engine of growth" and alleviate poverty. The expansion of IPSS coverage to informal workers and peasants, an important issue in the 1985 electoral campaign, received little or no attention in 1990. Conversely, privatization of social security became the main topic of discussion: the center-right coalition, FREDEMO, followed the Institute of Freedom and Democracy's ideas and endorsed the creation of a parallel private insurance system to eliminate the IPSS monopoly and infuse competition particularly in health delivery; the center-left and left parties either ratified the supplementary role of the private sector or rejected it altogether and requested a radical transformation of IPSS. Villa El Salvador was given as an example of how the state, even with a reduced role, could still help the informal sector to become the "engine of growth" ("La seguridad. . .", 1990; Annis and Frank, 1989). Because of its importance, Villa El Salvador's approach to health care is evaluated in a subsequent section.

General Review of Alternatives: Self-aid, Solidarity, NGOs

The vast majority of the poor who lack access to Ministry of Health services do not have enough savings or income to pay for private health care. They might resort to small loans from relatives or friends for that purpose; as most of them either live in the Andean highlands or come from there, they retain a tradition of extended family and intrafamily credit. It also has been reported that some of them are able to get "informal" care at IPSS services through their contacts with medical personnel. However, for the poor population of the Andean highlands, often the only available alternative is traditional medicine, or *curanderos*. The urban poor have many more options.

In Peru there is an informal protection system (also found in Jamaica) that reportedly has Indian roots; this mechanism, called *junta*, *bolsa* (purse), or *pandero*, can either be occasional or have some degree of permanence. For instance, informal shop-repair workers have organized into groups that raise funds with members' monthly contributions; the sum is awarded to those who suffer an accident or get sick or die. Another variation involves establishing a revolving fund awarded monthly in turns and through a lottery to the members, except when one of them faces exceptional expenses (usually for health care), in which case he or she has priority. In some neighborhoods such as San Martín de Porres and San Juan de Miraflores, there are written regulations concerning the fund and, in 1987, a meeting was held to promote it. Street vendors usually take up a collection in the area where they work to help one of them who is gravely ill or disabled, or to pay for a funeral. Leaders of two street vendor associations expressed their desire to establish a properly regulated solidarity fund to institutionalize the *juntas* and collections, but said they needed outside support for credit and training. These leaders were interested in holding a seminar on that issue, to which they would invite representatives of NGOs and insurance companies (Grompone, 1987; Mesa-Lago, 1990a).

There are very few mutual-aid organizations that provide health care. In the Hospital Francés, there is a "Health Club" that provides health care to members who pay a modest monthly fee set according to family size. An intriguing question is why there are no cooperatives or mutual-aid organizations to provide health care in Peru, as there are in Uruguay, despite a strong demand for low-cost health care services and an abundant supply of physicians, many of whom are either unemployed or underpaid. Some answers to that question were: distrust of the quality of the service, especially if the fee is low, a fear partly caused by previous cases of fraud (e.g., in Mutual Metropolitana, its administrators ran away with the funds); no credit and a lack of knowledge about

administration, accounting, and other necessary skills for establishing cooperatives; and cultural barriers, such as ethnicity, class, and status, between physicians and users. Several people interviewed suggested that the government or NGOs should provide credit and training to the physicians to enable them to start the co-ops. In 1988, it was reported that the Ministry of Health was planning to build consultation posts to be operated by young physicians, and that the Ministry of Housing was negotiating with the Medical Association to establish a credit program to fund them (Mesa-Lago, 1990a).

Very few of the country's 200 NGOs devoted to development, or the solidarity and mutual-aid groups, have health care as an objective. Some interesting examples are summarized below.

The Institute for Development of the Informal Sector is a private organization established in Lima in 1986 to promote credit, technical and managerial training, improvement of labor conditions, legal counseling, marketing, and health care and social security for informal workers. Since 1987, this Institute has operated a pilot project with UNICEF funding to train welfare assistants in health education and primary health care. Responding to a large number of requests from its 50,000 beneficiaries, in 1987 the Institute solicited bids from private insurance companies and one public insurance company for a popular family insurance package for the informal sector. The contract, awarded to the public company, offers protection to the workers and dependent relatives in case of death, disability, accident, and pregnancy, but not for illness. The premium is 2.38% of the minimum monthly income, equivalent to $US2 monthly, and pays from one to ten minimum monthly incomes according to the type of risk; the benefit is increased based on the minimum monthly income adjustment, and the insured is entitled to use the payment in various ways. For instance, a pregnant beneficiary can go to a Ministry of Health facility, to a private clinic, or to a midwife. Only government approval was needed to start this program, which was expected to cover 2,000 informal workers (Pinilla, 1987).

In 1988, the Center of Applied Economics planned to request from insurance companies the submission of group policies similar to the one above. The Center would select the two best policies and pass them to the most important federations of informal workers, which would democratically choose one for group coverage. The Center also considered, as a solution to the lack of sickness coverage, a program combining a private clinic, an insurance company, and a workers' association or union to provide health care for a reasonable monthly fee. Finally, there was the idea that existing credit cooperatives could manage popular pharmacies that would sell medicines at cost plus a small mark-up to guarantee the stability and growth of the program (Mesa-Lago, 1990a).

The Institute of Freedom and Democracy developed a project—which eventually became law—of "people's mortgage" (*hipoteca posesoria*); it allows squatters who possess a house but do not have legal ownership of the land where it is built, to receive mortgage loans using the house as collateral. Based on this credit program, insurance companies can offer policies including life insurance (to pay the mortgage in case of death of the insured), and sickness-accident insurance. These policies provide a basic minimum and offer additional benefits according to the insured's income and value of the collateral. From 60,000 to 180,000 families are expected to benefit from this program (Annis and Frank, 1989; Mesa-Lago, 1990a).

In 1981, the Program of Support to the Informal Sector organized the project *Alternativa* in San Martín de Porres, which has a population of 500,000, 40% of whom are informal workers, mostly street vendors. *Alternativa* offers programs of employment, training, legal counseling, aid to youngsters, and health care. In 1985, a federation of street vendors, the municipality of San Martín, and *Alternativa* established the Street Vendors' Health House (*Casa de Salud del Ambulante*), which provides disease prevention, health education, outpatient consultation, laboratory tests, training of health promoters, basic medicines at cost, control of TB and typhoid fever, treatment of some diseases (diarrheal, venereal and respiratory), infant-maternal care, and family planning. The medical personnel, three physicians and a midwife, are paid with donations from the Catholic Church, and the physicians, through personal contacts, arrange needed transfers of patients to Ministry of Health centers and hospitals.

Users report that there are no lines for consultations in the Health House and that its services are of higher quality than those provided by the Ministry post. And yet, initially, the number of users was low (a total of 100 consultations monthly for a daily average of one per physician/midwife), because the population did not know that the staff was made up of physicians and did not value the services because they were free. In 1988, physicians began to visit the street vendors' markets to interact with them and started to charge a symbolic nominal fee for their services: the monthly fee for the worker and his dependents was between 4% and 7% of that charged by private physicians for one consultation. *Alternativa* was planning a meeting on social security coverage of street vendors with the participation of their several federations as well as NGOs (Grompone, 1988; Mesa-Lago, 1990a).

The Example of Villa El Salvador

Peru has one of the fastest rates of urbanization in Latin America and the Caribbean, and in the last two decades, hundreds of "young towns" (*pueblos jóvenes*) have been established, mostly by rural migrants, and have grown rapidly. Usually, these shantytowns are pockets of poverty, although many of them have managed to gradually improve their living standards. Villa El Salvador is an outstanding case of a successful young town, not only for Peru but for many countries in the Region as well. It has earned a United Nations award and the prestigious Príncipe de Asturias award from Spain, was selected by Pope John Paul II for a much publicized visit, and is the recipient of significant international aid. In the field of health care, it is also a model that deserves analysis and replication.

History

Villa El Salvador began in 1971 when 500 families from an earthquake-ravaged city in the Andean highlands took over a parcel of land in the south of Lima, close to the current settlement. The military government at the time, led by Juan Velasco Alvarado, transferred the settlers to an 8,000-hectare stretch of beachfront desert that had been used for military maneuvers. The government designed the new community on the basis of self-government, democracy, and community participation at different levels: from the family, to the block, the neighborhood, the sector, and the district. The land was divided into four zones: an urban one for residences and commerce; a 1,000-hectare agricultural area for the cultivation of fruits, cotton, vegetables, tubers, and livestock forage; an industrial zone that initially was planned to hold large outside industries but which has been redesigned to relocate 1,000 small factories that operate in the community; and a recreational area along the beach.

Villa El Salvador's population rapidly organized an Urban Self-Governing Community (CUAVES) that basically governs the town. The basic CUAVES unit is the family, 24 families constitute a block, 16 blocks make up a residential group, 4 or 5 residential groups form a neighborhood (*barrio*), 22 residential groups compose a sector, and 4 sectors integrate a district. In addition, there are operational units in different functional areas, one of which is health. The representatives of each of these levels select their authorities, including an Executive Communal Council at the top of CUAVES. Supported by this strong central sociopolitical organization, the residents held meetings, organized marches to the presidential palace, and successfully demanded government help in building schools (200 at three levels), roads, and health care installations, as well as in hiring teachers and personnel. The community actively participated in the construction of many of these facilities.

UNDP, UNICEF, IAF, and many other international and charitable organizations, as well as foreign governments and national private organizations, have provided aid to Villa El Salvador. In 1983, it was granted municipal status, and the town elected its mayor, who has become a nationally known political figure. In 1985, Villa El Salvador elaborated a unified health plan that integrates all the town's health care activities. Finally, in 1988, the municipality developed a Popular Project of Integral Development that combines demographic, urban design, industrial, agricultural, commercial, educational, health, and nutritional policies (Equipo Técnico. . ., 1988; Robinson, 1988; Annis and Frank, 1989).

The Population of Villa El Salvador

The 2,000 people who founded the town in 1971 had increased to 250,000 inhabitants in 1988, and to 300,000 or 350,000 in 1990. The reasons for the growth in the 1980s have been the prolonged economic crisis, the heavy migration from poor departments (where guerrillas are active) such as Ayacucho, and the appeal of the town's success. In 1988, the Popular Project for Integral Development projected a population of 400,000 for 1996, but a more realistic projection is now 500,000 to 600,000.

Although the current population is not as poor as it was 20 years ago, one-fourth of its inhabitants still are close to indigence, and an additional unknown percentage are poor. According to a survey conducted by CUAVES in 1984 and a municipal review in 1988, 21% of the *families* earn less than $US360 annually—one-fourth of the national average *per capita* income in 1988—open unemployment and underemployment combined reach 60% of the EAP, 16% of housing is extremely poor, and 63% of family income is spent on food. About 71% of the population is under 25 years of age, 13% of the child population suffers from malnutrition, between 30% and 40% of the children have not been vaccinated against major infant diseases, most irrigation water is contaminated, almost 26% of deaths are caused by tuberculosis and pneumonia, and the most typical diseases are acute respiratory diseases and gastroenteritis. The labor force works either in Villa El Salvador or in metropolitan Lima, but very few have steady factory jobs or fixed salaries; most are in the informal sector, many of them working as street vendors or self-employed. There are about 500 microenterprises in the town that produce furniture, clothing, shoes, ceramics, or food, or are involved in repair and mechanical work (Equipo Técnico. . ., 1988; Grompone and Tuesta, 1988; Weber, 1989).

Health Facilities and Services

IPSS has no health care facilities in Villa El Salvador, an indication that very few of the town's inhabitants are insured. The Ministry of Health has four primary-level health centers and a health post, staffed by a total of 19 physicians and 10 nurses, plus an unknown number of health promoters from the community; local Ministry authorities have requested 10 additional physicians and 8 nurses, because the number of current personnel is considered grossly insufficient. Ministry services are predominantly curative, and include outpatient consultations; emergency and first aid; minor surgery; laboratory tests; special care of pregnant women and of children such as vaccination, growth monitoring, nutrition, and treatment of diarrhea; tuberculosis control and treatment; and family planning. Patients who cannot be attended to by the health centers are transferred to Ministry hospitals. The health centers do not provide child-delivery services (one of the centers has a delivery room but lacks the needed equipment); hence, most town women give birth at home aided by midwives, and those who need to be hospitalized must go to another town. User fees are charged by the health centers, but they are very low (Galindo, 1988).

The Villa El Salvador municipality does not provide curative care, but it operates three health posts that mainly offer prevention services; in addition, the municipality exercises sanitary control of commercial establishments that handle food (to control typhoid fever, hepatitis, and parasites) and provides milk to children (this program has been transferred to women's clubs); a tuberculosis asylum was being planned in 1988. At least two physicians work for the municipality (Injarte and Sattin, 1988).

Probably the most important health services in the town are those organized by CUAVES through 35 primary-level health care modules that were originally financed by UNICEF and were built in 1983–1984. The modules emphasize primary health care and target the infant-maternal population; they provide the following services: immunization against tuberculosis, polio, measles, and DPT, mostly to children and pregnant women; control of children's malnutrition, diarrhea, and respiratory diseases; and curative care, mostly for children. In addition, CUAVES has midwives who check pregnant women and care for them during childbirth. Medical personnel in the 35 units are supplied by various NGOs. Patients who require more complex treatment are sent to the Ministry health centers or to a nearby hospital.

Several NGOs provide health services in Villa El Salvador. One of the most important is the Institute of Health "Hugo Pesce," founded in 1982 as a private nonprofit association whose goal is to improve the health of slum dwellers in Lima's "young towns." This institution received financial aid from UNICEF and OXFAM (Great Britain) to launch successful community-managed health projects. In 1985, a group of four physicians who graduated from the medical school at Cayetano Heredia University, joined the Institute and later received support from IAF to pursue the following tasks at Villa El Salvador: integrate four technical teams, one physician and one nurse in each; train 40 residents selected by the community as health promoters to provide basic care; and participate in the community's public health campaigns. The Institute charges a very low user fee which is turned back to the community; one-half of its personnel have established residency in the town, have developed close links with the population and CUAVES, and have actively participated in the elaboration and implementation of the unified health plan. In late 1988, the Insti-

tute's team in the town consisted of four physicians, two nurses, one midwife, one nutritionist, and one health educator. At that point, they were sufficiently established in the community to form their own independent organization, the Institute for Support of Popular Health. One of its first activities was to organize a workshop in Lima to study affordable alternatives to offset the skyrocketing costs of medicines. With IAF support, the Institute for Support of Popular Health is now organizing a system of popular pharmacies in Villa El Salvador (Beirano et al., 1988; Weber, 1990).

Other NGOs that operate in the community are the Institute of Sciences for Health Development, organized by young Peruvian physicians and composed of six physicians and six nurses or paramedical personnel; the Institute for Ibero-American Cooperation, a joint operation between the Government of Spain and UNDP that has four physicians; the Latin American Lay Movement, a secular group that consists of two physicians and two nurses; Save the Children, a British organization with four physicians; and the Christian Community that operates several consulting posts with an unknown number of professionals. In addition, there are other minor Peruvian NGOs (CUAVES, 1986; Equipo Técnico..., 1988; Beirano et al., 1988).

In 1985, CUAVES, in cooperation with other organizations, elaborated the unified health plan to consolidate all the town's health services—Ministry of Health, CUAVES, Municipality, and NGOs—under a primary health care approach that aimed at avoiding duplication, maximizing existing facilities, evaluating past health activities, determining the health needs of the population, designing a program geared to families with high health risks, reducing infant-maternal morbidity and mortality, and improving the population's health standards. The town is divided into 15 health operation units, each one covering several residential groups of between 15,000 and 20,000 inhabitants. Each unit is served by about two health care modules and a technical team composed of one physician, one nurse, and several health promoters trained by the Ministry and by NGOs. The community is actively represented in each operation unit and, at the top, in the Health Council; medical personnel from NGOs are assigned to each of the units. The latter are expected to elaborate a diagnosis of the health needs and problems of the unit population and design a strategy to cope with them. In addition, there are topical commissions, integrated by representatives of all providers and popular organizations, that deal with specific issues such as pharmacy, nutrition, tuberculosis control, infant-maternal health, environmental sanitation, and development of human resources. These commissions elaborate concrete proposals to tackle specific problems and present them to the Health Council (CUAVES, 1986; Equipo Técnico. . ., 1988).

In the mid-1980s, the unified health plan conducted a census to classify all families into low, middle, or high health risk groups based on four factors: housing, food expenses, parents' education, and number of children under the age of 6. A system of points from zero (best) to 3 (worst) measured the degree of risk in each of the four factors. For example, a family living in a shanty house without water and with a very low food budget, illiterate parents, and three or more children was given 12 points and ranked as high risk. The census also gathered information on childrens' ages, weight, and vaccination record; pregnant women; and people with tuberculosis.

Based on the data gathered, the unified health plan developed several health programs. The child health program is geared to some 40,000 children below the age of 5 who are targets for vaccination (the Ministry supplies all the vaccines) and weight monitoring; since there is an unified system of immunization control cards, children who are not taken to health care facilities for vaccinations are immunized at home, and malnourished children are sent to a communal nutrition center for treatment and given nutritional supplements thereafter. In addition, the milk programs, now managed by women's clubs, provide milk powder and teach mothers to boil water to prevent diarrhea. The maternal health program is targeted to some 2,000 pregnant women who are also immunized; those at high obstetric risk are referred to Ministry facilities. The tuberculosis control program checks some 3,500 people suspected to have tuberculosis through laboratory tests, and refers those found to have the disease to Ministry facilities; an association of tuberculosis patients has successfully demanded jobs. A program to control diarrhea mobilized hundreds of students in an oral rehydration campaign. Finally, there is an antiparasitical program (CUAVES, 1986; Beirano et al., 1988).

Evaluation of Health Programs

The Villa El Salvador experience proves that relatively few health resources supplied by multiple providers can be successfully integrated to maximize their use and target the most urgent needs of the population. The public health sector in the community is primarily represented by the Ministry of Health, and, to a much lesser degree, by the Municipality; IPSS has no facilities. The Ministry plays a minor role in primary health care (8% of the health posts are municipal and only 2% are the Ministry's), but a fundamental role in curative care (75% of the installations belong to it). The Municipality emphasizes primary health care, but has few resources. There are no secondary or tertiary facilities in Villa El Salvador, and the closest Ministry hospital is in the neighboring town of San Juan de Miraflores. Conversely, the non-public sector emphasizes primary health care and operates 90% of the health posts or modules.

Slightly more than half of the community's medical personnel are furnished by the NGOs and emphasize primary health care; the remainder are in the public sector—mostly in the Ministry—and place more emphasis on curative care, except for the meager municipal personnel who focus on prevention and sanitation.

The town's human health resources do not compare favorably with national and departmental averages. For instance, Villa El Salvador has a ratio of 1.3 to 1.5 physicians per 10,000 inhabitants, compared with an IPSS ratio of 7.6 and a Ministry ratio of 4.3 (see Table 64). And yet, those scarce resources appear to be concentrated in primary health care, serving the needs of the population and targeting the groups at highest risk, such as children and pregnant women. Furthermore, a good number of community residents have been trained to serve as health promoters, filling some gaps in the professional staff. Practically all services are free or a very small user fee is charged and returned to the community. Finally, the community appears to be an active participant in health programs, identifying needs, proposing solutions, and managing key installations.

According to local reports, between 60% and 70% of all community children under 5 years of age have been immunized, and there is an ongoing effort to reactivate the vaccines and identify and immunize the remaining population. Acute diarrhea is reportedly reduced through the powdered milk supply, the increasing use of boiled water to prepare the formula, and the oral rehydration campaign. Significant efforts have been made to monitor and care for pregnant women, to identify and correct child malnutrition, and to control and treat tuberculosis.

Unfortunately, we do not have data to mea-

Table 64. Health care facilities and personnel at Villa El Salvador, by providers, Peru, circa 1988.

| Providers | Facilities at the primary level, with predominant: | | Medical personnel | | |
	Primary health care	Curative medicine	Physicians	Nurses	Others
Public	4	4	21	10	n.a.
Ministry of Health	1	4	19	10	n.a.
Municipality	3	0	2[a]	n.a.	n.a.
IPSS	0	0	0	0	0
Non-Public	36	1	23	11	7
CUAVES	35	0	0[b]	0[b]	0[b]
NGOs	0	0	23	11	7
Institute of Sciences and Health Development	0	0	6	4	2
Institute of Health "Hugo Pesce"/Institute for Support of Popular Health	0	0	4	2	3
Institute for Ibero-American Cooperation	0	0	4	2	2
Latin American Lay Movement	0	0	2	1	n.a.
Save the Children	0	0	4[a]	2[a]	n.a.
Others	1	1	3[a]	n.a.	n.a.
Total	40	5	44	21	n.a.

Sources: CUAVES, 1986; Equipo Técnico . . . , 1988; Beirano et al., 1988.
[a] Estimate.
[b] CUAVES' 35 health modules are staffed with NGO medical personnel and managed by the community.

sure the impact of all of these programs on the health care status of the Villa El Salvador population, particularly in the 1980s. We even lack accurate statistics on medical personnel and health promoters; data in Table 64 have been compiled from oral reports and estimates. It is, therefore, crucial to generate such data in order to assess the effects of this approach.

The town's health programs are not exempt from problems; most are related to the different health philosophies of the providers, the scarcity and quality of personnel, conflicts among organizations, and flaws in community participation. The insufficiency of medical personnel, lack of installations at the secondary and tertiary levels, and lack of child delivery care have already been noted. The Ministry health centers have a meager budget and a heavy load, making it difficult for their personnel to participate in the unified health plan; it also has been claimed that partisan politics has been a reason for such behavior. The Ministry's emphasis on curative medicine might be another reason for its lukewarm participation in the primary health care activities led by CUAVES and the NGOs. It has also been said that all Ministry physicians are from outside Villa El Salvador and none live in town or have close contact with the population. Some of the NGOs lack sufficient medical personnel, or they are improperly trained or have not become fully integrated into the unified health plan. The number of health promoters is insufficient and has declined in recent years. Furthermore, the Ministry and CUAVES frequently have been involved in confrontations; the former reportedly wanted the health modules operated by CUAVES and the latter is perceived by Ministry authorities as too militant and radical. The Municipality reportedly has accepted decisions without proper consultation with the community and other organizations. There have been communication problems between local leaders of residential groups and the Communal Executive Council, there are many residential groups without leaders, and there has been a lack of coordination in several activities (CUAVES, 1986; Beirano et al., 1988; Galindo, 1988; Equipo Técnico. . ., 1988). Even with these problems and with the need to have more accurate data to conduct a thorough assessment, the Villa El Salvador experience in health care emerges as a successful example of a community's mobilization to provide minimal health care for the urban poor.

DOMINICAN REPUBLIC

POVERTY: SIZE, TRENDS, AND CHARACTERISTICS

The ECLAC surveys on poverty in Latin America did not include the Dominican Republic. The only national data available are from two surveys on income and expenditures. The first, conducted in 1976–1977, fixed the poverty line based on income per capita; it estimated poverty incidence among households at 29% (15% urban and 40% rural) and among the total population, at 36% (20% urban and 47% rural) (Musgrove, 1986a).

The second survey, conducted in November 1984, did not estimate poverty incidence. The survey categorized households according to four income groups, the poorest 40% of which received less than 345 pesos per month ($US125) and, with an average of five members per household, per capita income was 69 pesos ($US25); the minimum monthly wage in November was 175 pesos ($US63). These figures indicate that about 40% of the households were below the poverty line; the proportion of urban households below the poverty line was 26.4%, while that of rural households was 54.4% (Del Rosario and Gámez, 1988). Although the 1976–1977 and the 1984 survey findings are not strictly comparable, they suggest that poverty was on the rise.

Surveys conducted in Santo Domingo, the capital city, in the early 1980s, also suggest that poverty incidence increased. In 1980, 38% of the *employed* EAP received an income below the minimum wage of 125 pesos ($US99) considered as the poverty line. In 1983, the incidence was about the same, but when the minimum wage was adjusted to inflation (151 pesos or $US94), the proportion below the poverty line increased to 48%. If the 21.4% of open unemployment in the capital city is added to that percentage, the potential EAP below the poverty line could have reached 69% in 1983 (Duarte, 1986; Kleinekathoefer, 1987).

A survey on household demand for health care conducted in Santo Domingo in October–December 1987, categorized households into three "socioeconomic residential strata" (low, middle, and high), according to characteristics such as the percentage of household expenditures for food and absence of piped water. In addition, the survey identified three household income groups: the lowest group, considered "very poor," had a monthly income below 400 pesos ($US105) or 85 pesos ($US22) per family member. In September of that year, the minimum wage had been raised to 350 pesos ($US92), a sum grossly insufficient to meet the basic needs of an average family of 4.7 members. More than half of the low stratum and 42% of all households had an income below that level (Gómez, 1988). According to the 1983 survey cited above, 48% of *individuals* received an income lower than the minimum wage, but the 1987 survey found that 42% of *households* had a combined income below that minimum. Hence, poverty incidence of the population must have been considerably higher in 1987, still another indication of growing poverty.

The World Bank has reported a poverty incidence in the Dominican Republic (at some point between 1977 and 1986) of 45% urban and 43% rural (Psacharopoulos, 1989), but did not specify the date, methodology, or source of such estimates. The urban poverty incidence given by the Bank is commensurate with the 1983–1987 estimates for Santo Domingo, as well as with other indicators of the country's development, but the rural incidence appears too low when contrasted with the 1976–1977 and 1984 estimates. To the best of my knowledge, there are no estimates of Dominican indigence.

The previous information on poverty incidence, when applied to the total population, results in very rough estimates of 1.9 million poor in 1976–1977, 2.4 million in 1984, and 2.9 million in 1986. Although accurate comparisons are not possible, the previous data indicate that poverty incidence in the Dominican Republic in the 1980s was higher than in eight of the ten Latin American countries surveyed by ECLAC.

In 1970–1980, the Dominican economy grew at a healthy annual GDP growth rate of 6.9% (4.2% per capita due to very high population growth), but the economic crisis brought on a slowdown to 2.7% in 1981–1989 (0.2% per capita). Open unemployment was quite high before the crisis, averaging 24% in the 1970s in Santo Domingo, and reaching 27% in 1985 (other sources report a decline in the second half of the 1980s), while underemployment jumped to 43%. In 1983, close to two-thirds of the labor force in the capital was either unemployed or underemployed. The annual rate of inflation, very low in the 1970s, increased to 7.4% in 1981–1983, and soared to 33% in 1984–1989. The real minimum wage declined 13% in 1980–1988.

As public social expenditures were cut and the public health budget was halved in real terms in 1982–1985, health standards deteriorated. The economic crisis of the 1980s had less of a negative impact on economic growth in the Dominican Republic than in most Latin American and Caribbean countries, and yet, the vigorous economic expansion of the 1970s could not significantly reduce unemployment or underemployment, nor increase the standard of living. The crisis aggravated social conditions and increased poverty incidence in the 1980s (Kleinekathoefer, 1987; ECLAC, 1989, 1989a, 1989b; Lewis et al., 1990).

The Urban (Informal) Sector

From 1960 to 1988, the proportion of the population living in urban areas increased from 30.5% to 52%; the annual growth rate of Santo Do-

mingo in 1960–1988 was the highest in the Region. Between 1960 and 1981, the percentage of the EAP engaged in agriculture and livestock declined from 66% to 24%, sparking a strong rural to urban migration that led to the rapid rate of urbanization. The proportion of the tertiary sector increased from 42% to 59% in 1970–1981. Most of the migrants joined the ranks of the informal sector, which rapidly expanded, particularly in Santo Domingo. The capital's share of the total population increased from 12% to 28.5% in 1960–1983, and in the last year, Santo Domingo's EAP employed in the tertiary sector was 69% (Duarte, 1986; ECLAC, 1989a; IDB, 1989; Reyes, 1990).

As noted, the urban poverty incidence was estimated at 20% of the population in 1976–1977 (less than one-half of the rural incidence) but at 45% between 1977 and 1986 (slightly higher than rural incidence). In Santo Domingo, poverty incidence ranged from 42% to 48% in 1983–1987. With the rapid process of urbanization and economic deterioration, the percentage of the total poor living in urban areas must have continued to increase.

According to PREALC, the informal sector grew from 8.5% in 1950 to 16% in 1980. In the latter year, 77% of Santo Domingo's poor—defined as those earning less than the minimum wage—worked in the informal sector (Tokman, 1980; PREALC, 1982). Surveys of the employed EAP in Santo Domingo estimated the informal sector at 38.6% in 1980, including 11.4% domestic service, increasing to 45% in 1983, with 11.6% domestic servants. Within the employed informal sector in 1983 (excluding domestic servants), 48.5% were self-employed (compared with 2% in the modern government sector), 18% were pieceworkers probably working at home, 14.3% were seasonal workers, 8.9% were salaried stable workers, 4% were unpaid relatives, and 6% were employers. Almost 82% of all domestic servants were wage earners. The distribution of the combined informal and domestic service sector in 1983 was as follows: 42.3% in services, including all domestic servants; 29.4% in commerce; 12.4% in manufacturing; 8.4% in construction; 4.7% in transportation; and 2.8% in other activities. About 89% of new houses in Santo Domingo in 1970–1980 were built by the informal sector.

In 1980, 49.4% of informal workers and 95.7% of domestic servants earned less than the minimum wage or were below the poverty line, compared with 28.7% in the modern sector; in 1983, the proportion had risen to 56% among informal workers and had declined slightly to

94.8% among domestic servants, compared to 39% in the modern sector (Duarte, 1986). The self-employed were, without a doubt, the largest segment of the informal sector in Santo Domingo in 1983, followed by pieceworkers, seasonal workers, employers, and domestic servants. There are no disaggregated income data for these groups, except for domestic servants. Even if one considers that a portion of the domestic servant's payment is in kind, this group probably suffered one of the highest poverty incidences.

Scanty available information also suggests that about one-fifth of employers are poor. In 1989, there were 145,000 microenterprises in the Dominican Republic that employed 400,000 workers, for an average employment of 2.8 workers: 50% of the enterprises employed only one worker and 21% employed two; 54% of these enterprises were in commerce, 31% in services, and 18% in manufacturing. More than half of the microenterprises lacked an official license or authorization, and neither paid taxes nor social insurance contributions (Reyes, 1990; Lizardo, 1990).

The 1976–1987 surveys provide information on the characteristics of the urban poor. In 1984, 32.5% of all urban poor in the EAP were openly unemployed, and of those employed in 1987, 44% were self-employed, domestic servants, or unpaid family workers. The remaining 56% were salaried employees; however, many of them had no labor contracts, hence, the large majority of the urban poor were in the informal sector. In 1981, about 59% of marginal urban workers in Santo Domingo were migrants, peasants, and landless farmers; in 1983, 41% of all employed males and 53% of all employed females were in the informal sector.

In 1976–1977, 44% of the poor were illiterate, and in 1984, 64% of the urban poor had no formal education. In the latter year, the urban poor lived in 82% of all existing "rustic" or "improvised" housing; 62% of urban poor homes lacked toilets (16% had neither toilets nor latrines); 78% of homes were not connected with a sewage system and 59% either used an outside rustic latrine or lacked any system of excreta disposal; and 45% lacked running water. In 1976–1977, the urban poor consumed 51% of the minimum recommended daily caloric intake and only 48% of the recommended level of protein (Consejo Nacional de Población y Familia, 1985; Duarte, 1986; Musgrove, 1986a; Kleinekathoefer, 1987; Gómez, 1988; Del Rosario and Gámez, 1988; Lewis et al., 1990).

The 1970 and 1981 censuses did not gather information on health status, which, combined with income, would have allowed us to describe the health status of the poor in urban and rural areas. However, the population's overall health standards in the Dominican Republic are among the worst in the Region (see the section on "Impact on Overall Health Standards," beginning on p. 168); therefore, health care for the poor would be expected to be below the national average.

The Rural Sector

Despite the rapid urbanization, in 1988, 41% of the Dominican Republic's population still lived in rural areas, proportionally the tenth largest in Latin America and the Caribbean. Rural poverty incidence was 47% in 1976–1977, and was roughly estimated at 54% in 1984; the 43% rural poverty incidence reported by the World Bank between 1977 and 1986, is probably an underestimation.

Income distribution data for 1976–1977 indicate that income was more even in rural than in urban areas; still, the average income of the rural poor was 20% lower than that of the urban poor; the lowest income in the rural sector was earned by those who only had income from agriculture, 76% of whom were poor. In 1981, there were 188,000 landless peasants and 61,000 small farms averaging 0.2 hectares that could not support the household for half of the year; about 83% of agricultural farmers owned only 13% of the total agricultural land. The 1984 national survey found that 54.4% of all rural households were in the lowest income category, compared with 26.4% among urban households.

In the early 1980s, the total rural population had the following standards, compared with the urban population (in parentheses): illiteracy 41.5% (18.4%), access to piped water 34% (85%), electricity 10.7% (76.3%), nutritional standards below PAHO-set levels 75% (25%), and underemployment 60% (43%) (Oficina Nacional de Estadística, 1980–1983; Moya, 1984; Consejo Nacional de Población y Familia, 1985; Musgrove, 1986a).

According to the 1984 national survey, the rural poor had a 27% unemployment rate, 98% of their homes lacked toilets and either used an outside rustic latrine or did not have a system of excreta disposal, and 67% lacked easy access to potable water. In 1976–1977, the rural poor consumed only 64% of the recommended minimum caloric intake and 54% of the recommended protein (Consejo Nacional de Población y Familia, 1985; Del Rosario and Gámez, 1988).

A comparison of the country's 30 provinces in 1986 showed that the least developed, most rural provinces had the lowest coverage by social insurance, the highest infant mortality rate, and the highest incidence of some diseases related to poverty such as gastroenteritis. The opposite was true of the most developed urbanized provinces (based on Oficina Nacional de Estadística, 1985–1987; Isuani, 1989).

HEALTH CARE COVERAGE OF THE URBAN (INFORMAL) AND RURAL POOR

Administrative Structure and Legal Coverage

Health care in the Dominican Republic is organized in three broad sectors: social insurance, public, and private.

The Dominican Institute of Social Security (IDSS) was established in 1947–1948, and it currently includes sickness-maternity, pension, and employment injury programs. The sickness-maternity program legally covers a tiny proportion of the population: private-sector blue-collar workers regardless of their wage level, and private-sector white-collar employees and employees of state industrial and commercial corporations whose salaries were not higher than 793 pesos ($US125) in 1989. The salary ceiling has been changed almost annually since 1985 due to rapid inflation, but remained unchanged from 1979 to 1985. The ceiling, therefore, excludes medium- and high-salaried white-collar workers, and, since the ceiling has lagged behind inflation, the segment excluded from coverage has steadily risen. Note that most civil servants, even those below the ceiling, are excluded from IDSS coverage. The active insured are divided into two categories: those with "stable" or fairly permanent jobs and those with "mobile," temporary, or seasonal employment. A large but declining proportion of the labor force is in the second category. There is no information on the average period of time that covered temporary workers have access to IDSS health care services, and the period without coverage could be significant.

The IDSS law includes domestic servants,

homeworkers, and apprentices, but in practice virtually all are excluded. Domestic servants working for enterprises and businesses such as hotels, are legally covered, but not those working in private homes. During IDSS's first decade of operation, several decrees temporarily postponed the mandatory incorporation of these workers, but the period of postponement set by the last decree expired in 1959. The self-employed are excluded from coverage, but the insured who become unemployed are protected for three months after dismissal. IDSS coverage of dependents, one of the most restricted in Latin America and the Caribbean, is limited to the legal wife on maternity (but not sickness) and the female insured's children on pediatric care and for only one year after birth. Most Dominican couples are not legally married, and common-law wives are excluded, as are all male spouses even if legally married and disabled. Children of male insureds whose wives are not insured also are excluded. Disabled pensioners are protected by the sickness-maternity program, but not old-age pensioners; the latter's average monthly pension in 1987 was 111 pesos ($US29), rendering them unable to pay for private health care. Because of this situation, some 40% of insured who are 60 years of age and older keep working beyond retirement age, thus reducing job opportunities in an economy with extremely high unemployment (Mesa-Lago, 1986b). The employment injury program is limited to occupational accidents and does not provide health care for labor-induced diseases.

The IDSS sickness-maternity program is essentially curative; it provides general and specialized outpatient consultation, surgery, hospitalization, medicine, and dental care and offers practically no prevention services. The insured are entitled to paid sick leave and, if female, to paid maternity leave, both at half salary. There is a nursing allowance payable for 12 months after the birth of the female insured's child. The law allows for free choice of health care in IDSS-owned facilities or in private clinics under contract, but given IDSS's poor record on reimbursement, practically no private facilities are currently under contract (Duarte, 1986; Isuani, 1989).

In 1982, under a new government administration, the President, three of the major trade unions, and the main employer association endorsed a legislative draft to expand IDSS health care coverage to all salaried workers in both the private and public sectors regardless of their salaries; the self-employed, domestic servants, home workers, unpaid family workers, and members of production cooperatives; and spouses (including common-law unions) and children below 18 years of age, as well as for occupational diseases. However, a last minute version of the legal draft restricted care to IDSS-owned facilities, which are notoriously insufficient and of very poor quality, thus eliminating free choice to use private facilities. The strong opposition of the private sector defeated the legal draft in Congress (see the section on "General Factors," beginning on p. 160), and since then, there has been no new serious attempt at expanding IDSS coverage.

Since 1982, the armed forces and the police have had an independent social insurance institution (ISSFAPOL), whose sickness-insurance program has broader coverage than IDSS's. It includes all active and retired members, as well as their dependent spouses, single children—males until they turn 18, or 25 if they are students and females with no age limit—and parents. Benefits are similar to those provided by IDSS, but the quality of these services is reportedly better.

The population not covered by social insurance and similar programs is entitled to health care by the Secretary of Public Health and Social Assistance (SESPAS). According to the Constitution, SESPAS must provide free medical and hospital care to the poor, but in practice, this institution lacks enough resources to do so. Furthermore, with the budget cuts suffered in the 1980s, user fees are being charged mainly for outpatient consultation and diagnostic services, but seldom for inpatient services (see the section on "User Fees," beginning on p. 171). Data to be discussed in the next two sections show that most of the poor are probably not covered by SESPAS.

The bulk of SESPAS expenditures has concentrated on curative medicine; however, in 1975–1986, SESPAS launched various programs that targeted rural and marginal urban areas and emphasized primary health care and prevention. With substantial external support, SESPAS built health subcenters in small towns, suburban clinics in large cities, and rural clinics. Taking advantage of a huge surplus of physicians, a compulsory one-year service was established for new graduates to work in the new SESPAS installations as *pasantes*; in addition, there were thousands of promoters from the communities, paramedic personnel, and supervisors hired by SESPAS. Unfortunately, these programs suffered from administrative inefficiencies, and it is unclear what effects they had (see the section on "Impact on Overall Health

Standards," beginning on p. 168). In addition, the 1982–1985 economic crisis caused the SESPAS budget to be severely cut. Although only a small proportion of the SESPAS budget was devoted to these new programs, the budget cuts probably damaged them (Ugalde, 1984, 1988; Gómez Ulloa, 1985; Lewis et al., 1990).

Other public-sector health-related institutions include the National Institute of Potable Water and Sewage; CARE, which distributes food in rural clinics and some nutrition centers; and the Program of Essential Medicines, established in 1984 as a separate but SESPAS-dependent agency to purchase drugs and medical supplies wholesale locally and abroad through a supposedly competitive bidding process. These products are distributed to SESPAS facilities nationwide, as well as to popular pharmacies (*boticas populares*). Medicines should be sold below the commercial price based on purchasing price plus operation expenses and a small profit, hence benefiting poor and low-income groups (see the section on "Public Sector (SESPAS) Viability," beginning on p. 164).

IDSS's low population coverage and the poor quality of its services, as well as those of SESPAS, have led to a remarkable development of the private health sector. The latter sector comprises three major types of providers: *Igualas*, payment plans similar to HMOs that provide diverse packages of services through affiliated clinics and physicians for a monthly fee; health insurance companies that reimburse health expenditures, based on different packages, for a premium; and NGOs such as the Dominican Red Cross and religious and charitable institutions. The first two types are basically inaccessible to the poor (but see) the section "Extending Coverage of the Poor through Private Pre-Payment Plans (Igualas)," beginning on p. 178), while the third usually provides free services to them.

Most civil servants, who are not covered by IDSS, are protected through the private sector largely financed by the state. For instance, in the mid-1980s, 63 state agencies were covered by HMOs. Some groups of well-organized workers such as teachers, port workers, drivers, and hotel and restaurant workers have their own health services or contracts with the private sector. In 1985, public-school teachers successfully opposed their incorporation into IDSS and exercised their power to obtain a special health care program that provides coverage to spouses and children below the age of 18; 75% of the program is financed by the Government. Skilled workers employed in large enterprises also have obtained medical insurance through collective agreements (Duarte, 1986; Isuani, 1989). A large proportion of the insured at IDSS also are covered by private services through collective agreements, *igualas*, or direct purchasing, because of the poor quality of IDSS services; consequently, they enjoy double coverage while a large proportion of the population, including the poor, remains unprotected (Duarte et al., 1989).

There is practically no coordination—much less integration—of health care institutions in the Dominican Republic. According to the law, SESPAS should have a coordinating role at least within the public sector, but in practice it has not exercised such leadership. There were national health plans elaborated from 1963 through 1986, but none were implemented. The law does not regulate the private health sector, and although theoretically private clinics and similar facilities should register with SESPAS, they have never done so; there might even be physicians who perform services without permission or registration (Oficina Nacional de Planificación, 1983; Gómez Ulloa, 1985; Guzmán, 1986).

To summarize, although the poor legally are entitled to health care coverage by SESPAS, this institution lacks the resources for this task, and the 1980s economic crisis reduced its capacity even more. The poor are not legally covered by IDSS—since all self-employed, most domestic servants, unpaid family workers, and home-workers are excluded—nor by special programs that protect civil servants and groups of the labor aristocracy, nor by enterprise medical insurance. The high cost of private services largely made them inaccessible to the poor, but, as will be seen, some are forced to make sacrifices and buy some of these services. Traditional medicine, quite important in the Dominican Republic, and a few charitable institutions may be the only alternatives for many poor.

Statistical Coverage

The Dominican Republic's statistics on health care coverage of the population are the worst among the five case studies and probably throughout the Region except for Haiti. Table 65 presents rough estimates for population coverage nationally and in Santo Domingo. The only available statistical series are from IDSS, and these have some problems: for instance, only the active insured (contributors) are reported, and the number of dependents is unknown, because there has been no registration of dependents for more than two decades. In some actuarial studies, dependents have been calculated at the national level with a ratio of 0.36 per one insured, but estimates for covered dependents in Santo Domingo, which are based on more

Table 65. Rough estimates of population coverage (national and Santo Domingo) on health care in the Dominican Republic, 1986–1987.

	National: circa 1986			Santo Domingo: 1987	
	(000)	% of population covered		(000)	% of population covered
Population	6,565	—	Population	1,743	—
Insured	1,932	19.9	Insured	601	34.5
IDSS[a]	276	4.2	IDSS[a]	153	8.8
ISSFAPOL[b]	262	4.0	ISSFAPOL[b]	62	3.6
Private[c]	1,394	11.7	Teachers[e]	24	1.4
Covered by SESPAS[d]			Private[c]	362	20.7
Lowest	2,626	40.0	Covered by SESPAS	663	38.0
Highest	3,939	60.0	Total covered	1,264	72.5
Total covered			Noncovered	480	27.5
Lowest	4,558	59.9			
Highest	5,333	79.9			

Sources: Author's estimates based on ECLAC, 1989a; Isuani, 1989; Duarte et al., 1989; La Forgia, 1990c.

[a]National includes active insured (266,102) and a rough estimate of 10,350 dependent wives and children. Santo Domingo's insured are 147,708 and the 5,744 estimated dependents were based on numbers of noninsured females' deliveries (2,200) and children born alive within the year (3,544). The ratio of dependents/insured in the capital (0.039 to 1) was used to estimate the national coverage of dependents.

[b]National includes insured and dependents. Santo Domingo probably only insured; using a hypothetical dependent/insured ratio of 2 to 1, the total number insured would be 186,000 or 10.7% of the capital's population.

[c]Insured and dependents; at the national level includes 210,000 civil servants; in Santo Domingo limited to the largest *igualas* and insured companies; the total should be much higher.

[d]Legally, SESPAS should cover all the noninsured population (80%), but most experts and officials report a "real" coverage of 40%; others report "real" coverage ranging from 50% to 60% of the population.

[e]Includes 7,960 insured and 13,368 dependents. In the national panel, this group is probably included under private insurance. In 1989, a total (national) of 103,000 teachers were reported.

Table 66.   Active insured in the IDSS sickness-maternity program, Dominican Republic, 1978–1986 (in thousands and percentages).

| | EAP (1) | IDSS insured | | | | | | % of EAP covered | | |
		Total (2)	%	Permanent (3)	%	Temporary (4)	%	2/1	3/1	4/1
1978	2,008	231	100.0	107	46.5	123	53.5	11.4	5.3	6.1
1980	2,112	244	100.0	138	56.4	106	43.6	11.5	6.5	5.0
1982	2,271	220	100.0	143	65.1	77	34.9	9.7	6.3	3.4
1985	2,529	274	100.0	181	65.9	93	34.1	10.8	7.2	3.6
1986	2,616	266	100.0	209	78.5	57	21.5	10.2	8.0	2.2

Sources: Author's estimates based on Duarte, 1986; Oficina Nacional de Estadística, 1987; ECLAC, 1989a; Isuani, 1989.

realistic data on child delivery, give a ratio of only 0.039 per one insured. It should be recalled that only legal wives are covered for maternity and female insured's children below one year of age for pediatrics. Table 65 shows that, in 1986, only 4.2% of the national population (but 8.8% of the capital's population) was covered by IDSS, probably the lowest coverage among all Latin American social insurance institutes (see Table 7).

Table 66 presents the IDSS series of active insured divided into permanent and temporary workers. The peak in total coverage was reached in 1980 with 11.5% of the EAP covered—tied with El Salvador for the lowest rank in the Region (Table 7)—but due to the economic crisis, coverage declined to 9.7% in 1982. The economic recovery during the second half of the 1980s induced a modest increase in coverage, but it did not reach the 1980 figure; apparently, there was a decline in the total number of active insured in 1986. The share of permanent insured in the total steadily increased from 46% to 78% in 1978-1986. Note that in the midst of the crisis, the number of permanent insured kept growing, although at a very low rate, but the number of temporary insured declined sharply; in 1986, the latter was less than half of what it was in 1978. Chances are that there are very few poor insured in IDSS, but if there are any, they should be in the temporary group, which steadily declined from 54% to 22% of the total in 1978-1986.

The distribution of active permanent insured in 1986 shows that 53% were in manufacturing; 20% in commerce; 18.7% in services, mostly government corporations, finance, and insurance; 3.7% in agriculture, mostly large modern plantations and agri-business; and the remaining 4.6% in mining, construction, and transportation. The low percentages in agriculture, construction, and personal services, where the poor are concentrated, indicate that they are largely excluded. This is confirmed by analyzing the degree of population coverage (active perma-

nent insured) by province in 1986. While the national average was 3.2%, the most developed provinces had considerably higher coverage: 11.7% in La Romana (site of a United States-owned sugar mill and tourist complex), 10% in San Pedro Macorís (one of the most developed provinces), 5.3% in the National District (Santo Domingo), and 4.9% in Santiago (where the second largest city is located). The 17 least developed, most rural provinces had degrees of coverage ranging from 0.04% to 0.9% (author's estimates based on Isuani, 1989).

Several studies have roughly calculated that armed forces personnel and their dependents covered in ISSFAPOL represent between 1.5% and 4% of the total population (Gómez Ulloa, 1985; Del Rosario and Gámez, 1988; Duarte et al., 1989; Rodríguez-Grossi, 1989). Table 65 indicates that in 1986 such coverage was 4% nationally and 3.6% in Santo Domingo; however, the latter probably excluded dependents. If they were included, ISSFAPOL's coverage of the population in · the capital should have been higher than 10%. Public teachers and their dependents added 1.4% to insurance coverage in Santo Domingo.

Private insurance coverage has been estimated from 10% to 12% of the total population, with the proportion of those in *igualas* being slightly higher than those covered by insurance companies (Del Rosario and Gámez, 1988; Gómez, 1988; Duarte et al., 1989). Table 65 gives a national estimate of 11.7% for 1986; however, for the capital city this figure was 20.7% in 1987, despite the fact that not all private providers were included and thus the actual proportion should have been higher.

The population insured by IDSS, ISSFAPOL, and the private sector is estimated in Table 65 as 20% of the total population and 34.5% of the capital's population, but the latter would be higher if dependents insured in ISSFAPOL and all private providers were accounted for. Therefore, there is a strong concentration of insured and of health resources in Santo Domingo. In

1987, the capital's population was 27% of the national population, but concentrated 55% of IDSS insured, 52% of expenditures, 65% of personnel, 51% of physicians, and 40% of hospital beds; 40% of SESPAS hospital beds and 58% of its physicians; 55% of ISSFAPOL physicians; and 64% of private clinical beds and 69% of private physicians (Duarte et al., 1989).

Legally, all of the uninsured population (80% nationally and 66% in Santo Domingo) should be cared for by SESPAS. Unfortunately, there are no statistics on SESPAS's actual coverage, but rough estimates range from 40% to 60% (USAID, 1975; Oficina Nacional de Planificación, 1983; Gómez Ulloa, 1985; Gómez, 1988). In 1986, SESPAS's Under Secretary for Administration candidly told me that SESPAS did not know what the actual coverage was, but that it might be between 40% and 60% (Guzmán, 1986). Data on SESPAS's coverage in Santo Domingo, where access must be higher, were given as 38% in 1987, below the lowest estimate of coverage at the national level.

Based on the above information, Table 65 roughly estimates the noncovered national population in 1986 as between 20% and 40% (the highest estimate probably being more realistic than the first) and 28% in Santo Domingo. Of those covered, from 80% to 85% were in the public sector and social insurance, and from 15% to 20% in the private sector. As we saw in the first section, between 1977–1986, poverty incidence was estimated at between 36% and 48% at the national level and between 38% and 48% in Santo Domingo. Although we cannot ascertain that all the poor are not covered, these figures strongly suggest that at least most of them are not. The lack of data makes it impossible to assess coverage of the poor separating urban and rural areas.

Real Access and Utilization

Some of the surveys conducted at the national level and in the capital have gathered data on access to health care by occupation or income group, which allows for a better evaluation of the protection of the poor. A 1981 survey found that large industrial enterprises mainly hired skilled workers; 94% of them were protected by collective agreements and 71% enjoyed medical insurance provided by the enterprise. Conversely, only 6% of construction workers had private medical insurance. A 1983 survey among home domestic servants (who are not

covered by IDSS) found that only 35% of them had health care paid by their employers (Duarte, 1986).

According to the four income groups used in the 1984 national survey classification, during the two weeks prior to the survey, 11% of the population—9% in the poorest income group—sought health care. Of these, 7.5% were insured at IDSS, ISSFAPOL, enterprises, and the private sector, a proportion considerably smaller than the 20% estimated as insured in Table 65. In the lowest income group (poor), only 3% of those who sought care were insured, 5% in the urban zone and 2% in the rural zone; that percentage increased with income, reaching 24% in the highest income group. Of the total who sought care, 63% received it in the private sector and 37% in the public sector, including social insurances; these proportions are the inverse of the 80%–85% public and 15%–20% private estimated in Table 65. In the lowest income group, the proportions in the 1984 survey were 42% private and 58% public, compared with 90% and 10% in the highest income group. Predictably, as income increased, a higher proportion of the population used private services, and as income decreased, a higher percentage of the population used public services. Still, it is surprising to find that 42% of the poor paid for private care, and that more did in the rural area (45%) than in the urban area (38%), especially considering that only 1.5% of all the poor who resorted to private services received free care through NGOs. The reason for the poor seeking private services no doubt was related to the unavailability or poor quality of public services, basically those of SESPAS. The lowest income group spent one-tenth of the highest income group's expenditures on health care, but still it cost the former 12% of its median income for a monthly average health expenditure of 20.66 pesos ($US7.54). Because few of the poor were insured in IDSS or by private companies, they only spent 0.14 pesos monthly for contribution/premium. The bulk of the contributions to IDSS (89%) was paid by the two middle income groups, while most of the premiums to insurance corporations and *igualas* (88%) were paid by the upper-middle and highest income groups (Del Rosario and Gámez, 1988).

Based on the 1987 survey of Santo Domingo, this city's population has been classified into three income groups. Almost 42% of the population reported to have some health problems two weeks before the survey; of those, 31% sought health care and 66% failed to do so for the following reasons: 51% considered it to be unnecessary or treated themselves and 21% said they lacked money and that services were unavailable or of poor quality. The proportion of those not seeking care because of poverty was estimated as 16% by one survey analyst and from 10% to 20% by another. Once the decision to seek care was made, the choice of which provider to use was more strongly influenced by income (Gómez, 1988; Bitran, 1989). According to Table 67, segment A, 24% of the capital's population was insured and 76% was not, a worse situation than the one depicted by the statistical estimates of Table 65, which gave figures of 34% and 66%, respectively. However, the proportions of the 1987 survey of Santo Domingo were better than those given for the nation by the 1984 survey, which found that only 7.5% were insured and 92.5% were not. Among the poorest income group, 15% were insured and 85% were not; as income increased, the proportion of those insured rose to 35% and that of the noninsured declined to 65%; of the insured poor, 7% were in IDSS, 3.8% in the private sector, 3.3% in ISSFAPOL, and 0.6% had double coverage (IDSS plus private). As income increased, the proportion of those with private insurance or in ISSFAPOL rose; the highest proportion of insured in IDSS was in the middle income group.

The proportion of the poor using consultation services was 43% from SESPAS, 27% from private providers, and 20% each from IDSS and ISSFAPOL. As income increased, the proportion of those receiving consultations from IDSS, ISSFAPOL, and the private sector also rose, while the proportion using SESPAS services decreased. The poor used SESPAS hospitalization services more than outpatient consultations (51% versus 43%), probably because the higher costs of hospitalization (free for the poor at SESPAS) precluded them from going to private hospitals. About 89% of all SESPAS users of consultation and hospitalization services were noninsured, and over 90% of SESPAS users were exempt from payment, while the remaining 10% paid user fees. These fees ranged from 35 pesos ($US9) for ambulatory care to 414 pesos ($US109) for hospitalization. A percentage distribution of the poor's utilization of hospitalization services by providers (not available for outpatient consultation) shows that 53% used SESPAS; 38%, private providers; 7%, IDSS; and 2%, ISSFAPOL. It was reported that the noninsured were often treated free of charge at IDSS and ISSFAPOL facilities, despite the fact that they were not entitled to that care; this, however, was usually the result of influence or bribes, resources that the poor obviously

Table 67. Real access and utilization by the poor to consultation-hospitalization services, by provider, Santo Domingo, Dominican Republic, 1987 (percentage distributions).

A. INSURANCE COVERAGE			
Coverage by monthly income[a]			
Less than 400	400–799	800 +	All
Insured[b] 14.7	24.9	35.0	24.0
IDSS only 7.0	9.2	8.8	8.1
Private only 3.8	9.8	19.4	10.5
IDSS and private 0.6	2.8	2.3	1.9
ISSFAPOL 3.3	3.1	4.5	3.5
Not insured[c] 85.3	75.1	65.0	76.0
Total 100.0	100.0	100.0	100.0

	B. UTILIZATION OF SERVICES[d]							
	Outpatient consultation				Hospitalization			
	Less than 400	400–799	800 +	All	Less than 400	400–799	800 +	All
IDSS	20.2	28.4	51.4	100.0	31.3	40.7	28.0	100.0
ISSFAPOL	19.6	13.0	67.4	100.0	26.5	30.7	42.8	100.0
Private	26.9	19.7	53.4	100.0	26.6	30.7	42.7	100.0
SESPAS	43.1	23.6	33.3	100.0	50.9	31.4	17.7	100.0

Sources: Gómez, 1988; Bitrán, 1989.
[a]At the 1987 exchange rate of 1 $US = 3.8 pesos, the brackets were $105, $105 to $209, and $210 and over. The minimum wage in September 1987 was 350 pesos (U.S. $92); the lowest household income bracket ($105) for an average family of five persons was grossly insufficient to meet basic family needs.
[b]Population (insured and dependents) with prepaid public or private health insurance or plans.
[c]Population not insured who might have been theoretically covered by SESPAS or bought health services from the private sector or other providers.
[d]Physician consultation and hospitalization by those who felt ill and sought care two weeks before the survey.

lacked. But, private services must be paid for, and a considerable proportion of poor used them, probably because of unavailable or poor quality SESPAS services (Bitran, 1989).

The following is a summary of the key information from the last two sections. Statistically, 20% to 40% of the national population and 28% of the population in the capital lacked any type of health care coverage; the population's percentage of noncoverage was lower than its poverty incidence (36%–45% nationally and 38%–48% in the capital), suggesting that two-thirds of the poor were unprotected; the proportion of the insured population estimated statistically (20% nationwide and 34% in the capital) was much higher than that found by the surveys (7.5% nationwide and 24% in the capital); and insurance coverage of the poor, as reported in the surveys, was higher in the capital (15%) than in the nation (3%), but it was quite low in both. Of 66% of those who failed to seek care when they experienced health problems, 31% did so either because of poverty (10%–20%) or lack or low quality of services; statistical estimates of the noncovered population (20%–40% nationally and 28% in the capital) are probably low because of the above reasons. According to the surveys, 58%–62% of the poor utilize public services (basically SESPAS) and 38%–42% use private services (the latter range is twice as high as the statistically estimated national coverage by private insurance); and according to the survey, 89% of SESPAS users are not insured and 90% do not pay user fees (at least in Santo Domingo). Hence, the buying of private services by the poor (at an average of 12% of their median income) suggests that about two-fifths of them either do not have access to SESPAS services or these services are of very poor quality.

REASONS FOR LACK OF OR VERY LOW COVERAGE OF THE POOR

The Dominican Republic shares some of the characteristics seen in Costa Rica and Uruguay that facilitate universalization of health coverage: small size (the third smallest country in Latin America, about the same size as Costa Rica), a single language and culture, few topographical barriers, and a good communications system. And yet, health care coverage of the

Dominican Republic's population, particularly of the poor, is perhaps the worst among the five case studies, or at least as bad as that in Peru. In this section, we analyze two types of reasons that could explain that phenomenon.

General Factors

The Dominican Republic is one of the poorest countries in the Region; according to the World Bank, in 1988 it had the lowest GDP per capita after Haiti and Bolivia. Although accurate comparisons cannot be made, the country's poverty incidence appears to be worse than in eight of the ten countries surveyed by ECLAC in the 1980s, and possibly similar to that of Peru. In terms of literacy, sanitation, protein consumption, infant mortality, and life expectancy, the Dominican Republic ranks among the seven least developed countries in Latin America and the Caribbean. Although its territory is the third smallest in Latin America, its population is the 12th largest in the Region, hence, population density is very high (three times higher than in Costa Rica and Mexico), and the population growth rate, although declining, was the sixth highest in the 1980s. Hence, this population's demand on the country's scarce resources is enormous.

In 1980, the country's informal sector was proportionally one of the smallest in Latin America, while the rural traditional sector fell about midway within the Region. And yet, the annual growth rate of Santo Domingo in 1960–1988 was the highest of all capitals in Latin America and the Caribbean, and the combination of rapid urbanization and slow economic activity in the 1980s brought on a very rapid growth of the labor market's informal sector. Thus, in 1983, the informal sector in the capital was 45% of the EAP, and close to two-thirds of the labor force was either unemployed or underemployed. Differences in living standards between urban and rural areas are significant.

Government Leadership and Social Security Policy

Given that more than half of the labor force is constituted by salaried employees—only seven Latin American countries had a higher percentage in the early 1980s—and that the country has one of the lowest percentages of salary contributions in the Region, one would expect that, even with a traditional social insurance system, the proportion of the labor force covered by the sickness-maternity would be higher than 10%, the lowest in Latin America and the Caribbean, with the possible exception of El Salvador. Countries with lower proportions of salaried EAP have higher social insurance coverage than the Dominican Republic: Bolivia with 38% salaried EAP has 21% coverage and Peru with 45% salaried EAP has 32% coverage; Dominican percentages are 51% and 10%, respectively (see Tables 7 and 8).

IDSS has been unable to extend insurance coverage to the salaried labor force due to several reasons: most civil servants and private white-collar workers earning more than $US125 monthly are excluded; IDSS administration is notoriously inefficient and its services are of poor quality, leading to high rates of evasion; and the necessary political leadership to thrust expansion forward has been lacking. The absurdly low salary ceiling (gradually shrinking due to inflation, despite periodic adjustments) has deprived IDSS of the critical resources from high-salaried employees that are necessary for extending coverage. The exclusion of most civil servants also is a great loss, because it would be relatively easy to collect from this group. Finally, the largest enterprises that pay the highest salaries, are the easiest to control and collect from.

The failure of the 1983 draft legislation to extend IDSS coverage is a good example of poor political leadership. As noted previously, the draft was elaborated by a new administration, and had substantial union and employer support and the endorsement of ILO. A commission composed of representatives of all interested parties, including private health care organizations, reviewed the draft that allowed the insured the freedom to choose between IDSS and the private sector, a necessary compromise given the poor quality of social insurance health services and the inability of IDSS installations to absorb a greater population. Furthermore, this choice would have eliminated the costly duplication of coverage by IDSS and private insurance and would have fostered competition that may have led IDSS to improve its services. Finally, it was the only politically viable alternative, at least at that time, due to the enormous power of the Dominican Medical Association and the private health sector.

And yet, the final version of the draft was changed at the last minute to read that ''health care will be provided only at IDSS-owned facilities'' and that ''only in the cases and conditions set by IDSS could such care be offered in private clinics and other centers contracted with and under the fees and tariffs set by IDSS.'' Thus, the draft rendered the participation of the private sector an exception, and left its regulation exclusively in the hands of IDSS officials. The last-minute amendment provoked an acrimonious debate in Congress, prompted the strong opposition of the private sector, split the government party, and led to the eventual defeat of the draft. Apparently, most civil servants opposed the final version of the draft because it would have forced them to join IDSS and use its facilities, rather than the private clinics provided to them by the *igualas*. High-salaried private employees, who would also be incorporated into IDSS after the projected elimination of the salary ceiling, also opposed the amendment because they would be paying contributions but not using the IDSS services. The defeat of the draft strengthened the private health sector and contributed to the further erosion of IDSS prestige (Mesa-Lago, 1986b).

A political leadership that is incapable of taking advantage of favorable factors to extend social insurance to the salaried labor force, would be even less able to go beyond the existing structural barriers for making coverage to the urban marginal and rural poor universal. Last but not least, the percentage of the uninsured population is so high in the Dominican Republic (80% in the best of cases), that the government would have to make an extraordinary effort to cover it through SESPAS, an institution that has been traditionally underfunded and inefficient and whose problems worsened in the 1980s. These issues will be discussed in the next section.

FINANCIAL VIABILITY OF SOCIAL INSURANCE AND THE PUBLIC SECTOR TO COVER THE POOR

Probably less than one-tenth of some three million poor in the Dominican Republic are insured either by social insurance or the private sector, and SESPAS probably covers only about two-fifths of the uninsured. This section evaluates the ability of IDSS and SESPAS to extend effective health care protection to the noncovered poor.

Social Insurance (IDSS) Viability

IDSS is financed by salary contributions: 9.5% from employers (7% for pensions and sickness-maternity and 2.5% for employment injury) and 2.5% from the insured. The state is legally bound to contribute an additional 2.5%, but it has seldom met that obligation. In the first four decades of IDSS's existence, the state paid a fraction of its contribution for only five years, bringing the cumulative state debt to IDSS to $US95 million in 1980, equivalent to the combined IDSS expenditures in 1978–1980. In 1982, 78% of all IDSS revenue came from employers, 19% from the insured, and 3% from investment returns. Funds for the employment injury program are not separated from the rest; the former has generated steady surpluses and a good portion of them have been used to cover expenses, mostly of the sickness-maternity program (a total of $US43 million in the 1970s). In 1985, 70% of the IDSS revenue came from salary contributions, 27% from surpluses of the employment injury program, and 3% from investment returns.

The bulk of IDSS expenditures go to the sickness-maternity program. Although there is no separate account for the three IDSS programs, in 1980 it was roughly estimated that 66% of total expenditures went to sickness-maternity. In 1985, 56% of expenditures went to health care, 27% to administration (most of which is related to sickness-maternity), 8% to capital expenditures (most investment is in health facilities), and 7% to monetary benefits (a portion of which are sickness and maternity paid leaves); at least three-fourths of all these expenditures were related to sickness-maternity (Pan American Health Organization, 1983; IDSS, 1985; Duarte, 1986; Mesa-Lago, 1986b; Duarte et al., 1989).

In 1976, 1979, and 1985, IDSS (all programs combined) ended in a deficit ($US6.6 million in 1985), mainly brought on by a serious imbalance in the sickness-maternity program. IDSS physicians went on a two-week strike in 1985, and received generous salary increases that aggravated the deficit. Congress quickly lifted the salary ceiling by 75%, but despite a projected revenue increase of 29% for 1986 (estimates of the increase actually ranged from $US8 million to $US45 million!), financial difficulties persisted. By mid-1986, IDSS did not have funds to pay its employees' salaries, was delaying payment of monetary benefits, and was borrowing to meet its obligations. According to IDSS actuaries, the institution's statistics have been chaotic since 1984—there are no separate accounts for the three major programs, making it impossible to conduct a serious financial evaluation, let alone an actuarial study, and no data are gathered on collected revenue, but rather on what should be collected, thus including the unpaid state debt and other sums that do not materialize due to evasion and payment delays. Actuaries have tried three times to introduce a proper statistical system, but failed because the IDSS Director changed three times between 1982–1986 and the chief actuary was sent abroad for training, only to come back and "do nothing for two years." IDSS reserves amounted to $US10 million in 1980, but once IDSS's debt to banks was subtracted, they decreased to $US8 million. The actuaries report that in June 1986, the IDSS reserves were equal to or smaller than the IDSS debt, amounting to no reserves at all. The latest actuarial study (as of 1986) had been conducted in 1980 with 1979 data. I could not obtain a copy of this study but was told that the actuarial deficit was enormous (Pan American Health Organization, 1983; IDSS, 1985; Romero and Quesada, 1986; Mesa-Lago, 1986b).

Reasons for the IDSS deficit from the revenue side are evasion and payment delays, state debt, low and declining investment yields, and maturation of the pension program. From the expenditure side, the reasons are high administrative expenditures, growing share of pensions in total expenditures, provision of free services to the uninsured, and hospital inefficiency. The total percentage salary contribution paid to IDSS is one of the lowest in Latin America and the Caribbean, but an increase would not solve the problem unless the institution's serious inefficiencies are resolved.

The chief actuary estimated evasion at between 30% and 35% in 1986 and rising after the increase in the wage ceiling. This is partly due to poor registration, control, and collection; lack of accurate statistics; absence of individual accounts; and ineffective enforcement mechanisms. Sanctions on evaders are very lenient, such as $US34 to $US343 for payment delays (*mora*) by registered employers, and $US3 to $US34 for unregistered employers (evaders), hence stimulating clandestine enterprises. Interest charged for *mora* is 12% yearly, which has been below the inflation rate since 1984. Reportedly, some employers have raised salaries just above the ceiling to exclude their employees from IDSS coverage and avoid paying contributions if savings from the latter offset the wage increase. As mentioned before, the state seldom pays its dues as a third party contributor. IDSS investment is mostly in unprofitable health care facilities; investment revenue as a percentage of total IDSS revenue declined from 8% in 1970 to 4% in 1976, and to 2.4% in 1982. Investment yields are reportedly lower than the inflation rate, particularly since 1984 (Duarte, 1986; Mesa-Lago, 1986b; Romero and Quesada, 1986; Isuani, 1989).

IDSS is one of the least efficient social insurance institutions in the Region. Administrative expenses took up from 22% to 30% of total IDSS expenditures in 1978–1985, but this figure excludes "other administrative expenditures"; when the two categories are added, the total amounts to 33.5% in 1985, undoubtedly the highest percentage in Latin America and the Caribbean. These figures exclude medical personnel salaries, which could add another 40% or 50% to the total. The number of IDSS employees increased 69% in 1975–1985 (from 3,693 to 6,250); in the same period, the number of employees per 1,000 active insured rose from 19.7 to 22.8, a historical record for the Region; 65% of the personnel are concentrated in Santo Domingo. About 60% of IDSS employees are in the health sector, and the ratio of physicians per 10,000 active insured was 34.8 in 1985, one of the highest in the Region. In 1980, about 57% of IDSS expenditures went to salaries of and fringe benefits for medical personnel, and this was before the 1985 doctors' strike that resulted in a 58% salary increase. Officially, IDSS physicians work four hours daily, but in practice, their work schedule is one-half that (Pérez Montas, 1974; Duarte, 1986; Nadal, 1986; Mesa-Lago, 1986b; Isuani, 1989).

Reportedly, about 40% of IDSS health services are provided, without any record, for the uninsured through political patronage, bribery, and other illegal means. From 10% to 15% of IDSS patients are officially treated for "scientific interest," a very high percentage indeed. All of these practices raise costs and reduce the availability and quality of services to the insured (Nadal, 1986; Betances, 1986).

The percentage of IDSS expenditures going to pensions increased from 4% to 20% in 1961–1982, as the number of pensioners increased twelvefold in that period. The maturation of the pension program has contributed to the financial disequilibrium of IDSS (Duarte, 1986).

In 1985, IDSS operated 16 hospitals, 22 polyclinics, and 122 outpatient consultation centers. The number of total installations remained basically the same as ten years earlier: two more hospitals and four more clinics, but fifteen fewer centers. The centers, located in marginal urban areas and on the outskirts of cities, provide ambulatory primary health care; few have general practitioners and are staffed by *pasantes* and auxiliary personnel, none perform laboratory tests, and they have a limited supply of drugs. Polyclinics are second-level facilities located in high-density areas: they offer general and specialized outpatient consultations and emergency, dental, and psychiatric services, and are staffed by general practitioners and specialists. Hospitals are located in the capital and major cities, and provide tertiary-level care such as surgery, as well as outpatient consultations. Referrals are usually ignored by physicians in hospitals and, in general, there is little communication among the three levels. There were 1,511 hospital beds in 1985, an 11% decline from the 1974 level; the number of IDSS-owned beds did not significantly change in that period, but the number of beds contracted with the private sector fell from 200 to 25. In 1976, 90% of emergency cases were allowed to use private facilities, but, by 1985, that proportion had declined dramatically. The cut in contracted services has been due to the refusal of many private clinics to provide services to IDSS, because the latter seldom reimburses them or delays its payments.

Although the IDSS insured population increased 20% in 1974–1985, the stagnation or small decline in IDSS facilities does not appear to have led to overcrowded services. In the first quarter of 1985, the overall hospital occupancy rate was 51.7% (41% in maternity hospitals and 28% in pediatric hospitals), one of the lowest in Latin America, while the average hospital length of stay was 10.4 days, quite high and rising. The problem, therefore, is not lack of capacity, but poor quality of services that forces the insured to go elsewhere. IDSS facilities were evaluated by PAHO in 1983 as being of "very poor" and "low quality," and the situation has deteriorated since. Polyclinics and centers have averages of two to three outpatient consultations per hour. Medicine supply has been called "awful," since a significant proportion of drugs are wasted through spoilage or misplacement. A 1984 private survey found that 92% of the insured were critical of IDSS services, and would not want to use them if they had an alternative. It is because of these reasons that many insured in the IDSS have duplicate coverage through enterprise plans or *igualas* (Pérez Montas, 1974; Pan American Health Organization, 1983; IDSS, 1985; Nadal, 1986; Mesa-Lago, 1986b; Duarte et al., 1989).

The small, almost-stagnant percentage of population covered by IDSS, and the institution's financial and actuarial disequilibria and other serious inefficiencies reported above, demonstrate IDSS's inability to significantly extend health care coverage. The costs of universalization with the current IDSS structure would be astronomical; in Table 12, it was projected that it would cost 16.7% of GDP, the fifth highest proportion among 22 Latin American and Caribbean countries. The 1983 failed attempt to extend IDSS coverage demonstrated not only poor political judgment but also an inability to calculate the costs of the extension. For instance, three different estimates were made of the necessary increase in salary contributions to finance the extension; the number of insured to be incorporated ranged from 808,000 to 1.7 million (more than a 100% difference); and the estimates of the increase in annual revenue resulting from the 1985 rise in the salary ceiling varied by 442% (Molina, 1983; IDSS, 1983; Conte Grand, 1985). Certainly, the poor cannot expect health care protection from the IDSS in the future unless that institution is radically transformed.

Public Sector (SESPAS) Viability

A 1985 evaluation of SESPAS rated it as one suffering from "overall inoperativeness"; other technical reports have used terms such as "terrible" and "non-working." The economic crisis has accelerated the deterioration of SESPAS. A thorough assessment of this institution is difficult because of the lack of data: none of its facilities keep cost information; administrators often do not know their facility's monthly expenditures by major categories or even how many patients are treated annually; patient records are poor or nonexistent; data on hospital beds and physicians, average days of stay, and occupancy are spotty and contradictory; the Program of Essential Medicines does not keep records of drugs sent to hospitals and their costs; and for years, there have been no statistics kept on hospital discharges, morbidity, outpatient consultation, etc. (Gómez Ulloa, 1985; Skolnik, 1986; Lewis et al., 1990).

SESPAS is highly centralized, but has no effective powers for coordinating its various levels or for carrying out supervision, control, and evaluation; an attempt at regionalization failed, and local officials lack authority. The public health system is structured in three levels—clinics, subcenters, and hospitals—and there also is a National Laboratory. Clinics are first-level facilities located on the periphery of urban areas and in rural communities with fewer than 3,500 inhabitants; they offer primary health care, especially general outpatient consultation and infant-maternal care, emergency services, and oral rehydration, and are staffed by a *pasante*, a nurse, an assistant, and a supervisor. In rural clinics, promoters selected from the community perform primary health care services for which they receive a token compensation; the health promoter program began in 1976, and by 1984 there were about 5,289 promoters, an average of one for every 80 families (Ugalde, 1984, 1988). Serious deficiencies keep demand for clinic services very low, and only one-third of the consultation time is used. The population distrusts the *pasante's* skills and he or she, being transitory, does not establish relations with the community (see the section on "Impact on Overall Health Standards," beginning on p. 168); most clinics operate in rented houses with terrible conditions and two-thirds of them lack running water, even a washstand; in the first half of 1985, there were practically no supplies delivered.

Subcenters theoretically are second-level facilities (some of them have beds), but in practice they operate as first-level facilities; they function in more populated cities and offer outpatient consultations, infant-maternal care, basic laboratory services, emergency services, minor surgery, and a popular pharmacy. Subcenters are staffed by several physicians, nurses, and other administrative personnel. The quality of these services is usually as poor as those in the clinics: only 25% of potential consultation time is used, there is not enough room for consultations, and often several physicians share one room or see their patients in the halls; only half of the subcenters have diagnostic services; they charge user fees without any regulation; and supplies are irregular, at best. The above-mentioned evaluation concluded that neither the SESPAS clinics nor the subcenters appear to have played a significant role in increasing health standards.

There are three levels of hospitals: local, regional, and national. The last are tertiary-level facilities located in Santo Domingo and other major cities that offer complex, specialized care and that have laboratory and X-ray services and pharmacies. As will be seen later, hospital occupancy is at about one-half of installed capacity, and the average length of stay is too long because of a lack of control of patient histories, unnecessary delays in tests and surgery, and overall inefficiency. Supplies are poor or nonexistent, including basic materials for surgery, medicine, food, linen, china, and silverware, all of which usually have to be supplied by the patients or their relatives. Funds allocated by SESPAS were drastically cut in the 1980s, and user fees are charged in most hospitals without standardization or regulation. Finally, the National Laboratory, probably the most efficient institution in the public health sector, performs all sorts of diagnostic tests on patients referred from SESPAS facilities, as well as on users who approach it directly (Gómez Ulloa, 1985).

Because of the deficiencies and the poor quality of services offered by clinics and subcenters, 65% of outpatient consultations and 86% of laboratory tests are done in the hospitals. However, 90% of these services could be offered at the first or second level at lower cost, if these facilities were properly funded, staffed, and equipped. Because of enormous public demand, lines start to form at 5:00 a.m.; consultations are expected to begin at 8:00 a.m. and end at noon, but in practice, they are reduced to three hours—schedules are seldom met, and physicians spend about two minutes with each patient. Appointments for specialties such as for gastroenterology take several months, and appointments for outpatient consultations and

hospital admissions are often sold or obtained through connections (Gómez Ulloa, 1985; Guzmán, 1986; Torres, 1986).

Between 1974 and 1985, SESPAS hospitals increased from 45 to 47, subcenters increased from 38 to 55, and clinics, from 0 to 23 in urban areas and from 109 to 348 in rural areas. This significant growth of primary and secondary facilities resulted from a primary health care program that will be discussed later. The number of SESPAS hospital beds is not easy to determine, but it apparently declined from 7,038 in 1979 to 6,509 in 1985; one expert believes that official figures are inflated. The number of physicians is even more difficult to assess; it was reported as 2,756 in 1983 and 2,518 in 1985 (SESPAS, 1983, 1984; Consejo Nacional de Población y Familia, 1985; Gómez Ulloa, 1985; Oficina Nacional de Estadística, 1987; Lewis et al., 1990).

A comparison of SESPAS facilities and resources, nationwide and in the capital, with those of other providers in 1985–1987 shows that the former are the worst (see Table 68). At the national level, SESPAS ratios per person covered were estimated using 80% and 40% of population coverage. Based on the highest coverage, SESPAS resources were about one-half of the national average and those of ISSFAPOL, one-third those of the private sector, and one-fourth those of IDSS; based on the lowest coverage, SESPAS resources were above the national average, but still below those of other providers except for private sector physicians. The comparison in Santo Domingo in Table 68 is based on an estimated SESPAS coverage (53%) of the capital's population minus a small proportion

Table 68. Comparison of health care facilities and resources by provider in Santo Domingo and the Dominican Republic, 1985–1987.

Providers	Santo Domingo (1987)							National (1985)	
	Percentage distribution			Ratios per person covered				Ratios per person covered	
	Population covered[a]	Hospital beds	Physicians[b]	Hospital beds (x 1,000)	Physicians[b] (x 10,000)	Consultations	Expenditures ($US)	Hospital beds (x 1,000)	Physicians[b] (x 10,000)
SESPAS	53.4	33.8	20.3	2.9	12.0	1.8	9.54	1.3–2.5[h]	4.9–9.8[h]
IDSS	12.4	10.1	24.8	3.7[e]	44.4	3.2	46.32	5.4	37.4
ISSFAPOL	5.0	6.5	10.0	5.9	44.6	n.a.	n.a.	2.5	10.4
Private[c]	29.2	49.6	44.9	7.6	34.1	12–36[f]	27.72[g]	3.5	8.8
Total[d]	100.0	100.0	100.0	3.4	20.3	n.a.	n.a.	2.1	7.9

Sources: Author's calculations based on Oficina Nacional de Planificación, 1983; SESPAS, 1983, 1984; IDSS, 1985; Consejo Nacional de Población y Familia, 1985; Gómez Ulloa, 1985; Duarte, 1986; Del Rosario and Gámez, 1988; Isuani, 1989; Duarte et al., 1989; Lewis et al., 1990.
    [a]Excludes population covered by private nonprofit organizations and special groups such as teachers; see also [c].
    [b]Based on positions, not physicians, as the latter have multiple employment.
    [c]Private for-profit institutions; includes only part of the total, hence, actual percentage of population should be higher. Facilities and resources are total (except expenditures), hence, percentages and ratios actually should be smaller.
    [d]Ratios refer to total population and facilities.
    [e]In 1983 was reported as 5.2.
    [f]Range of part of total *igualas* and insurance companies.
    [g]Part of cost is not shown as it is paid by insured as copayment.
    [h]Lowest estimate based on SESPAS coverage of 80% of the population; highest estimate based on a 40% coverage. Other estimates based on a reported higher number of beds and physicians are in 1983, 1.5–2.9 and 5.6–11.2, respectively, and in 1985, 1.4–2.9 and 6.0–11.9, respectively.

covered by NGOs and a few special groups. Once again, SESPAS resources are the worst, all well below the overall average, and from one-fourth to one-half those available from other providers. Note that the private sector has proportionally three times more beds and physicians than SESPAS and offers from seven to twenty more consultations per person, but at three times the cost per capita. IDSS has slightly more beds, four times more physicians, and offers twice as many consultations per capita as SESPAS, but spends five times more per capita, another indication of IDSS waste and inefficiency.

At first glance, the above data indicate that SESPAS facilities and personnel are insufficient to cover the assigned population, including the poor. And yet, it has already been noted that only from 25% to 35% of the capacity of outpatient consultation is actually utilized because of inefficiencies and poor funding at first- and second-level facilities. Furthermore, hospital occupancy in the 1980s was systematically below 60%—56.7% in 1980, 55.7% in 1985, and 54% in 1986. The national average length of hospital stay was 23 days in 1980 and 21.2 in 1982; no data are available thereafter. In the provinces in 1986, occupancy of subcenters and local hospitals ranged from 3% to 58%, and that of area and regional hospitals from 15% to 77%. In general, the lower the level of the facility, the lower the occupancy; in some specialized hospitals of the capital, beds have to be shared by two patients and some beds are placed in the halls for lack of space, while some provincial hospitals are almost empty. Although existing resources may indeed be insufficient to properly cover all the uninsured population without resources, there is considerable unutilized capacity due to inefficiency and poor quality of services, which forces the poor to pay for private services (SESPAS, 1983, 1984, 1986a; Consejo Nacional de Población y Familia, 1985; Gómez Ulloa, 1985; Guzmán, 1986; Duarte et al., 1989).

The only figure I was able to locate on SESPAS employment was 10,723 for 1983; based on it, the ratio of employees per 1,000 persons covered ranged from 2.2 to 4.3, depending on whether an 80% or a 40% population coverage figure is used. These figures, particularly the low one, are not high by Latin American and Caribbean standards, but are certainly minuscule when compared with those of IDSS, 18 to 22 employees per 1,000 insured. But, once again, the issue here is not quantity but quality. In general, SESPAS personnel have low-level skills; are not in a civil service career;

lack stability and labor incentives; and are hired, assigned, promoted, fired, and paid by the Ministry, usually with no regard to performance and with no input from local units. Medical professionals receive the same basic salary regardless of differences in skills and seniority, and there is an abundance of physicians and a serious scarcity of nurses and other paramedic personnel (Gómez Ulloa, 1985; Lewis, 1987; La Forgia, 1989).

The national surplus of physicians and their powerful association pose some of the most serious problems for SESPAS and the entire public health sector. In 1986, there were 13 medical schools that were not subjected to any regulation, and career lengths varied from three to seven years. There were 10,000 students registered and 1,000 graduated annually; the country's ratio of medical students to population was the second highest in the Region. About half of the graduates emigrate, representing a $US20,000 loss per migrant, but the rest stay, expanding the surplus and pressing for jobs. With PAHO's cooperation, a special commission was established in 1983 to regulate all medical schools; it elaborated a legal draft, which was defeated by the powerful university lobby. An initial measure would be to make the entry exam stricter, since reportedly few candidates fail, but because universities are autonomous, a law would be needed to make that change.

More than 1,000 physicians are unemployed, and the pressure to hire them is intense. They are paid high salaries for services that could be provided by paramedical personnel at a lower cost, and they resort to strikes to get raises. Physicians are expected to work four hours (eight, since 1986), but they actually work two and spend an average of two minutes per patient; they only see a few patients daily. In addition, they are frequently absent, delay hospital dismissals, violate rules, and reject any effort to introduce planning, set work schedules and targets, and enforce the budget.

The Dominican Medical Association (AMD) is the most powerful union in the country. It systematically defends physicians whether they are right or wrong; as a result, they have become untouchable and it is impossible to dismiss them. In 1962, a law removed from SESPAS the power to discipline its employed physicians, and transferred this authority to a council controlled by the Dominican Medical Association, which always rejects charges and orders the reinstatement of a suspended physician with retroactive payment of his/her salary. Physicians usually have multiple jobs and cut down their public sector work as much as possible in order to devote more time to private practice. Nurses work an average of 15 days per month, 4 to 20 hours weekly; many of them are on permanent paid leave and others work for two or three employers and minimize the time spent at SESPAS. One-third of the nurses' time is wasted on activities not related to their jobs, and there is neither control of attendance nor evaluation of nursing performance. As a result, the patients' relatives often must feed, bathe, and assist them (USAID, 1975; SESPAS, 1983; Gómez Ulloa, 1985; Calventi, 1986; González Gatreaux, 1986; Gúzman, 1986; Mendoza, 1986; Torres, 1986; Ugalde, 1988).

Maintenance and repair of SESPAS equipment are deplorable. In the mid-1980s, 90% of the incubators, 75% of X-ray and laboratory equipment, 72% of intensive care units, and 50% of autoclaves and anesthesia equipment did not work. In Santo Domingo, four-fifths of the hospitals needed urgent repair of their physical plant and substitution or repair of washing, boiling, kitchen, sterilizing, and surgical equipment (Oficina Nacional de Planificación, 1983; Gómez Ulloa, 1985; Skolnik, 1986; Duarte et al., 1989). The following revealing anecdote was told to me by the director of the principal maternity hospital in the capital. In 1979, an agreement was signed with a French bank to buy equipment valued at $US240,000 to supply two hospitals and six clinics; the equipment arrived in 1982 and sat on the docks for three years. In mid-1986, equipment for the maternity hospital sat in boxes at the hospital's warehouse waiting for the required installation, which was estimated to cost $US14,000, but SESPAS had not provided the funds (Calventi, 1986). The situation during the rest of the 1980s apparently deteriorated further, and in January–July 1990, most operating rooms in the Dominican Republic were shut down due to constant strikes (La Forgia, 1990b).

The Program of Essential Medicines is the main supplier of drugs and medical goods to the public sector. Initially, it bought and distributed 165 generic medicines at relatively low prices, hence benefiting the poor; reportedly, this competition also led to a drop in prices in the private sector. The Program's revolving fund was practically depleted by 1986, and buying fell to 15% of previous levels. A major reason for that decrease apparently was the state's failure to reimburse or payment delays to the Program, but a lack of knowledge of demand that resulted in stockpiles and the loss of a preferential ex-

change rate to import medicines that cut the agency's purchasing power by half also were responsible. The Program of Essential Medicines also has been criticized for lacking a warehouse, adequate distribution, and adequate consultation with local units to assess their demand, and for irregular supply; inconsistent bidding that results in fraudulent commissions and higher prices for medicines; an inability to control the prices of medicine and to guarantee their quality; and administrative inefficiency and excessive profits that also raise the price of medicines (Calventi, 1986; Gómez and Gross, 1986; González Gautreaux, 1986; Hernández Llamas, 1986; Mendoza, 1986; Mesa-Lago, 1986b).

In 1981, the central government's per capita expenditure in health in $US (basically related to SESPAS) was the ninth highest among 23 countries, and was higher than the per capita expenditures of more developed countries such as Argentina, Brazil, and Mexico. This surprising fact makes even more evident the waste and inefficiency in the use of SESPAS resources. However, by 1984 the country's per capita expenditure had been halved, and this cut was the largest among 14 countries for which data are available (Musgrove, 1986, 1989a). As a percentage of the central government's budget, SESPAS's share declined from 8% to 5% in 1982–1985; as a percentage of GDP, SESPAS's expenditures were halved from 2.2% to 1% in 1979–1987.

From 73% to 94% of the SESPAS budget is provided by the central government, and the remainder comes from user fees and international aid and loans; as government funds have shrunk, user fees have risen. SESPAS expenditures are distributed as follows: 91% to the tertiary level (mostly to the five major hospitals in the capital), 6% to the secondary level, and 3% to the primary level; less than 1% of the budget is spent on prevention and sanitation and most of the budget goes to curative specialized care. As the SESPAS budget was cut in real terms in the 1980s, personnel salaries were the least affected (this item increased from 58% to 68% of the budget in 1980–1984), while all remaining expenses, as well as capital expenditures, sharply declined (SESPAS, 1983; Bartlett, 1983; Isuani, 1989; Duarte et al., 1989).

The above figures reinforce previous statements made here regarding the fact that SESPAS services steadily deteriorated in the second half of the 1980s and that its funds are irrationally allocated vis-à-vis the health needs of the population. If SESPAS facilities and resources were more efficiently utilized, targeted on vulnerable population groups such as the poor and infants and pregnant women, and less concentrated on curative medicine and the tertiary level, that institution could effectively provide health care to the poor. Unless there is a radical transformation of SESPAS, the poor will have to search for alternative ways.

THE IMPACT OF THE PUBLIC HEALTH SYSTEM ON HEALTH STANDARDS

This section evaluates SESPAS services, particularly those programs implemented in 1975–1986 on behalf of low-income groups, and their potential impact on the overall health standards of the population. There are no data to evaluate the potential effects on health standards among the poor; however, the redistributive impact of state health subsidies on this group will be reviewed briefly.

Impact on Overall Health Standards

In the mid-1970s, a study conducted in the Dominican Republic by a USAID official indicated that curative health services had not been as effective as expected in reducing child morbidity and mortality, because almost half of all diseases, such as gastrointestinal and respiratory infections, were related to socioeconomic and environmental factors. The study concluded that programs emphasizing prevention and nutrition would significantly reduce morbidity and mortality, and would cut health costs (Marx, 1978). This study may have prompted a shift in the country's health policy with the aid of external funding.

In 1975–1986, the Dominican Republic, primarily SESPAS, received at least $US39 million, and possibly $US42 million, from several international and regional organizations to expand primary health care and prevention coverage of the population, particularly the poor: $US17.5 million from USAID in 1975–1986, $US15.6 million from IDB in the late 1970s and early 1980s, $US3.8 million from PAHO/WHO in 1982–1986, and $US2.5 million from UNICEF in 1982–1986; UNDP planned to give an additional grant of $US2.5 million in 1987–1991, and in 1986, IDB was studying another grant for remodeling and

rehabilitating many SESPAS facilities. Although the specific objectives of all these grants and programs may have differed, all focused on prevention and sanitation—except for the IDB grant that was for the expansion and equipment of clinics, subcenters, and hospitals—and there was significant overlap among them.

The grants specifically aimed at improving nutritional levels and access to potable water (hand pumps) and excreta disposal (latrines), particularly in rural areas; reducing contagious diseases through malaria control campaigns and immunization campaigns against tuberculosis, polio, DPT, and measles; decreasing deaths caused by diarrhea and parasites through rehydration and antiparasitic campaigns; improving health care in the infant-maternal group; expanding health care services, mostly preventive, for the poor in urban marginal and rural areas (the latter partly through 6,000 health promoters); creating a system of providing and/or selling medicines at low cost; and improving the organization and promoting the integration of the public health system. Expected end results of these programs were a decline in infant mortality, an increase in life expectancy, and an overall improvement in health standards (USAID, 1975; Bartlett, 1983; Pan American Health Organization/UNDP/UNICEF, 1986; Early, 1986; Lewis et al., 1990).

To the best of my knowledge, there is no comprehensive or thorough evaluation of the results of these grants and programs. As has been said, in 1974–1985 there was a threefold increase in the number of SESPAS rural clinics, plus the creation of urban clinics and the addition of two hospitals. However, as the previous discussion clearly showed, in this period coverage of the population did not expand significantly, SESPAS hospital beds and physicians remained stagnant or declined on a per capita basis, and the quality of public health services and managerial efficiency deteriorated.

An important evaluation of the program of rural clinics and promoters was conducted in 1982–1983 by a team of United States social scientists who spent nine months in a small rural community conducting interviews, collecting data on morbidity and family budgets, and testing pilot plans. The community had a clinic with 22 employees and spent $US7 per capita annually, or $US9 if the cost of referrals is added; the last figure was similar to the SESPAS average per capita expenditure in Santo Domingo in 1987 (Table 68). Despite the large infrastructure and high costs, services offered were inefficient and of poor quality, and as a result, two-thirds of the community's out-of-pocket expenses on health care went to the private sector. Surprisingly, user fees for outpatient consultation in the clinic were slightly higher than those of private physicians.

The team found several causes for the inefficiency of the public services. A major flaw was the performance of the *pasantes*, recent graduates without primary health care training who stay for only one year and who lack interest in the community, minimize their services, are frequently absent, and do not gain the community's trust. Medicine was free, but the supply was very irregular; when medicines arrived at the clinic, patients came for the medicines, rather than for consultation with the *pasante*; overprescription of medication also was a common problem. The *pasante* spent an average of less than three minutes per patient, ended consultations at 10 a.m., and did nothing else for the rest of the day. *Pasantes* also failed to order spare parts and maintain the equipment, let alone to educate the community on better health practices. Although based on a single community, the team felt that the evaluation had national value and recommended that *pasantes* be replaced by permanent experienced physicians with specialized training (taking advantage of the surplus of physicians), who should devote part of their time to train health promoters and educate the community; that rural posts served by the rural clinic be established to maximize the physician's time; that administrative practices be improved (which would have to come largely from above); and that communal pharmacies that would charge a fee (exempting the poor) and use a revolving fund to buy medicine when SESPAS's supplies fail be established (Ugalde, 1984, 1988).

There is little or no information on the outcome of other programs. In 1983, USAID attempted to evaluate the impact of the programs it had helped to finance, but due to the lack of data, the assessment could not be done properly (Early, 1986). During my 1986 visit, I heard contradictory opinions from Dominican health officials and experts on the effectiveness of the SESPAS programs under review. The SESPAS Under-Secretary for Administration told me that the immunization campaign had been successful and had reduced the incidence of contagious diseases and eliminated bottlenecks in the outpatient consultation in children's hospitals (Guzmán, 1986). On the other hand, a well-known physician maintained that the antiparasitic campaign and the effort to expand the number of latrines and hand pumps in rural areas failed due to wasted funds and inefficiency (Gautreaux, 1986).

Statistics for the needed assessment are scarce and contradictory. A Dominican source reports that immunization coverage of children under 1 year of age declined in 1978–1982: from 98% to 54% for polio and from 93% to 41% for DPT (Consejo Nacional de Población y Familia, 1985). A World Bank study claims that in 1984–1987, the immunization rate for polio and diphtheria in the same population group was 28% (indicating a further decline), while for measles it was 24%; these rates were the lowest among six countries compared, including Costa Rica and Mexico (Pfeffermann and Griffin, 1989). Conversely, a United States-based study claimed that in 1981–1985, immunization rates for polio increased from 42% to 80%, and from 17% to 81% for measles (Lewis et al., 1990).

According to one Dominican source, institutional child delivery declined from 73% to 67% in 1979–1982, but another domestic source reported an increase from 76% to 85% in 1975–1980; among institutional child deliveries the proportion handled at SESPAS rose from 56% to 61%. Care of pregnant women was given as 21.4% in 1982 (SESPAS, 1984; Consejo Nacional de Población y Familia, 1985). Nevertheless, the 1987 survey of Santo Domingo found that "virtually all women requiring prenatal care obtain such services," with over 80% reporting more than one consultation (Bitran, 1989).

Analyzing the evolution of health facilities and standards also is hindered by inconsistent statistical series. Table 69 shows that the ratio of hospital beds per 1,000 inhabitants declined from 2.6 to 2.1 in 1970–1985; in the latter year, however, the Dominican ratio ranked 13th among 24 Latin American and Caribbean countries, well above that of relatively more developed nations such as Mexico (see Table 12). The ratio of physicians per 10,000 inhabitants was basically stagnant throughout the period; on this indicator, the Dominican Republic ranked lower, 18th among the 24 Latin American and Caribbean countries. Given the reported surplus of physicians, this figure and ranking are puzzling. It is possible that the figure is underestimated; Table 68 reports a ratio of 7.9 physicians per 10,000, which would rank the Dominican Republic 13th in the Region, but that ratio was overestimated due to multiple employment of physicians.

For mortality rates and life expectancy, Table 69 offers two different series: the first is given by ECLAC and is systematically more favorable than the second, based on domestic data, except

Table 69. Health care facilities and standards in the Dominican Republic, 1960–1990.

| | Hospital beds per 1,000 inhabitants | Physicians per 10,000 inhabitants | Mortality rates[a] | | | | Life expectancy[a] | |
| | | | General | | Infant | | | |
			(1)	(2)[b]	(1)	(2)[c]	(1)	(2)[b]
1960	2.3	n.a.	n.a.	18.5	132.2	142.6	51.0	49.1
1965	n.a.	5.8	14.7	15.4	117.0	n.a.	53.6	52.6
1970	2.6	n.a.	12.1	13.1	105.0	170.6	57.0	55.4
1975	2.5	n.a.	9.8	11.0	93.5	[39.4][d]	60.0	57.8
1980	n.a.	5.6	8.4	9.1	84.3	n.a.	62.1	60.2
1985	2.1	5.7	7.5	n.a.	74.5	[37.6]	64.1	62.6
1988–1990	n.a.	5.7	6.8	n.a.	65.0	n.a.	65.9	n.a.

Sources: Oficina Nacional de Planificación, 1983; Oficina Nacional de Estadística, 1965–1987; Gómez Ulloa, 1985; Consejo Nacional de Población y Familia, 1985; ECLAC, 1989a; IDB, 1989; World Bank, 1990.

[a]Five-year estimates, except for a few cases. Column 1 comes from ECLAC and is systematically more favorable than data in column 2 (from domestic data) except for infant mortality in 1970 and 1985.

[b]From Consejo Nacional de Población y Familia (National Council for Population and Family).

[c]1970 from population census; 1975 from Oficina Nacional de Estadística (National Office of Statistics); 1985 from IDB.

[d]1976.

for infant mortality in two years (shown in brackets). PAHO has reported an underregistration of infant mortality as high as 50% (Gómez Ulloa, 1985). Indeed, the 1970 census gave a rate of 170.6, 62% above the ECLAC rate of 105. Conversely, official estimates are often half the ECLAC figures, such as 37.6 and 74.5, respectively, for 1985. According to the ECLAC series (column 1), the average annual rate of reduction of infant mortality in five-year periods steadily declined from 3.04 in 1960–1965 to 1.84 in 1975–1980, but then increased to 1.96 in 1980–1985 and slowed down to 1.90 in 1985–1990. However, the 1960 and 1970 observations (column 2) show an increase in infant mortality, while the 1975 and 1985 observations indicate an annual rate of decline of only 0.2. The ECLAC series, therefore, shows a modest acceleration of the rate of decline at the time that the above-mentioned SESPAS programs were implemented, but without reaching the rates of decline of the 1960–1975 period; furthermore, such improvement is questionable.

The ECLAC series of life expectancy at birth exhibits a declining trend in the average rate of annual increase (in years), from 0.68 in 1965–1970 to 0.36 in 1985–1990. Actually, in 1976–1985, the period when the SESPAS programs were in force, this rate declined sharply. The second series of life expectancy also indicates a declining trend in 1960–1970, but stagnation thereafter at the time the programs were implemented. Even using the more favorable ECLAC series, in 1985 the Dominican Republic ranked 20th among Latin American and Caribbean countries in terms of the infant mortality rate (only four countries had higher rates; see Table 12), and ranked 16th in life expectancy (eight countries had a lower life expectancy). And yet, at the beginning of the 1980s, the

country's per capita expenditure for public health was the ninth highest among those countries. Although the Dominican Republic's per capita expenditures on health were almost as high as Mexico's, the latter's immunization coverage of the population tripled that of the former (Pfeffermann and Griffin, 1989).

Changes in morbidity ratios and causes of death are the most difficult to assess because there are no accurate comparable data for the mid-1970s and the 1980s. However, available information for the early 1980s gives very high ratios of contagious diseases and of "underdevelopment diseases" as causes of death. For instance, the ratio of malaria was 49 per 100,000, and this disease was the fifth cause of morbidity among all ages; the ratio for tuberculosis also was above 40 per 100,000. Acute diarrhea was the leading cause of death among those under age 15 and above age 50. Among infants under 1 year of age, perinatal diseases caused 21% of deaths; diarrhea and intestinal infections, 14%; respiratory diseases, 13%; and malnutrition, 11%. About 35% of preschoolers suffered from malnutrition (SESPAS, 1983; Consejo Nacional de Población y Familia, 1985; Gómez Ulloa, 1985).

Access to piped water reportedly expanded in 1969–1985, from 75.8% to 85% in urban areas and from 9% to 34% in rural areas. In the latter, the increase occurred in 1969–1980; thereafter, the proportion was almost stagnant. I estimate that at the national level, the expansion was from 35.7% to 62.5% in 1969–1985. Urban houses connected with a sewage system increased from 19.5% in 1973 to 41% in 1985 (ECLAC, 1989a). These figures indicate an important expansion of sanitation facilities in urban areas, but still the levels in the mid-1980s were quite low and the overwhelming majority of poor families lacked those facilities. No data are available on the results of the program to expand the number of latrines and pumps in rural areas. Furthermore, the situation seemed to deteriorate in the second half of the 1980s. Most of the diseases are related to unsafe water. Frequent power shortages interrupt the water supply, and the quality of piped water has deteriorated because the water sits stagnant for long periods in faulty pipes; in addition, the quantity of chemicals used to treat the water has declined. The sewer system in Santo Domingo has insufficient capacity to handle the wastewater; hence, most city sewage is discharged untreated into rivers and the ocean. In 1986, close to one-half of the residents did not have frequent garbage collection, and the situation worsened thereafter (Lewis et al., 1990).

Although the above analysis does not permit solid conclusions, it suggests that the substantial funds invested in SESPAS programs had not yielded the expected results by the mid-1980s, with the possible exception of an expansion of piped water in urban areas, due to waste and inefficiency. Health standards appear to have deteriorated in the second half of the 1980s. The health status of the poor no doubt has worsened as well.

Effects of Income Distribution

In 1982, a survey was conducted in the Dominican Republic to measure the impact of state subsidies to social services on income distribution. State subsidies to health were the only subsidies found to have a progressive distributive effect; subsidies to other social services (housing, pensions, education, water) were found to be regressive.

The poorest population quintile received 41% of the health subsidy, but the second quintile received only 16%, while the third quintile received 20%; the wealthiest two quintiles were allocated 23% of the subsidy. After adding the subsidy, income distribution became slightly more equal: 1.4 percentage points from the richest two quintiles were transferred mostly to the poorest two quintiles (see Table 17). Although the state subsidy to public health care had a progressive effect, its effect on improving the distribution and the poor's income was minor. This finding of the survey suggests that a small proportion of funds was allocated to health, but we found contradictory evidence in the previous section.

The same survey also was conducted in four other countries. The Dominican Republic's distribution of income, both before and after receiving the health subsidy, was the most unequal of all the countries but one. Furthermore, the subsidy's impact in reducing income inequality (measured by the Gini Coefficient) was the smallest in the Dominican Republic: −0.0154, compared to −0.0182 in Argentina, −0.0205 in Uruguay, −0.0290 in Chile, and −0.0575 in Costa Rica (Petrei, 1987).

PUBLIC AND PRIVATE ALTERNATIVES TO EXPAND ACCESS AND QUALITY OF HEALTH CARE FOR THE POOR

The previous sections indicate that some of the poor do not have access to health care and that some, who have such access, do not utilize SESPAS services due to their poor quality and, hence, are forced to pay for private care. It also has been demonstrated that if SESPAS managerial efficiency and quality of services were improved, existing facilities could provide adequate health care to a significant portion of the poor who are currently unprotected. This section examines two alternatives to improve coverage and utilization by the poor: user fees in SESPAS facilities and prepaid private plans (*igualas*) for low income groups.

User Fees[2]

Under good management conditions, user fees can be an effective financial mechanism to improve the quality of health care services, which could lead to increased utilization of such services by the poor. (Herein, quality improvement usually refers to improving facility operation and medical care organization). Conversely, charging fees within a poorly managed environment, coupled with poor quality of care, may

---

[2]This section is basically a summary of a report specifically prepared for this study by Gerard M. La Forgia: "User Fees, Quality of Care, and the Poor: Lessons from the Dominican Republic," Santo Domingo, September 1989. La Forgia's report is supplemented herein with my own observations (Mesa-Lago, 1986b) and a previous study (Lewis, 1987). All information in this section, unless otherwise specified, comes from La Forgia, who technically is its author, although I take responsibility for any errors that might have resulted from summarizing his report.

reduce utilization of services by the poor and low-income groups. There is at least one public facility that has been successful in reaching those objectives in the Dominican Republic, but most have failed to improve the quality of services, although they have been able to maintain basic quality in the midst of economic deterioration.

Legal Base and Policy

The Dominican Constitution stipulates that "[the state] will provide free medical assistance and hospitalization to those who have scarce economic means and request such services." The Constitution implicitly prohibits charging user fees to the poor, but permits fees to be charged to those who have economic means. And yet, decrees and regulations enacted in the 1940s set prices for inpatient, outpatient, and diagnostic services in SESPAS facilities. Furthermore, in 1982–1986 the government allowed the charging of user fees for some medical services. The Dominican Medical Association has opposed user fees based on the Constitution, and the government has refrained from regulating the fees, fearing a negative political reaction. According to SESPAS officials, fees for inpatient care are prohibited, but most hospitals charge fees for some outpatient services. Because of the absence of a clear policy on outpatient charges, there is no standardized practice of user fees, but rather different responses to hospital directors' initiatives and perceived needs.

Despite the ambiguous government policy, a general pattern of user fees has emerged. Most SESPAS facilities provide outpatient physician consultations and inpatient care free of charge. However, large hospitals charge for diagnostic services for outpatients, but inpatients receive these services free of charge. The National Laboratory charges for diagnostic services, but not for patients hospitalized in SESPAS facilities. At least two hospitals charge for a medical record card for the first outpatient visit; cast setting and expensive drugs for cancer treatment; and endoscopic surgery and some types of eye surgery. Most of these practices encourage the use of emergency services or admittance to hospitals in order to avoid charges, and they subsidize inpatient services by outpatients.

Depending on the region, small maternity/children's hospitals (subcenters) in the countryside may charge outpatients for some diagnostic services. And yet, in 1989, three subcenters that were visited for this study in the eastern region of the country, did not charge fees for any ser-

vice. Nevertheless, SESPAS officials claim that subcenters in the southern region do collect user fees. Small outpatient facilities (clinics) do not charge fees, but neither do they provide diagnostic services (Mesa-Lago, 1986b; Lewis, 1987; La Forgia, 1989).

Facilities Investigated

In 1986, while seeking user-fee information, I visited and interviewed the directors of the National Laboratory and three hospitals in Santo Domingo: general hospital Aybar, maternity hospital Altagracia, and children's hospital Reid Cabral (Mesa-Lago, 1986b). The first thorough study on user fees, conducted in 1986, selected the National Laboratory, five hospitals in Santo Domingo (Altagracia, Aybar, and Reid Cabral, general hospital Bellini, and trauma hospital Contreras), and four regional hospitals, in San Pedro de Macorís, Barbados, Santiago, and San Cristobal (Lewis, 1987). La Forgia's study, conducted in April–June 1989, was limited to three hospitals in Santo Domingo (Altagracia, Aybar, and Reid Cabral) plus the National Laboratory. Hence, four of the facilities investigated by him were previously visited by me and studied by Lewis, which allows for some continuity in the information.

The four selected facilities have had extensive experience with user fees and keep financial records. In terms of the number of hospital beds and patient flow, the three hospitals sampled are the largest in Santo Domingo; they account for 50% of beds, 80% of hospital discharges, and 50% of outpatient physician consultations in all SESPAS facilities in that city. With a few exceptions, these three hospitals also are the largest in the nation; they are national referral centers and thus receive patients from all over the country. The National Laboratory only performs laboratory exams and accepts patients referred from public and private facilities as well as walk-ins.

Financial Importance of User Fees

Facilities receive personnel funds and supplies from the SESPAS personnel budget and operational subsidies, drugs and medical supplies from the Program of Essential Medicines, user-fee revenue, and donations. Administrators of the facilities have no control over personnel—SESPAS hires and pays them directly—nor over medical supplies—the Program of Essential Medicines manages them based on available stocks and standing orders from the facilities (which may or may not be completely filled).

More important are operational subsidies and user fees because they are managed by the facility and have the greatest potential to affect the quality of care. SESPAS regulations distribute operational subsidies according to use (e.g., medicine and salaries), but there is considerable flexibility to alter such distribution.

SESPAS and the Program of Essential Medicines allocations to the facilities have been insufficient to cover needs and, by 1986, the facilities had the following debts: Aybar Hospital, $US87,400; Altagracia Hospital, $US61,000; and National Laboratory, $US4,600. Reid Cabral Hospital did not have any debt largely because of a successful foundation that collects contributions from local enterprises and individuals, as well as external donations; unfortunately, there are no data on the amount of these donations. The National Laboratory also receives domestic donations, but these are negligible in the other two hospitals (Mesa-Lago, 1986b; Lewis, 1987; La Forgia, 1989).

Table 70 presents the sources of revenues for the four facilities, excluding donations. In the three hospitals, revenues from SESPAS represent from 98% to 99% of total revenue, but only 56% in the National Laboratory. Consequently, user-fee revenue appears to be significant only

Table 70. Charges, revenues, expenditures, and waivers of user fees in four public health facilities, Dominican Republic, 1989.[a]

	Public Sector				Private sector
	Hospitals			National Laboratory	
	L. Aybar (General)	Reid Cabral (Children)	Altagracia (Maternity)	National Laboratory	Private sector
1. Revenues by source (%)[b]	100.0	100.0	100.0	100.0	—
SESPAS	97.8	98.2	98.8	56.4	—
Personnel budget	78.5	85.2	88.4	48.3	—
Operating subsidies	19.3	13.0	10.4	6.1	—
User fees (outpatient consultation)	2.2	1.8	1.2	43.6	—
2. Outpatient fees ($US)[c]					
Laboratory exams	0.47–3.93	0.16–2.36	0.16–3.14	0.78–5.00	0.78– 12.60
X rays	3.14–6.30	0.78–3.14	n.a.	n.a.	6.30– 31.50
Sonograms	5.50–7.87	n.a.	0.0	n.a.	31.50– 55.18
Electrocardiograms	0.0	0.78–3.14	n.a.	n.a.	19.68– 47.24
Encephalograms	3.14	n.a.	n.a.	n.a.	102.36–125.98
3. % of waivers[d]	100.0	100.0	100.0	100.0	—
Fee waived	35.0	36.1	1.0	0.0	—
Fee reduced		9.3	0.02	50.0	—
Fee fully paid	65.0	54.6	98.98	50.0	—
4. % distribution of user-fee expenditures	100.0	100.0	100.0	100.0	—
Personnel	2.8	56.3	42.3	20.8	—
Skilled salaries	0.0	0.0	8.3	14.1	—
Unskilled salaries	0.0	48.4	27.9	2.2	—
Incentive pay	2.2	7.9	5.6	2.6	—
Overtime	0.6	0.0	0.5	1.9	—
Services	34.4	8.5	46.1	6.5	—
General	7.6	2.2	8.5	4.7	—
Construction	0.0	0.0	14.3	0.0	—
Diagnostic	1.1	3.1	1.0	0.0	—
Maintenance/repair	25.7	3.2	22.3	1.8	—
Supplies	61.1	34.1	9.4	70.9	—
Medicine	17.9	6.2	0.6	0.0	—
Medical supplies	16.1	2.8	0.0	61.8	—
Nonmedical supplies	20.3	2.1	0.1	6.7	—
Food	2.8	23.0	1.2	0.0	—
Fuel	3.2	0.0	1.3	0.8	—
Equipment	0.8	0.0	6.2	1.6	—
Other	1.7	1.1	2.2	1.8	—

Sources: La Forgia, 1989; Lewis et al., 1990.
[a]Based on data gathered in April–June 1989, except for waivers that are partly based on 1986 data collected by Lewis.
[b]Includes SESPAS personnel budget and operating subsidies and user fees; excludes donations; domestic donations represented 3% of revenue in the National Laboratory but were negligible in the hospitals.
[c]The table uses the 6.35 pesos for $US1 exchange rate given by La Forgia.
[d]Aybar based on 1989 data; the rest based on 1986 data from Lewis; percentages of those who paid less than the full fee (given by La Forgia, 1989) are: 30% in R. Cabral, 10% in Altagracia, and 10% in National Laboratory.

for the latter (44% of total revenue). But, if we focus on facility managed funds, such as operational subsidies and user fees, the latter become more important: about 10% for the hospitals and 87% for the National Laboratory. Furthermore, in 1984–1986, increases in user-fee revenue exceeded growth in SESPAS funding (Lewis, 1987). Those trends continued in 1986–1989, with one exception (increases in the operational subsidies and user-fee revenue are given for each facility): National Laboratory, 9% and 321%; Reid Cabral Hospital, 47% and 688%; Aybar Hospital, 50% and 328%; and Altagracia Hospital, 50% and 52% (La Forgia, 1989). The National Laboratory collected 69% of the total user-fee revenue in the April–June 1989 period, while the rest was almost equally divided among the three hospitals.

User Fee Prices

Due to the Government's ambiguous policy, each facility uses a different formula to set fees: the three hospitals use informal criteria to set prices, whereas the National Laboratory has established prices based on specific cost criteria. In Altagracia Hospital, fees are determined according to estimates of a patient's ability to pay. Aybar Hospital sets prices at 20% to 30% of estimated private sector charges. In Reid Cabral Hospital, prices are fixed according to approximations of material costs and a patient's ability to pay. The National Laboratory sets fees according to three criteria: current costs of supplies, a percent surcharge to pay for incentives to technicians, and a percent surcharge to compensate for reduced-fee services to patients who are unable to pay.

Table 70 presents fee schedules for similar services in the four facilities and in the private sector. There is relatively little variation in prices charged for most laboratory exams at the three hospitals. Fees at the National Laboratory average 40% to 50% higher than at the hospitals and are comparable to the lower spectrum of private sector fees. Fees for X-ray exams at Aybar Hospital are twice as high as the charges of Reid Cabral Hospital, but less than half the price of private sector charges. Fees for other diagnostic services, mainly offered at Aybar Hospital, are only a fraction of the private sector's prices. For instance, the price of an encephalogram in the private sector is from 32 to 40 times higher than in Aybar Hospital. Unless covered by insurance, the poor simply cannot afford private sector charges for these services.

Means Tests and Waivers for the Poor

The four facilities analyzed use an informal means test to waive fees for the poor. Patients who cannot pay the full price may pay a lower fee or none at all, depending on the judgment of a social worker who supposedly assesses the patient's socioeconomic status. Some facilities keep accounts of these efforts and of the final decision; others do not keep records on waived or reduced fees. According to the 1987 survey of Santo Domingo, over 90% of SESPAS users were exempt from payment, while the remaining 10% paid user fees (Gómez, 1988). The studies by Lewis and La Forgia found a considerably lower percentage of waivers. In 1986, 36% of Reid Cabral Hospital's outpatients did not pay a fee and 9% paid a reduced fee, but the proportions were negligible in Altagracia Hospital (99% paid full fees); in the National Laboratory, there were no waivers, except for inpatients hospitalized at SESPAS facilities, but half of the outpatients paid a reduced fee (see Table 70). There are data on two other hospitals (not shown in the table) from the 1986 study: in Contreras Hospital, 26% of patients were granted waivers and 34% paid reduced fees, while in a regional hospital, half of the outpatients were eligible for a waiver and 20% were granted a fee reduction (Lewis, 1987). In 1989, 35% of Aybar Hospital patients either were granted waivers or paid a reduced fee, compared to 30% in Reid Cabral Hospital, 10% in Altagracia Hospital (much more than in 1986), and 10% in the National Laboratory (much less than in 1986).

According to La Forgia's observations of the socioeconomic assessment conducted at one hospital, the process appeared quite arbitrary and somewhat dehumanizing, and the fee that was ultimately paid was not really based on the patient's income or other criteria, but rather was arrived at through a bargaining process between patient and social worker. This negotiation was carried out in the midst of numerous onlookers who interjected comments on the negotiation process, and often, a social worker negotiated with more than one patient at a time. Since a price list is not available, the social worker often is accused of arbitrarily setting the fees. Furthermore, it is evident that friends or relatives of hospital workers and patients with sufficient political contacts receive waivers. These individuals also receive prompt appointments, while others—including patients who pay the full fee—may have to wait several weeks or months. The medical director of the hospital estimates that revenues would increase by half if fees were collected from those who are able to pay.

In other facilities, the environment may be less chaotic, but fees are set by a similar process; price lists are not displayed and there are no formal criteria for determining eligibility for a discount. At the National Laboratory, managers have an unwritten policy whereby all patients must pay something. Each morning, before services begin, a social worker addresses the patients in the waiting area and requests their cooperation in paying the full fee, explaining the high cost of services. An ''economic evaluation'' form is completed for all patients who request a price reduction, and discounts must be approved by the facility administrator or subdirector. Most patients requesting a discount receive a 10%–25% reduction. Although the process is less dehumanizing at the National Laboratory, it does increase the waiting time.

Do user fees deter the poor from seeking services and/or are they an unfair burden to them? The above information points to the fact that the means test is ineffective in identifying those who can afford to pay a full fee, and that a significant portion of patients either receive a waiver or pay a reduced fee. However, as has been pointed out, in 1986, 99% of patients paid full fees in one hospital, and this also was true at the National Laboratory, where 90% of patients paid full fees in 1989. Because no data are available on the characteristics of the population that does not pay or that receives discounts, Lewis (1987) shows that those who benefit are not necessarily those who cannot pay. La Forgia (1989) reaches a more optimistic conclusion— few are denied care because of their inability to pay but those requesting a waiver or a discount usually have to wait longer and endure a humiliating evaluation (see the section on ''Effects on the Poor,'' beginning on p. 176).

How User-Fee Revenue Is Spent

Revenues from user fees are mainly used as stopgap expenditures directed at critical operational needs that vary from facility to facility. Only at the National Laboratory is this revenue spent according to a general plan that utilizes it to improve the quality of services.

Table 70 presents a breakdown of user-fee fund expenditures for the four facilities by major expenditure categories (personnel, services, and supplies) subdivided according to the more important line items. No expenditure pattern emerges from the data, because each facility spends the revenues according to specific needs, but these needs often are related to erratic SESPAS hiring practices, the vagaries of the Program of Essential Medicine's supply system, devalued SESPAS subsidies, and facility-level management practices. Increasingly, user-fee revenues are allocated to items that were previously covered by SESPAS and the Program of Essential Medicine. These allocations will be discussed by category of expenditure.

With the exception of Aybar Hospital, in the other facilities from 21% to 56% of expenditures went to personnel: the bulk of these funds were used to hire unskilled personnel in Reid Cabral and Altagracia hospitals, but to hire skilled personnel at the National Laboratory. In 1989, Reid Cabral Hospital faced a serious lack of manpower in housekeeping, laundry/linen services, and in the central supply room. Because SESPAS did not provide the needed personnel, the hospital's administration was forced to hire them to avoid paralyzing those general services; a similar situation occurred in Altagracia Hospital. As did the hospitals, the National Laboratory spent part of the user-fee revenue to hire manual laborers and technicians to fill vacancies and provide stability, but unlike the other facilities, it appointed professionals who have been instrumental in creating and maintaining effective accounting, auditing, purchasing, and materials-management systems. Aybar Hospital did not spend user-fee revenue on personnel, because its director was appointed by the current government, and he managed to obtain greater control over personnel from SESPAS. All facilities paid incentives and most provided overtime pay, but the National Laboratory expenditure on these two items was 60% higher than in the other three facilities; on the average, incentive earnings were one-third of the Laboratory technicians' base salary. A higher proportion of revenue from user fees, combined with supervision and labor incentives, allowed the National Laboratory to retain its best workers, require a full day's work, and demand high performance, characteristics absent at SESPAS hospital laboratories.

Regarding services, Aybar and Altagracia hospitals allocated approximately one-fourth of total expenditures on repairs and maintenance, mostly for nonmedical equipment and infrastructure; in the past, these activities were mainly financed by SESPAS operational subsidies. On the other hand, the National Laboratory relied on user-fee revenue to pay for service and maintenance of medical and scientific

equipment. Construction involving the remodeling of a storage room took 14% of expenditures in Altagracia Hospital. All facilities
spent a small portion of user-fee revenue on
general services such as printing, prescriptions,
and administrative forms, and the hospitals
spent even less on sophisticated diagnostic services not offered at SESPAS facilities.

Supplies represented approximately two-
thirds of total revenue expenditures at Aybar
Hospital and the National Laboratory, and one-
third in Reid Cabral Hospital. Because of the
Program of Essential Medicine's irregular supplies of drugs and medical materials, Aybar
Hospital used most of the user-fee revenue to
buy these items. Reid Cabral Hospital, in turn,
used one-fourth of all user-fee revenue to buy
food. Conversely, the National Laboratory does
not depend on the Program for Essential Medicine, but purchases them from private vendors;
hence, almost two-thirds of expenditures went
to this line item. This facility, however, has developed efficient systems of supply and distribution that allow it to avoid scarcities and to
assure that the right item arrives at the right
place at the right time. Although not shown in
the table, fuel expenditures were rising rapidly
due to frequent and prolonged blackouts that
required increasing purchases of diesel fuel for
electrical generators. This situation worsened in
May 1989 and deteriorated further by August
1990.

Effects on the Poor

User fees charged to hospital outpatients have
been instrumental in maintaining a basic level of
health services, but probably have not improved the quality of such services. As has been
seen, user-fee revenues are mainly used by the
hospitals to fill crucial gaps created by
SESPAS's shrinking operational subsidies and
the Program of Essential Medicine's irregularities in supply. These allocations have been
instrumental in keeping performance from falling below a maximum standard or even in keeping medical services from stopping altogether.
However, in hospitals user fees probably have
not been an effective mechanism for extending
coverage to or increasing utilization by the poor.
The major problems there are unfavorable administrative conditions and SESPAS inefficiencies under which hospitals operate. User fees do
not generate a significant portion of hospital
revenue and the gap between their needs and
available resources is expanding rapidly. To

close that gap, and to improve the quality of
services, will require not just quantitative increases in resources (which user fees alone cannot provide) but qualitative changes in the hospitals' administrative environment.

Conversely, user fees at the National Laboratory have been successfully used to develop and
maintain a positive management environment
and to improve the quality of services which, in
turn, has fostered increased utilization. Furthermore, only at the National Laboratory do user
fees constitute a large portion of total revenue.
Before the introduction of user fees, the few laboratory tests that were performed there took as
long as three months, patients had to wait in
long lines, and the test results were unreliable.
Now the services are performed quickly (usually results are available in the same or the next
day), there are no waiting lines, and results are
highly reliable—even high-income individuals
use the National Laboratory when needed
(Mesa-Lago, 1986b). But once again, the fees
without administrative improvement would not
have yielded the same results.

According to La Forgia, the inability to pay
does not appear to deter access to the services
for which fees are charged. In general, prices
are considerably lower than in the private sector. Although the means test is an ineffective
screening device—especially for identifying patients who can pay—it probably does not dis-
criminate against the poor. In 1989, a significant
percent of users at all facilities were granted
waivers or paid a reduced price. Furthermore,
given that only modest fees are charged and
that these are restricted to outpatient diagnostic
services, it is unlikely that user fees burden the
low income users who do pay or that they represent a deterrent to utilization. Furthermore,
data from the National Laboratory suggest that
increases in prices have not affected utilization.
In 1986–1988, the number of laboratory exams
performed increased by 56%. Yet, over this
same period, the fees for most "simple exams"
increased by 50%, and the fees charged for
"complex exams" doubled. The rise in utilization is related to the high quality of services provided at the Laboratory, as well as to the deterioration of laboratory services offered by
SESPAS hospitals.

The poor clinical and operational quality of
many services offered at SESPAS hospitals may
strongly influence utilization and may create
greater financial hardship for the poor than the
fees charged for these services. Perceived quality of care may be more influential than price on

an individual's choice of provider. Rather than endure the inadequate conditions of SESPAS facilities, many turn to the private sector. As we saw in a previous section, the 1987 survey demonstrated that approximately one-fourth of households with a monthly income below $US105 utilized private facilities, and, as seen in Table 70, private sector charges dwarf SESPAS user fees for similar services. Furthermore, users of private facilities also must pay physician honoraria and other types of fees such as hospitalization, which are free of charge at SESPAS facilities.

Faced with medical bills equal to or greater than a family's monthly income, the poor's use of private facilities may aggravate poverty. Improvements in the quality of SESPAS services, including reducing waiting periods, would probably increase utilization by the poor, significantly reducing their out-of-pocket medical expenditures.

Raising user fees at SESPAS facilities without a concomitant improvement in quality could reduce utilization of services by the poor or could delay this group's presentation at SESPAS facilities until an illness episode reaches a severe stage. The current management environment will limit whatever effort is undertaken to improve quality through user-fee revenues. Under different conditions, however, user-fee revenues could be used to improve quality and perhaps to increase utilization (extend coverage) by the poor.

The National Laboratory is an exception: it has made an impressive effort to humanize treatment, reduce congestion, present an attractive physical plant, organize work environments, and provide an excellent service that is also of high technical caliber. As such, it offers a rudimentary model for improving operational and clinical quality through user fees. That model is the basis for the recommendations in the next section.

Recommended Changes

In order to improve the quality of hospital services and increase their utilization by the poor, the following changes are necessary. SESPAS should permit hospitals to directly contract a limited number of professionals, such as material and inventory managers, and accountants, as well as general service personnel. SESPAS also should provide the base salary for these personnel, which, in turn, should be supplemented with substantial incentive payments fi-

nanced by user fees. Department heads, directors of diagnostic and medical services, head nurses, and other key professionals should be properly rewarded through both salary and incentives. Hospital management must have the final word concerning assignments of employees hired through SESPAS, and training should be provided to increase the skills of old employees. Using user-fee revenue, professional staff should conduct scientific and operational research to improve health care at the hospitals; a materials management system for medical and nonmedical supplies also must be developed.

An additional source of revenue for the purchase of drugs and medical supplies would be derived if the hospitals took over popular pharmacies (*boticas populares*). These are supplied by the Program of Essential Medicines, and most of them sell their drugs to hospital users at inflated prices. The hospitals could operate these pharmacies, retain a percentage of their earnings, and introduce items that are currently sold only in private pharmacies. Hospitals also could establish snack bars as a way to take advantage of thousands of patients and visitors who currently purchase food and beverages from street vendors.

Hospitals should develop a standardized, more effective, and less dehumanizing means test that avoids deterrents to those unable to pay, such as increased waiting time, and abuses by those able to pay. User fees should be set according to the costs and volume of materials, and all prices should be posted. Each facility must develop a fixed price-reduction scale based on patient income, and income and employment records should be kept and updated on all patients requesting discounts and waivers. Economic evaluations should be conducted in private, and the final decision to grant a waiver or a discount should be made by at least two facility officials; this will reduce waivers for friends and family of facility workers. Finally, the facilities should make it known that services will not be denied due to inability to pay the full fee, but they should require that all patients pay something.

Given the proper mix of leadership, administrative conditions, and political will, user fees can become an effective financial mechanism to improve the operational and clinical quality of SESPAS services and to increase utilization by the poor. The National Laboratory has proven that such a task is feasible and other SESPAS facilities should follow its example.

Extending Coverage of the Poor Through Private Pre-payment Plans (Igualas)[3]

Due to lack of access to or poor quality of SESPAS services, in 1984–1987, a significant proportion of the poor nationwide and in Santo Domingo paid for expensive private health services. A further erosion of the quality of public services in the late 1980s and 1990, due to continual strikes and a lack of supplies and shrinking funds, probably forced an increasing number of poor to seek private health sector care. Most residents of impoverished neighborhoods in the capital cannot afford to pay fees for health care, and yet, they prefer to borrow money or sell off possessions to pay a private physician rather than go to SESPAS facilities. This section discusses the potential for covering a portion of the poor and low-income groups in the informal sector in Santo Domingo through low-cost *igualas*. For his report, La Forgia investigated seven *igualas* in Santo Domingo.

General Review of Igualas

Most *igualas* are private HMO-type companies that provide comprehensive health care coverage equally to all subscribers for a monthly fee (the term *iguala* comes from the word *igual*, meaning equal). Currently, there are 20 *igualas* in the country that focus on group plans and cover 450,000 subscribers, most of them employed in relatively small and mid-sized enterprises.

All *igualas* provide services at designated providers and facilities, but assume different forms. Owners of the *iguala* can be a small group of physicians who also own the principal provider facility or they can be a large group of physicians (who are the shareholders) more or less grouped into a single facility usually contracted by the *iguala*. *Iguala* owners can negotiate contracts with a network of independent physicians and facilities, or the *iguala* can have its own facility and salaried physicians. One of the investigated *igualas* is a nonprofit organization that covers public-school teachers and contracts with a wide range of hospitals, which, in turn, contract physicians. With few exceptions, the main

[3]This section is a summary of Gerard La Forgia's, ''Health Services for Low-Income Families: Extending Coverage Through Pre-Payment Plans in the Dominican Republic,'' Washington, DC, US-AID HFS Technical Report, No. 1, October 1990. Unless otherwise specified, the information in this section comes from that source. La Forgia is the author of this section, but I take responsibility for any errors resulting from my summary of his report.

purpose of the *igualas* is not so much to earn a profit, which is usually low, averaging 4.7% in 1989 (Duarte et al., 1989), but to channel a large volume of patients to a limited number of physicians and usually to a single hospital.

For an enterprise to qualify for a plan, most *igualas* require a minimum number of employees varying from 15 to 50; one *iguala* requires a minimum of 500 enrollees to qualify for its basic low-income plan. Inflation is driving most *igualas* to exclude small firms with fewer than 50 employees because of the high risks involved. Monthly premiums vary between $US5.50 and $US9.50 per person; the teachers' *iguala* charges $US1.90. Employers cover between 50% and 100% of the premium, and the remainder is deducted from the employee's salary; most employers pay 75% of the premium for minimum wage workers. Without the substantial employer contribution, few employees could afford the premium.

Except for preventive care, the *igualas* offer comprehensive coverage of both outpatient and inpatient services. Most *igualas* offer two or three plans, depending on the coverage desired and employee salary levels. Enrollees incur no or few out-of-pocket expenses for routine curative care, within predetermined utilization limits, but normally pay for special services; there are payment ceilings and various services require a copayment. Providers are paid directly by the *igualas*. About 75% of the health insurance market is controlled by the *igualas*, which successfully compete with insurance companies because *igualas* do not have the same administrative and marketing requirements as insurance companies, they pay lower fees to physicians and hospitals, their profits are lower, and they offer a similar range of services as insurance companies for one-third less the cost.

The Population Covered and Possibilities of Expansion to Incorporate the Poor

From two-thirds to three-quarters of enrollees in *igualas* earn between $US79 and $US190 monthly. According to a 1989 study, the poverty line for a family of five was $US115 monthly; therefore, some enrollees may be below the poverty line and are covered because their employers pay 75% of the premiums. Without this contribution, the premium for a family of four would take from 27% to 48% of the low-level salary and from 12% to 20% of the high-level salary that most *iguala* enrollees earn. Due to the deterioration of SESPAS and IDSS services, both low- and middle-income employees are putting pressure on their employers to enroll them in *igualas*.

Informal workers are currently not covered by either social insurance or private health insurance. In 1988, there were 400,000 workers employed in 145,000 microenterprises in the nation, and, because microenterprises have an average of only 2.8 employees, these workers have not been able to join the *igualas*. Since the latter have increased the minimum number of employees needed for enrollment, the possibility of coverage for that large population group is increasingly remote.

Two associations of microenterprises, ADEMI and ADOPEM, currently provide services and loans to 3,500 microenterprises that employ 22,500 workers who have 86,000 dependents; if past beneficiaries of the services of these associations are added, the potential population may be twice as high.

ADEMI maintains a network of salaried field promoters in specific neighborhoods who seek out new businesses, arrange for all loans, and collect monthly payments. The promoters report that 80% of microenterprise owners and employees are very interested in joining *igualas*. ADEMI is willing to provide the needed administrative base to extend coverage to present and past loan recipients. ADEMI leaders estimate that 75% of affiliated microenterprises can afford the standard premium charged by most *igualas* for a basic plan. Furthermore, they claim that the majority of the employees earn above the minimum wage and can pay a portion of the premium. Finally, according to ADEMI, a pilot program could enroll 10,000 owners and workers and 40,000 dependents; ADEMI promoters would play a key role in enrolling enterprises and collecting the premium.

ADOPEM clients are mainly small groups of two or three women, vendors of foodstuffs and clothing. Since these are "subsistence" type microenterprises, they cannot afford the standard *iguala* premium. ADOPEM executives argue that health problems are the main reason for loan defaults among the association's borrowers, and have recommended a reduced benefit plan that would cost between $US3 and $US6 monthly per family and would emphasize preventive care, health promotion, and infant-maternal care. ADOPEM also has offered to manage the plan and collect the premiums; the latter would be added to the principal of each microenterprise loan, thus increasing the monthly payments accordingly.

Most *iguala* executives have responded favorably to extending coverage to a collective of microenterprise owners and employees managed by ADEMI and ADOPEM. However, they require that these owners and employees be constituted in a group; microenterprises, in particular, have never received coverage, and hence, it is difficult to estimate their utilization rates.

Models of Extension

Based on the previous findings, La Forgia proposes three extension models to cover an approximate population of 100,000 people. The first is for those microenterprises affiliated with ADEMI that can afford current *iguala* premiums ($US6 to $US8 per person monthly). Through a bidding process, ADEMI would negotiate contracts with one or more *igualas* that would specify benefits, premiums, and provider networks. *Igualas* would, in turn, contract with hospitals and physicians; *igualas* with limited providers would have to secure additional facilities close to the residence of the new enrollees. For a minimum number of enrollees, the *igualas* would grant a 10% discount on premiums; these funds would remain with ADEMI to pay for administrative costs and provide incentives to their promoters to collect premiums.

The second model, based on an *iguala* that covers public-school teachers, is geared to a population with lower income, and would provide a similar package of services as the first model at approximately half the cost ($US3 to $US4 per person monthly). ADEMI or ADOPEM would contract directly with single facilities and, through bidding, would assign a minimum number of enrollees—about 5,000—to each facility; the premium would be based on the number enrolled. The facility would be responsible for providing the services stipulated in the contract; hence, only those facilities with operational referral and utilization control systems, along with low fees, would be eligible. A variation of this model would involve establishing links between the main facility and outpatient clinics located in the neighborhoods where the low-income population lives. The clinics would provide basic curative, infant-maternal, and preventive services, while the hospital would offer specialist, diagnostic, and inpatient services for patients referred from the clinics.

The third model, most relevant for the poor, focuses on owners and employees of subsistence microenterprises who could not afford even the reduced premium of the second model—premiums in the third model would be $US0.80 to $US1.50 per person monthly. Services would be limited to basic curative care, routine diagnostic tests, infant-maternal care, essential medicines, and preventive and promotional services such as immunization and treatment of diarrhea and parasites. ADOPEM would contract with outpatient clinics located in impoverished areas that, in turn, would provide the needed personnel and services. ADOPEM would gather information on enrollees and utilization rates, and identify, assess, and select providers.

Needed External Aid

None of the above models would be able to function without external technical assistance and a minimal start-up investment. Assistance is required from USAID for ADEMI and ADOPEM to become efficient administrators in training, management, and information systems, as well as for start-up funds for staff, supplies, and equipment. It is expected, however, that the program would become financially sustainable after several months in operation.

Technical assistance is also required for *igualas* interested in bidding for microenterprise coverage, in order to improve their efficiency. USAID should provide credit to develop utilization control, management information systems, and quality assurance, as well as to upgrade the physical plant and equipment. Finally, technical assistance will be needed to help *igualas* add preventive and promotional services to their benefits package.

Since 1985, USAID has considered the expansion of coverage to low-income population groups in the Dominican Republic through *igualas*, and has commissioned at least eight studies to that end (Mesa-Lago, 1986b). La Forgia's study is the most sophisticated so far, and shows the feasibility of this approach. Although he does not provide a cost figure for the project, it obviously would be a fraction of the $US17.5 million invested by USAID in 1975–1986 to try and improve SESPAS services. A small investment in this project might ultimately provide better health care services for the poor in the Dominican Republic.

5.
FINDINGS, LESSONS, AND POLICY RECOMMENDATIONS

POVERTY: SIZE, TRENDS, AND CHARACTERISTICS

Clearly, the greater a country's poverty, the more difficult it is to provide health care for the poor. It might also be expected that the degree of development would be inversely correlated with poverty, and yet, based on GDP per capita, Mexico ranks slightly better than Costa Rica in terms of development, but has a much higher poverty incidence. Costa Rica's more equal distribution of income, particularly of social services including health care, largely explains this discrepancy. Although data on the Dominican Republic's poverty are not comparable with those of the other four selected countries, we found the lowest national poverty incidence in Uruguay and Costa Rica (respectively, second and third lowest among the ten countries surveyed by ECLAC, which is to say in Latin America); Mexico's poverty incidence ranked midway within the group (the lower fifth); and the poverty incidence in the Dominican Republic and in Peru were the highest (respectively, the second and third highest). In the mid-1980s, Peru's poverty incidence tripled that of Uruguay, doubled that of Costa Rica, was 1.5 times higher than that of Mexico, and was probably somewhat higher than the Dominican Republic's. The effort required to provide health care for the poor in Peru and the Dominican Republic must be greater than in Uruguay and Costa Rica.

The economic crisis of the 1980s probably led to an increase of national poverty incidence in all five countries. Increments in percentage points between 1977–1981 and 1984–1988 were: 11 to 20 in the Dominican Republic, 7 in Peru, 5 in Uruguay, and 3 in Costa Rica. Mexico's poverty incidence reportedly declined 3 percentage points, but the latest available estimate for that country is for 1984, at the beginning of the crisis; our analysis indicates that poverty rose in Mexico during the rest of the 1980s. In absolute terms, the number of poor experienced growth in all countries, ranging from 8% in Mexico to 52% in the Dominican Republic. The rapid expansion of poverty combined with the 1980s crisis made it even more difficult to provide health care for the poor. The countries that suffered the greatest losses in economic growth in the last decade were Peru and Mexico, followed by Uruguay and Costa Rica; the Dominican Republic's economy had a small cumulative increase for the period. And yet, Costa Rica appears to enjoy the steadiest, although modest, economic recovery since 1983; Uruguay's (except for 1986–1987) and Mexico's economies remain sluggish; the Dominican Republic's economy suffered another decline in 1984–1985 and was stagnant in 1988–1989; and Peru's economy has been in the midst of a serious crisis since 1988. The most optimistic outlooks do not anticipate a strong economic growth for Latin America and the Caribbean in the 1990s, as there was in the 1960s and 1970s; hence, at best poverty will likely persist, and it might continue to increase.

In all five countries, the poverty incidence was much higher in rural than in urban areas, ranging from 25% higher in Costa Rica to 70% in Mexico. Due to rapid urbanization, poverty incidence in urban areas exhibited a strong rising trend in the 1980s, with the largest increases being registered in the Dominican Republic and Peru. In rural areas, there was either a decline of poverty incidence (Mexico and Peru), stagnation (Costa Rica), or small increases (Uruguay and the Dominican Republic). And yet, today poverty still is concentrated in rural areas in most countries: in Peru almost three-fourths of the rural population is poor; in the Dominican Republic and Mexico, more than one-half; and in Uruguay and Costa Rica, less than one-third.

The provision of health care for the rural poor not only is more difficult because of the magnitude of poverty, but also because of the population's isolation and dispersion, its lower living standards, and, consequently, the higher costs to supply health services. One-half of the urban population in Peru and in the Dominican Republic is poor, one-third in Mexico, one-fourth in Costa Rica, and one-fifth in Uruguay. In the future, the greater problem will be urban poverty, unless strong growth occurs, which is an unlikely prospect.

In the urban area, poverty is concentrated in the informal sector, and this sector is largely excluded from protective labor and social insurance legislation. Although not all informal workers are poor—many employers are not—most are; for example, in the Dominican Republic and Peru, 77% and 86% of the urban poor, respectively, work in the informal sector. The larger the informal sector, the more difficult it is to provide health care for its population. Proportionally, the largest informal sectors at the beginning of the 1980s were found in Peru and Mexico (respectively, third and sixth largest in Latin America), followed by Uruguay and the Dominican Republic; the smallest was found in Costa Rica (the smallest in Latin America). Most informal workers work in tertiary activities, such as personal services and commerce, and to a lesser extent in manufacturing, construction, and transportation. Available data from all countries (except from Mexico) show a significant increase of approximately 6 percentage points in the size of the informal sector during the 1980s. Currently, Lima is the Western Hemisphere capital with the highest percentage of informal sector—from 50% to 60% of its labor force is engaged in informal activities.

Informal-sector workers are mainly self-employed, followed by wage earners employed in usually clandestine microenterprises, domestic servants, and, to a lesser extent, unpaid family workers and small employers; pieceworkers constitute the second most important group in the Dominican Republic. At the beginning of the 1980s, the nonsalaried sector of the labor force equaled 55% in Peru and 49% in the Dominican Republic, but only 30% in Uruguay and 25% in Costa Rica; there are no sound data for Mexico. Since the Bismarckian model of social insurance basically covers salaried workers, the larger the nonsalaried labor force, the more difficult it is to cover it.

The average income of informal workers was found to be between one-third and one-half that of formal workers in Uruguay and Costa Rica,

and three-fourths of the informal workers in Peru and more than half of those in the Dominican Republic earned less than the minimum wage. In Mexico, the proportion of informal workers earning less than the minimum wage was seven times higher than that of formal workers. Domestic servants have the lowest income among informal workers.

Living standards, including health, among informal workers are considerably lower than among formal workers. Most of the former are youngsters and women, and most have no education, very low-level skills, very little access to credit, and the worst housing. This group, which likely suffers from a higher sickness incidence than the population average but has no social insurance coverage, is supposedly covered by public health services. However, these services are often insufficient, and informal workers have meager resources to purchase health care in the private sector.

Because Latin America's rural population usually has lower living standards than the urban population, the countries with the highest proportion of their populations living in rural areas would be predictably more afflicted with poverty. As expected, the Dominican Republic and Peru, which have relatively large rural populations, have the highest rural poverty incidence; Uruguay, the least rural, has the lowest incidence. Mexico's rural share of the population is relatively lower than its rural poverty incidence. Conversely, Costa Rica is the most rural of the five countries, but has the second lowest rural poverty incidence, which is largely explained by the fact that Costa Rica has both the lowest traditional rural sector (most of the agricultural labor force is modern-salaried or landowners) and the smallest differences in living standards between urban and rural areas among the five countries, with the possible exception of Uruguay.

In some countries, living standards of the rural population were found to be about half of those of the urban population. Although overall living standards in Uruguay are five times better than in the Dominican Republic, in both countries the rural population has twice the illiteracy rate than the urban population. In three countries, the average income of the rural poor is about one-half that of the urban poor. The rural population has worse housing; considerably less access to potable water, excreta disposal systems, and health care; and lower nutritional levels than the urban population. Hence, it is not surprising to find considerably higher levels of malnutrition and infant mortality, as well as lower life expectancy in rural than in urban areas. In all five countries, we found that the poorest states, departments, or provinces, which usually are the most rural and, in Mexico and Peru, those where the Indian population is most concentrated, have the worst health resources and standards. Therefore, the provision of health care for the rural poor is more urgently needed, but as noted, it is a most difficult task.

HEALTH CARE COVERAGE OF THE POOR

In this work, a distinction was made among legal entitlement, statistical coverage, and real access to and utilization of health services by the poor. In all of the countries, three health sectors were studied—social insurance, public (essentially the Ministry of Health), and private. In Uruguay, Collective Institutions of Medical Aid (IAMCs) also were analyzed.

Legal Coverage

It should be recalled that legal coverage does not necessarily mean that the law is enforced. Enforcement is relatively simple in large urban enterprises and in the public sector, but it is much more difficult to carry out for small enterprises, the self-employed, and rural workers. In all five countries, the social insurance sickness-

maternity program legally covers the urban salaried labor force, but there are significant differences among them concerning legal coverage of the urban informal and rural sectors where the poor are concentrated (see Table 71). When covered, these groups of poor are registered in the country's main social insurance institute. Very few or no poor are protected by separate or special health programs that cover the armed forces, civil servants, or other groups of the labor aristocracy; such programs exist in all countries except in Costa Rica.

Costa Rica has the most comprehensive insurance coverage; it extends compulsory coverage to domestic servants, employees of microenterprises, rural workers, the unemployed insured for a period after dismissal, and pensioners. In addition, there is voluntary coverage for the self-employed, small urban and rural employers, and unpaid family workers. Furthermore, all the poor (indigent) population that are not insured is entitled to free care in social insurance facilities. Finally, the dependent family (spouse and children) of the insured, indigents, and pensioners are entitled to health care as well.

Uruguay's social insurance ranks second in coverage; it is legally obligatory for all the groups in question, with the exception of the self-employed, unpaid family workers, and pensioners. (It should be recalled that the legal incorporation of those groups only began in the mid-1980s.) The self-employed without a fixed place of work are totally excluded from legal coverage, and this also is true of unpaid family workers, except for spouses of small rural em-

Table 71. Comparison of legal health care coverage, by social insurance, of labor groups potentially poor in the five countries, 1988–1989.

	Costa Rica	Uruguay	Mexico	Peru	Dominican Republic
Domestic servants	M	M	V	M	N[g]
Self-employed	V[b]	M/N[c]	V	V	N
Rural workers, peasants	M	M	[f]	V	N
Agricultural producers	V[b]	M	V	N	N
Employees microenterprises	M	M	M	M	M
Employers macroenterprises	V[b]	M	V	N	N
Unpaid family workers	V[b]	N[d]	V	N	N
Unemployed[a]	M	M	M	M	M
Pensioners	M	N[e]	M	M	N[h]

Sources: Country analyses.
M = Mandatory; V = Voluntary; N = None.
[a]Temporary protection for the insured who become unemployed.
[b]Those not insured are entitled to welfare coverage, if indigents.
[c]Self-employed without a fixed place of work are excluded.
[d]Except spouses of small rural employers.
[e]Except for maternity.
[f]A tiny group of rural workers is mandatorily insured; a very significant proportion is covered under COPLAMAR.
[g]Except for those employed in businesses.
[h]Only for the disabled.

ployers; pensioners are eligible for maternity care, but not for sickness insurance. Furthermore, Uruguay's legislation does not provide social insurance coverage for indigents as does Costa Rica's. Finally, legal coverage of dependents in Uruguay is the second worst among the five countries: it is limited to spouses for maternity care only and to infants under 3 months of age; after that age, no curative services are provided for children, but primary care is available until 6 years of age. The poor cannot afford supplementary coverage of dependents, available through IAMCs.

Mexico's social insurance mandatorily covers employees of microenterprises, some rural groups that might include poor such as salaried plantation workers and members of credit associations and *ejidos*, the unemployed insured, and pensioners. In addition, it offers voluntary coverage to domestic servants, the self-employed, small-business employers, and unpaid family workers. A few urban informal groups such as lottery vendors and street musicians have been incorporated through collective agreements with their associations, but in practice, legal, economic, and administrative barriers tend to exclude the poor. The country's scope of coverage of insured dependents is the broadest of all countries—in addition to spouses and children, it includes parents. However, the most important social insurance program to cover the poor in Mexico is IMSS-COPLAMAR, which offers primary health care to the dispersed poor rural population; a previous program (Social Solidarity) was expected to cover the urban poor as well, but in practice has been limited to rural areas.

Peru's social insurance coverage is legally obligatory for domestic servants, employees of microenterprises, the unemployed insured, and pensioners. Voluntary coverage is available for the self-employed, rural workers, and housewives; the rest of the groups are excluded. Several laws that have mandated coverage of all groups that were previously excluded from or with optional coverage, remain unenforced, as the required administrative regulations have not been enacted. In the mid-1980s, coverage was extended to the insured's dependent spouse and children.

The Dominican Republic's social insurance has the narrowest legal scope among the five countries studied and probably for the entire Region. It excludes all the groups under discussion, with the exception of mandatory coverage of employees of microenterprises, unemployed

insured, domestic servants employed by businesses (but not the majority of domestic servants who work in homes), and pensioners for disability (but not for old age). Coverage of the insured's dependents is the most restricted as well; it is limited to the legal wife for maternity (not sickness) and to children of female insured's for pediatric care for 1 year after birth.

In all five countries, the poor who are not legally covered by social insurance are entitled to public health care, mainly through the Ministry of Health. In a few countries, municipal health services are available for the poor, particularly in the capital city. All public health services, with the possible exception of Costa Rica's, charge user fees; in Uruguay and Costa Rica, all or most of the poor are exempt from paying those fees after passing a means test; in other countries, the poor pay a reduced fee for some services. In Costa Rica, the Ministry of Health manages primary health care programs aimed at the poor living in isolated rural areas and in urban marginal areas where social insurance services may not be available; when needed, the poor are referred to higher levels of care provided by social insurance facilities that offer free services for indigents. In Mexico, COPLAMAR patients that require tertiary level care are referred to Ministry of Health facilities. Finally, in all countries, the poor legally benefit from general public health programs such as immunizations, control of contagious diseases, sanitation, and nutrition that are managed mainly by the Ministry of Health.

Private health care is legally available but, in practice, closed to the poor due to its high cost. Yet, in some countries, such as the Dominican Republic, lack of accessibility and/or low quality of social insurance or public health services force the poor to resort to expensive, private-sector services.

An obstacle for the expansion of coverage to the poor has been the lack of integration and/or coordination of social insurance and public-sector health services. Although the Ministry of Health has the legal authority to accomplish this task in all the countries, in reality, little progress has been made except in Costa Rica. In this country, social insurance owns and manages all hospitals, while the Ministry of Health is responsible for primary health care, prevention, and other general health services; some integration has been achieved at the local level. Costa Rica's unique combination of universal social insurance, supplementary services by the Ministry of Health, and good coordination between the two agencies offers the most comprehensive legal coverage for the poor among the five countries.

Statistical Coverage and Real Access

This study amply demonstrates the serious gap in reliable statistics on the population covered and its characteristics. The best available data are those from Costa Rica, with Uruguay's and Mexico's lagging behind; the worst data are from Peru and, particularly, from the Dominican Republic. This statistical vacuum has been the subject of international studies and recommendations for decades, but there is no significant improvement. In fact, the economic crisis has worsened the availability and reliability of data in some countries, such as the Dominican Republic and Peru.

Although social insurance statistics are better than those of the Ministry of Health, they are still seriously flawed; worse data exist for the private sector and other public programs. Countries that have multiple institutions and a large private sector, such as Uruguay, face more obstacles in producing sound statistics than do those with one or two central institutions, such as Costa Rica. In Peru, the number of active insured does not come from registration records—which need to be updated, among other things, to exclude those registered who have died, left the labor force, or migrated—but from projections of the EAP based on the 1981 census and the erroneous assumption that all those legally covered are actually incorporated; a very high rate of evasion and a jump in the proportion of the informal sector in the 1980s make such projections virtually worthless. Furthermore, in Peru dependents are estimated on a ratio per active insured, assuming, again incorrectly, that the extension of legal coverage to dependents has materialized. As a result of these problems, social insurance coverage in Peru is overestimated by 35%—about two million people. In the Dominican Republic, dependents are estimated by ratios per insured that have fluctuated from 0.04 to 0.36 (a ninefold difference!). Overestimation is not a serious problem in the Dominican Republic, given its tiny coverage of dependents, but it is in Peru, where the dependents/insured ratio jumped from 0.07 to 1.0 in less than one year.

Few ministries of health generate sound data on population coverage, and we have only rough estimates from ministry of health officials and independent experts. In the Dominican Republic, such estimates range from 40% to 80%; in Peru, officials acknowledge that only half of the reported population legally covered has real access, representing a difference of 6 million people; and in Uruguay, percentages of coverage fluctuate from 20% to 35%. In countries where the population covered by the ministry of health is a minority, as in Uruguay, such uncertainty is less of a problem than in those countries where the large majority of the population lacks "institutional coverage" or insurance and is reported as a "residue" theoretically covered by the ministry of health, as in the Dominican Republic. Because the poor are undoubtedly included in that "residue," it is impossible to seriously assess whether they are actually protected.

Since this work concerns only the poor, data on coverage by the private sector are only important in order to know how many persons in the "residual" population without institutional coverage can pay for private services, so as to determine who are those left at the mercy of public services; and in those countries, such as the Dominican Republic, where the quality of Ministry of Health services is so poor that the poor are forced to go to the private sector. It should be noted that estimates on private coverage often vary enormously: in Peru, for 1984, one source gave a figure of 350,000 and another between 4 and 10 million, depending on whether 6 million poor were excluded or included in the private sector.

With such poor ingredients, the resulting stew cannot be good. In Mexico, when one adds the scattered official data on coverage by all the public and social insurance institutions, the total population covered in 1988 was 5.6% higher than the country's total population, and this figure did not even include the private sector. Even in Costa Rica, where data are best, the overlap of social insurance and public sector services produces a total coverage of 36% above the actual population, again after omitting the private sector.

Population censuses could be used to fill the statistical vacuum, but data on health care coverage by income groups were not gathered by the censuses in the selected countries. Fortunately, population surveys, which began to be conducted in the 1980s, provide some information on real health care access and utilization by the poor, at least for Costa Rica, the Dominican Republic, and Uruguay. And yet, published survey data are usually incomplete and not standardized, impeding proper analyses and comparisons.

This long introduction is necessary in order to present Table 72, which attempts to summarize the most relevant available information from statistics, surveys, and experts on health care coverage of and real access to health services by the poor in the five countries. The statistics invariably give a much more optimistic view than do survey and expert data. Statistically speaking, in the mid-1980s, the population not covered by social insurance, the Ministry of Health, or other public and private institutions was zero in Costa Rica, 11% in Mexico, 12% in Uruguay, 32% in Peru (based on a high estimate of private coverage), and 40% in the Dominican Republic. Note that in Mexico, all the private sector and some public institutions are excluded; if they were included, everyone would be covered. In the Dominican Republic, the lowest estimate of

coverage by the Ministry of Health was used; if the highest estimate had been used, all the population would be protected.

Using survey data or adjustments by experts, the picture is gloomier but more realistic: still zero uncovered in Costa Rica (but see below), 20% in Uruguay, 21% in Mexico, 51% in Peru (based on a low estimate of private coverage; see below), and 92% in the Dominican Republic. In the last country, the figures actually are on the "uninsured" population; if a 40% statistical coverage by the ministry is used (probably an optimistic estimate), 52% of the population would be without protection. The survey data on Costa Rica that has been available to me, do not tell how much of the population was unprotected, but show which services were used by those who were sick and sought medical care. Still, the survey is useful because it shows a more comprehensive integrated picture than the statistics on the distribution of users by pro-

Table 72. Comparison of health care coverage and access (statistics and surveys) of total population and the poor among five countries, 1982–1988.

	% of population covered					
	Social insurance	Ministry of Health	Others[a]	Total covered	Uncovered	Poverty incidence
Costa Rica[b]						
Statistics (1987)	83	53	n.a.	136	0	—
Survey (1983)						
Population	81	4	15	100	0	—
Indigent	83	10	7	100	0	9 (1988)
Poor	89	4	7	100	0	27 (1988)
Uruguay[c]						
Statistics (1987)	47	27	14	88	12	—
Survey (1982)						
Population	45	24	11	80	20	—
Poor	26	40	7	73	26	20 (1986)
Mexico[d]						
Statistics (1987)	65	23	4	89	11	—
Adjusted (1987)	55	12	12	79	21	37 (1984)
Peru[e]						
Statistics (1984)	15	26	27	68	32	—
Statistics (1984)	15	26	8	49	51	60 (1986)
Dominican Republic[f]						
Statistics (1986)	4	40	16	60	40	—
Survey (1984)						
Population	n.a.	n.a.	n.a.	8	92	—
Poor	n.a.	n.a.	n.a.	3	97	49 (1980s)

Sources: Tables 2, 29, 34, 37, 43, 48, 60, 65 and discussions in the text.

[a]Private, armed forces, and other small public institutions.

[b]Statistical overlap in coverage results from different services. Survey does not specify the percentage of population covered; the distribution by provider is of those who were sick and sought care.

[c]Statistics on social insurance include IAMCs (the large majority). Survey coverage refers to those with "institutional coverage"; part of the uncovered probably buys private services directly.

[d]Statistics exclude the private sector and a small public sector; social insurance includes COPLAMAR. Adjusted figures by Wilkie, 1990.

[e]Both are rough statistical estimates of 1984 before inflation of social insurance coverage worsened, and include adjusted figures of the Ministry of Health. The first is based on a private coverage of 4 million and the second on a private coverage of 350,000; in addition, "others" includes 850,000 in public and charitable institutions.

[f]Statistics on the Ministry of Health are based on lower estimates of coverage. Survey refers to those who were covered by social insurance, armed forces, enterprises, and the private sector, excluding the Ministry of Health. The 1987 survey of Santo Domingo found that 76% of the total population and 85% of the poor were not covered (excluding coverage by the Ministry of Health).

vider; they eliminate the overlap between the ministry and social insurance, reducing the former's coverage, and add the private sector.

A disaggregated analysis of coverage by social insurance is possible in four of the five countries for the three most important groups of the labor force where the poor are concentrated—excluded are employees in informal microenterprises for whom data are not available (see Table 73). Although we lack statistics on the Dominican Republic, those three labor groups are excluded from legal coverage there, except for a tiny proportion of domestic servants employed in enterprises. Only rural workers in Mexico and, to a lesser extent, in Uruguay and Costa Rica, and the self-employed in Costa Rica and, to a lesser extent, in Uruguay, reach a sizable proportion of the total insured. All the self-employed are practically covered in Costa Rica; one-third are covered in Uruguay, but such coverage includes small-business employers and excludes the self-employed without a fixed place of work; and only a fraction are covered in Peru and Mexico. Note that the self-employed are voluntarily covered in all these countries except for Uruguay, but only in Costa Rica do they appear fully protected, partly because the uninsured are entitled to care if indigent.

Although the table does not provide information on coverage of employees in microenterprises (mandatorily covered in all countries), we found that most of them are not actually covered because of the enormous difficulties in controlling evasion. In Peru, a survey found that 42% of salaried workers who were supposed to be insured were not covered, and most of them were probably employed in microen-

terprises. About half of rural workers are covered in Mexico, Costa Rica, and Uruguay. The last two countries have mandatory coverage for the entire group, but in Mexico only a tiny proportion—plantation workers and members of credit associations—are covered. Practically all rural workers covered in Mexico are under the COPLAMAR program. In the case of Costa Rica, the table shows only rural workers who are insured, but the noninsured who are poor are eligible for indigent care.

Finally, less than one-fourth of domestic servants are covered in Costa Rica and Uruguay, but a tiny fraction of them is covered in Peru; practically none are covered in Mexico. It should be recalled that domestic servants have the lowest income among all informal workers, even when payment in kind is taken into account. Once again, all domestic servants who are not insured are entitled to indigent care in Costa Rica. The law stipulates that all domestic servants be covered in Costa Rica and Uruguay, as well as in Peru; however, statistics show a high coverage in the first two countries but a very low coverage in the third. Mexico offers voluntary coverage to this group but in practice covers none. To summarize, Table 73 confirms that Costa Rica has the highest statistical coverage of potentially poor groups in the informal and rural sectors, closely followed by Uruguay, except for the self-employed; Mexico's coverage of the rural sector is up to the level in these two countries, but coverage of the informal sector is nil; Peru does not cover any in practice; and the Dominican Republic excludes all of these groups from legal coverage.

The previous information and the analysis

Table 73. Comparison of degree of coverage of potential poor labor groups by social insurance in four countries, 1986–1988.

Countries[a]	Percentage of total insured			Degree of coverage[b]		
	Self-employed	Domestic servants	Rural workers	Self-employed	Domestic servants	Rural workers
Costa Rica	25.2	0.9	11.0	93–100[e]	24[g]	49[g]
Uruguay	11.3[c]	2.7	16.6	34[f]	21	55
Mexico	0.1[d]	0.1[d]	27.9[d]	0.4–1.0	0.1	56[i]
Peru	4.3	2.3	n.a.	4.1	3.1[h]	[j]

Sources: Tables 31, 38, 48–50, 61.
[a]Data for the Dominican Republic are not available.
[b]Percentage of the EAP group covered by social insurance.
[c]Includes small-business employers.
[d]Rural workers based on total insured (including COPLAMAR); self-employed and domestic servants based on total insured minus COPLAMAR; if the latter is included, the percentages become negligible.
[e]Includes both insured and indigents.
[f]Coverage of the self-employed with fixed place of work plus small-business employers equals 53%; the self-employed without a fixed place of work are not covered.
[g]Those who are not insured are covered as indigents.
[h]Lima.
[i]Mostly peasants and their families living in dispersed marginal rural areas.
[j]Negligible.

done in the preceding chapters allow us to do a more detailed assessment of the poor's health care coverage and real access in the five countries. In Costa Rica, survey data in Table 72 show that the overwhelming majority of the population uses social insurance services, with the poor and the indigents using them slightly more than the nonpoor: 89%, 83%, and 80%, respectively. Indigents use the Ministry's services more than twice as much as the nonpoor (10% and 4%, respectively), while the opposite is true of private services (15% use by the nonpoor versus 4% by the other two groups). It has been reported that 17% of the population not covered by social insurance can pay for private services, and this is roughly confirmed by the survey. In addition, 91% of all births and 88% of all pregnant women are said to be taken care of at social insurance facilities and the remainder either at Ministry of Health or private sector facilities; the Ministry immunizes 85% of the children.

These figures indicate that very few poor, if any, lack health care at least at the first level of attention. However, one official said that 20% of the urban poor visited by Ministry of Health personnel, do not use the facilities to which they are referred; if this is true, such a percentage should be higher in rural areas. It should be recalled that the Ministry of Health targets the poor; its services cover 48% of the total urban population (twice the urban poverty incidence of 24% and seven times the urban incidence of indigence of 6.7%), and 58% of the total rural population (twice the rural poverty incidence of 30% and five times the indigence incidence of 11.6%). Therefore, it appears that all the poor are covered at least at the first level of attention, but perhaps one-fifth of them do not use the higher-level services to which they are entitled.

The survey reported that 55% of the indigents and 64% of the poor did not seek medical care when feeling sick, but these proportions, particularly the poor's, were not significantly higher than among the nonpoor (66%). Reasons related to accessibility or costs given for not seeking medical help, such as lack of a nearby facility, poor quality of services, and high cost, were proportionally similar among the three groups: 14% of nonpoor offered that explanation, compared with 16% and 18% among the poor and indigents, respectively. Considering that the poor do not pay for public or social insurance services, only cultural barriers, lack of transportation, or perceived poor quality of services may explain the nonutilization of services.

Finally, during the economic crisis, social insurance coverage declined 8 percentage points, but the number of indigents served increased sharply, showing that anticyclical mechanisms to protect the poor worked; by 1987, the previous peak of insurance coverage was almost recovered. Ministry of Health coverage declined 11 percentage points during the crisis, but priority was given to rural services that declined less; by 1987, rural coverage had fully recovered. Conversely, urban services in 1987 were far behind the peak, but the urban poor probably had easier access to social insurance than the rural poor. The above discussion and the low percentages of indigence (9%) and poverty (27%) in Costa Rica allow us to conclude that the poor are protected by health care in that country, although there may be minor problems with access and, perhaps, quality of services that could be solved with better education, communication, and efficiency.

In Uruguay, the statistics and the survey data for the overall population are fairly close. However, Ministry of Health coverage is three percentage points lower in the survey than in the statistics, which confirms our selection of the lowest statistical estimate of coverage by the Ministry; this also is true for both social insurance and "other" coverage. As a result, the uncovered segment of the population increases from 12% in the statistics to 20% in the survey. However, the 1982 survey was conducted in the first year of a serious recession that caused a decline in overall population coverage of about two percentage points. Conversely, the higher statistical coverage in 1987 possibly reflects both the vigorous economic recovery of 1986–1987 and the expansion of social insurance coverage to low-income groups that caused a three percentage point increase in coverage and surpassed the previous peak. Unfortunately, we lack recent survey data to test this assumption.

Survey data show that the proportion of poor covered by social insurance/IAMCs and private services was 40% lower than the overall population, while the proportion of poor who used Ministry of Health services was 66% higher than the overall population. We also found statistical indications that, at the time of the crisis, social insurance/IAMC coverage declined, but that of the Ministry of Health that covered the poor expanded; however, it was not possible to check if such coverage was effective. Lack of institutional coverage—meaning no right or access to services—among the poor was 26% in 1982, compared with 20% in the overall population and 13% among the wealthiest third. The uncovered poor face some type of inaccessibility to the Ministry of Health services, be it cultural, administrative, or related to transportation problems, such as inadequate hours for outpatient consultation. A survey reported that non-coverage in Montevideo was 14%, compared with 29% in cities with fewer than 10,000 inhabitants, suggesting that coverage of the poor was better in the capital than in small towns and rural areas. The percentage of the overall population covered increased with age: children 14 years old and younger had the lowest coverage, reflecting the limited legal coverage of this group. Based on the survey data of 1982, we conclude that in the midst of the crisis, 5% of the poor were not covered by health care. That percentage is equal to the 5% incidence of indigence estimated by ECLAC for Uruguay. But the situation should have improved with the economic recovery and the expansion of coverage to low-income groups that occurred in the second half of the 1980s.

Mexican statistics of total population coverage are inflated and the adjusted figures, shown in Table 72, indicate that the uncovered segment of the population is twice as high as the official figures, 21% versus 11%. The statistics exclude the private sector and some public institutions, but the adjustment figures include both; hence, we can assume that in the adjusted figures, most of the uncovered population are poor. To the best of my knowledge, there are no survey data available on health care protection of the poor in Mexico. According to ECLAC, in 1984, at the beginning of the crisis, the national incidences of poverty and indigence were 37% and 13%, respectively, and both incidences probably increased due to further economic deterioration during the rest of the decade. All this leads us to believe that virtually all indigents and one-half of the poor are not protected by health care.

Mexico's informal sector is the sixth largest in the Region, but few labor groups in the informal sector are covered by social insurance; the degree of coverage of the self-employed and domestic servants is below 1%, and exhibits a declining trend. Furthermore, most of the apparent informal workers who are insured, probably are not poor; for example, 40% are employers and 16% are owners of taxis. The urban poor (30% of the urban population) are entitled to care by the Ministry of Health and other public and charitable institutions; although unable to evaluate the urban poor's real access, we know that public services are grossly insufficient to meet the demand and are of poor quality. In 1987, the proportion of potential rural poor *insured* by social insurance was also very

small, about 3% of the total number of insured. Conversely, at that time, 57% of the rural population was covered by COPLAMAR-Social Solidarity, plus the health services transferred to the states. These programs target the poor: 97% of the locations covered have fewer than 2,500 inhabitants, 69% of subsistence agriculture, and 87% of Indian groups are protected, and poor mothers and children are the primary users. Half of the population covered and half of the facilities are concentrated in nine states that have the lowest social insurance coverage, a very high proportion of Indian population, and the worst health and sanitary standards. In 1984, rural poverty incidence was 50% and coverage by COPLAMAR and similar services was 49% of the total rural population, but was concentrated on the poor; therefore, most of the poor rural population should have access to primary health care services. Access to secondary and, especially, tertiary-level care is much more limited.

Peruvian statistics on total population health care coverage are even worse than Mexico's. Data for 1984 in Table 72 show social insurance coverage prior to the statistical burst resulting from the legal inclusion of dependents, and data on the Ministry of Health are estimates of real access. The two different sets for 1984 result from diverging estimates of private sector coverage. The first row is based on the ten million "residue" (uncovered) that included six million poor (Zschock, 1988); for reasons already explained, we consider those six million as uncovered and, hence, estimate that only four million were covered by the private sector. The second row is based on a lower estimate of 350,000 covered by the private sector. In both cases, an additional million covered by other public and charitable institutions were included under "other." The uncovered population in 1984 was 32% or 51%, depending on whether the high or low estimate for private coverage is used. Even rougher estimates for 1988 (not shown in the table) suggest a small improvement, as the uncovered population declined to 28% or 47%, respectively. That improvement could have resulted from the 1986–1987 strong economic recovery and the expansion of social insurance coverage to dependents (possibly an increase of 5 percentage points), but these figures should be taken with extreme caution. National poverty incidence was 60% in 1986, hence, possibly one-half (in the best of cases) or four-fifths (in the worst scenario) of the poor were not covered. Peru has the largest informal sector in the Region, but only a tiny fraction of it is covered by social insurance: 3% to 4% of the self-employed and domestic servants are covered, and most of the self-employed insured are professionals with relatively high incomes. We also have noted that most employees of microenterprises in the informal sector are not covered. From 36% to 41% of the urban population (the poorest) are not covered, contrasted with an urban poverty incidence of 52% (19% indigence). The situation is worse in rural areas, where more than half of the population is not covered on health care, contrasted with a rural poverty incidence of 72% (46% indigence).

Dominican Republic data are the worst, but despite that, it can be stated that health care coverage of the poor in that country is similar or worse to that in Peru. Statistically, from 20% to 40% of the national population and 28% of the capital's population lack any type of health care coverage, and these figures are probably underestimated. Compared with poverty incidences of 36% to 49% nationally and 38% to 48% in urban areas, it appears that about two-thirds of the poor are not protected. The proportion of the population with institutional coverage—by social or private insurance and *igualas*—is estimated as 20% nationwide and 34% in the capital. But the surveys found much lower proportions (8% and 24%, respectively) meaning that 92% and 76% of the national and capital populations are expected to be covered by the Ministry of Health, except for those who can afford private services. Among the poor, however, surveys found that 97% nationally and 85% in the capital were in that situation. Half of the population who were sick and failed to seek medical help did so either because of poverty (as much as one-fifth), because of lack of access, or poor quality of services. Furthermore, three-fourths of the poor utilized Ministry of Health facilities (where 90% of patients do not pay user fees), but the remaining one-fourth bought private services (at a cost of 12% of their median income). The above discussion indicates that two-thirds of the poor are not effectively protected by health care, and many of them are forced to buy private services at great financial cost and sacrifice.

Predictably, surveys in three countries found that health care coverage of the population and quality of services are positively related to income: the highest income group mainly uses private services that tend to be better than the rest (very few poor utilize these services); the middle income group (and, to a lesser extent, the high income group) is mainly protected by social insurance services (through IAMCs in Uruguay) that usually are better than public services, and the poor are the group with the least access to these services, except in Costa Rica where there is no significant difference in access by income (in Uruguay those poor recently insured have gained access to IAMCs); and the poor basically rely on public services (fundamentally the Ministry of Health) that tend to be the worst in quality (once again, Costa Rica is an exception).

Substantial evidence was also found in all five countries on geographical differences in social insurance health care coverage and facilities related to poverty. The most developed, urban, and wealthier states, departments, provinces, and counties have the highest coverage, while the least developed, most rural, and poorest units, where most Indians live, have the lowest coverage. The following comparisons give the highest and lowest coverage by geographic units in each country: Montevideo 72% and Rivera 19% in Uruguay; Federal District 100% and Oaxaca 17% in Mexico; Lima-Callao 27% and Apurimac 2% in Peru; and La Romana 12% and Elías Pina 0.04% in the Dominican Republic. There is a very high concentration of social insurance coverage and services in the capitals that goes beyond the logical need for concentration of tertiary level facilities. For instance, the Central Region in Costa Rica, where the capital is located, has 50% of the total population but 80% of hospital beds, physicians, and nurses; Santo Domingo, with 27% of the total population, has 55% of the insured, 65% of personnel, and 40% of hospital beds; and Lima, with 31% of the population, has 56% of the insured and hospital beds, and 70% of personnel. For these reasons (at least in Costa Rica and Uruguay) the ministry of health coverage is higher in poor regions and ministry facilities target the poorest areas, which partly offsets social insurance gaps. In the same vein, Mexico's COPLAMAR facilities are concentrated in the poorest states, such as Oaxaca and Chiapas.

REASONS FOR LOW/HIGH COVERAGE OF THE POOR

General Factors

Costa Rica and the Dominican Republic, the smallest of the five selected countries, have the same territorial area. Neither has significant topographical barriers, and their small size combined with good to fair communications systems makes practically all their territory accessible. Costa Rica and Uruguay have almost the same population (about three million), while the Dominican Republic has about twice these two countries' population and three times the population density of Costa Rica. Consequently, pressure on scarce resources is higher in the Dominican Republic than in the rest. All of the people in these three countries speak the same language (Spanish), and there are no significant cultural differences within each country. However, the illiteracy rate in Uruguay and Costa Rica is very low (respectively, second and fourth lowest in the Region) while the Dominican Republic's rate is four times higher. Given these factors, Uruguay and Costa Rica have advantages over the Dominican Republic.

Mexico, the largest of the five countries, encompasses a territory that is 50% larger than Peru and much greater than the other three countries. Both Mexico and Peru have significant topographical barriers, and there are vast areas that are isolated or difficult to reach. Furthermore, significant portions of these countries' populations do not speak Spanish and are physically and culturally isolated. Illiteracy rates in Mexico are twice as high as in Costa Rica and Uruguay, but one-third lower than in Peru. For these reasons, access to health care by the poor is more difficult in Mexico and Peru.

Uruguay's per capita income is 50% higher than Mexico's and Costa Rica's, twice as high as Peru's, and 3.5 times as high as the Dominican Republic's. Uruguay and Costa Rica have more equal income distributions and fewer inequalities in living standards between urban and rural areas than do the other countries. And, as has been seen, poverty incidence in these two countries is lower than in the other two; Uruguay has the smallest rural sector of the five and Costa Rica the smallest informal sector (although it has the largest rural sector). The percentage of the nonsalaried labor force in these two countries is one-half of that in Peru and the Dominican Republic, hence, making easier the extension of social insurance. To summarize, Uruguay and Costa Rica share a combination of physical, cultural, and socioeconomic advantages over the other three countries that facilitate the health protection of the poor, but the disadvantages faced by the rest are not insurmountable, as Mexico has shown with COPLAMAR.

Uruguay and Costa Rica have been blessed with political stability and a long democratic tra-

dition, although Uruguay's was temporarily interrupted by the military. Both countries have a multi-party system in which two powerful parties have alternated in power; one party has been in control for longer periods and has been mainly responsible for enacting social legislation that the other major party has usually supported. Uruguay and Costa Rica have many strong workers' and farmers' associations that are relatively independent from the government and that have pressured to obtain social gains. Elected officials have usually responded to pressure from below or have taken the initiative in social security. In Uruguay, they have granted a succession of social security concessions in order to get re-elected; in Costa Rica, political leaders introduced and rapidly expanded social security. The early development of mutual aid societies in the 19th century in Uruguay set the stage for the unique expansion of IAMCs as major providers of health care in that country. On the other hand, a proliferation of institutions and a relatively weak central government in Uruguay prevented adequate coordination of the public and social insurance health systems. Conversely, the Costa Rican Government has been sufficiently powerful to effectively coordinate and promote local functional integration of the health system.

Mexico has enjoyed political stability for half a century, but it is a less pluralistic democracy than the previous two countries. One party has complete control, hindering true political competition; at least until very recently, popular organizations have been traditionally coopted by the government or the party, and the political leadership has been much less responsible to the electorate than in Costa Rica and Uruguay. In the 1950s, possibly responding to increasing agricultural union organization and outbreaks of rural rebellion, the Government tentatively began to extend social insurance coverage to the countryside, a movement accelerated in the 1970s with Social Solidarity and COPLAMAR. But extension of coverage to the urban poor has been basically rhetorical or symbolic, with little practical progress.

Peru and the Dominican Republic have suffered from long dictatorships, control by political caudillos, or frequent military interventions. Both countries, particularly Peru, are less stable politically than the other three, and have a much less democratic tradition than Uruguay and Costa Rica. The Dominican Republic's political leadership has been unable to enact legislation to extend coverage of social insurance, missing a unique opportunity to do so with union and employer support, due to political mishandling. In Peru, however, several laws have been enacted to extend such coverage, but none have been enforced, either for lack of political will or power, technical know-how, or resources.

A combination of favorable physical, cultural, socioeconomic, and political factors can largely explain the universalization of health care in Costa Rica and Uruguay; conversely, a combination of adverse factors may explain the failure in Peru and the Dominican Republic. Mexico, endowed with the most abundant resources of the five countries, has not been able to replicate the success of Costa Rica and Uruguay, and yet, political will combined with economic means allowed the country to break down the Bismarckian model of social insurance and produced COPLAMAR, despite physical, human, and administrative obstacles. The two poorest countries have different performances in this respect: Peru, with 45% of the labor force as salaried workers, has expanded social insurance to 32% of it, while the Dominican Republic, with a higher percentage of the labor force as salaried workers (51%), has only 10% of this group covered; despite favorable physical and cultural factors, the latter figure is the second lowest in the Region. Finally, a greater amount spent on health care does not necessarily assure wider coverage and better standards. For instance, the Dominican Republic and Mexico spend a similar per capita amount on health, but the record of the latter is much better than that of the former; targeting resources and their efficient use largely explain such differences (Pfeffermann and Griffin, 1989).

Social Security/Health Policy and Other Factors

Different social insurance and/or security policies to reach the poor in the informal and rural sectors may partly explain divergent outcomes. This section will focus on the financial aspects of such policies, administrative difficulties to extend coverage, and weak mobilization of the poor.

Financing

Clearly, the poor's low income and low health standards hinder their incorporation into a traditional model of social insurance; the poor cannot fully finance their protection, and they are more likely to use the public or social insurance services than are those with higher incomes, because of a higher sickness incidence and little or no possibilities of buying private services. We have demonstrated that most workers in the informal and rural sectors have the lowest national incomes. And yet, the percentage contribution imposed on informal workers is often higher than that charged to salaried workers with higher incomes.

Table 74 shows that the percentage contribution of the self-employed is three times higher than that of salaried workers in Peru and Mexico. The range of the contribution in Costa Rica is from 5% to 12%, depending on income, but most of the self-employed declare a lower income than they actually earn, making the average contribution 6%, only slightly higher than the salaried contribution. The burden of the contribution is alleviated for this group because the taxable base is less than the full compensation or salary. For instance, it is 75% of the minimum agricultural wage in Costa Rica and the minimum insured compensation in Peru, but in Mexico, it is 1.6 times the minimum wage in the Federal District. Although accurate comparisons are difficult to make, the self-employed in Costa Rica proportionally pay the least among the three countries and less than salaried employees in their own country, which leads salaried workers to register as self-employed. It is not surprising, therefore, that the highest coverage of the self-employed is achieved in Costa Rica. Including indigent coverage, practically all the self-employed are protected in Costa Rica, but only a fraction are in Mexico and Peru. Social insurance officials in Uruguay consider that the cost of extending coverage to the self-employed without a fixed place of work would be very high, and do not plan to incorporate them. In Peru, draft regulations of the 1987 law that mandated the incorporation of this group, stipulate a reduction by more than half of the contributions of the self-employed, with the state helping to finance the extension through 1% of the total wage bill; because the latter has not materialized, the regulations have not been approved.

As should be recalled, coverage of domestic servants is mandatory in Costa Rica, Uruguay, and Peru, but voluntary in Mexico. The contribution of domestic servants is the same as that of salaried workers in the four countries, but twice as high in Costa Rica (5.5%) than in the rest (3%). Furthermore, in Uruguay the taxable base is 85% of the minimum wage, and in Peru it is one-third of the minimum insured compen-

Table 74. Comparison of percentage contributions to social insurance sickness-maternity paid by salaried, informal, and rural workers in four countries, 1988–1989 (as percentage of salary or income).

Countries[a]	Insured			Salary base for contributions			
	Salaried and domestic servants	Self-employed	Rural workers/peasants	Salaried	Domestic servants	Self-employed	Rural/peasants
Costa Rica	5.5	5–12[b]	5.5	TC	TC	75% of agricultural MW	n.a.
Uruguay	3	—	3	TW	85% of MW	—	n.a.
Mexico	3	7.8	3	TW	MW	1.6 times Federal District MW	n.a.
Peru	3	9	4–9[c]	TC	1/3 of MIC	MIC	MIC

Sources: Tables 32, 40, 52, 62.
MIC = minimum insured compensation; MW = minimum wage; TC = total compensation; and TW = total wage.
[a]Dominican social insurance excludes the self-employed, home domestic servants, and rural workers/peasants.
[b]Average for all is 6%.
[c]The lower percentage is for economically depressed areas.

sation. However, in Mexico the taxable base is the minimum wage and, since employers can choose whether or not they register their servants and are expected to pay an 11.4% contribution if they do, most employers do not register their employees, which explains why only 0.1% of domestic servants are covered. Despite its highest percentage contribution, Costa Rica has the largest proportion of insured domestic servants (24%), closely followed by Uruguay (21%), which could be explained by the fact that in Uruguay, the burden of the pension contribution is the highest in the Region, and stimulates evasion. Only 3% of domestic servants are covered in Peru, probably because of poor enforcement. Two projects are being considered by Mexican social insurance to extend coverage to the informal sector. Coverage for domestic servants would become mandatory, but would be limited to high-income urban areas; the contribution would be equally divided between workers and employers (the latter cut by half) and benefits would be reduced. Coverage for the self-employed would remain optional, but their contribution would be reduced to one-third (upon a taxable base cut by one-third), and the state would finance half of the program.

Coverage of all rural workers is mandatory in Costa Rica and Uruguay, and in Mexico it is mandatory for only a small group; in Peru it is voluntary, mostly for peasants organized in associations. The percentage contribution for rural workers is the same as for other salaried workers in all countries except Peru, where it is higher. Mandatory coverage and a relatively wealthy agricultural sector appear to be the most important factors explaining why half of this group is covered in Costa Rica and Uruguay. Conversely, voluntary coverage, a poor agricultural sector, and the requirement to be part of an association explain the negligible percentage of coverage in Peru. Coverage of more than half of the rural population in Mexico is achieved through COPLAMAR, which does not require a cash contribution from peasants.

In the Dominican Republic, extension of social insurance coverage has been obstructed by the exclusion of civil servants and by an absurdly low ceiling ($US125 monthly) that practically excludes employees that earn mid-level and high salaries. These excluded groups can contribute much more than those covered, and it would be easier to detect, register, and collect from the former (the Government and large enterprises) than from those currently covered. Still, coverage of the informal and rural sectors would be difficult to finance with that additional contribution alone.

In Costa Rica, the state fully finances coverage of indigents. Although the portion of the state debt due to this sort of social insurance coverage is certainly sizable, without state financing, it would never have been accomplished; moreover, the debt is being paid, albeit under adverse terms. In Uruguay, social insurance coverage of low-income groups is subsidized by the state. In other countries, such as Mexico, the state contribution has declined, or, as in the Dominican Republic and Peru, it is stipulated by a law that has not been enforced.

The higher the percentage of the poor not covered by social insurance (an occurrence usually concurrent with a higher poverty incidence), the higher the proportion of the poor that is under the care of the Ministry of Health. The Ministry often operates with meager, dwindling resources from the central government, and if the bulk of the assigned population is poor, the possibility of collecting sizable revenues from user fees is nil.

Coverage of the poor in rural areas is often more expensive than in urban areas, because the population is scattered and isolated, transportation costs are higher, and cultural barriers pose obstacles. Furthermore, the possibility of earning substantial revenue from contributions or user fees is remote. Once again, Mexico's COPLAMAR and Costa Rica's indigent programs prove that coverage can be extended to the rural poor, but those two countries have more resources than Peru and the Dominican Republic.

The informal sector also presents serious administrative difficulties for incorporation. For instance, the cost of detecting, inspecting, and collecting microenterprises can be higher than the contributions actually paid. For example, in Peru, between about 35% and 40% of contributions do not materialize for that reason; in Lima, 66% of all registered enterprises have fewer than six workers, employ 10% of the total number of insured, and pay 4% of total contributions. In 1985–1988, an attempt to computerize registration and payments achieved some progress, but this effort ended for lack of funds. In the Dominican Republic there are 145,000 microenterprises that employ an average of 2.8 workers each.

The number of self-employed is many times higher than the number of microenterprises, and the difficulties and costs to register and collect from the former are higher. To cope with these problems, social insurance institutes have entered into agreements with associations of self-employed workers, whereby the responsibility for registering and collecting from members falls on the associations. However, this solution is not always successful. For instance, in Mexico, an agreement with a street-vendors association has not come through because a minimum of 2,000 members are required, and the leaders of the association are reluctant to become financially responsible for payments. Agreements have been more successful in Costa Rica, but they have been used by middle-income self-employed to pay a lower contribution; in addition, the lower contribution has been an added incentive for salaried workers to register as self-employed.

Inefficiencies in public health agencies, such as long waits for consultations, poor quality of services, absentee personnel, and lack of supplies, often alienate even the poor. In Peru, admission to public hospitals often requires "contacts" with relatives and friends, and in some Dominican hospitals, appointments are "sold" to users.

Weak or Ineffective Mobilization of the Poor

In most of the selected countries, the first labor force groups to be covered by social insurance were the most powerful and best organized, and the last to be covered, if at all, have been the least powerful and most poorly organized in the informal and rural sectors. In rural areas, a scattered population, cultural barriers, and physical isolation can help explain a weak or lack of organization, but this is not true of many informal workers who are well organized. In Peru, street vendors are members of several federations, but their major concerns, rather than health coverage, are to obtain security in their public stands and markets. Fragmentation and rivalries among these associations, as well as lack of a well thought out long-range plan and sustained action have determined the failure of the few attempts to force authorities to provide street vendors with health coverage.

EFFECT OF POOR COVERAGE ON OVERALL HEALTH STANDARDS AND INCOME DISTRIBUTION

A lack of sufficient and comparable data in the five countries prevented the measurement of the potential impact of health care coverage of the poor on the health standards of the overall population and of the poor. It was possible, however, to review the experience of three countries: the Ministry of Health programs for the poor in Costa Rica, the COPLAMAR program for rural poor in Mexico, and the Ministry of Health programs for rural and urban marginal populations in the Dominican Republic. In addition, survey data on Costa Rica, the Dominican Republic, and Uruguay allowed an evaluation of the impact of state subsidies to health care on income distribution.

Health Standards

Table 75 presents a comparison of two significant indicators of health standards—infant mortality and life expectancy—among the five countries within a 28-year span (1960–1988). The lack

Table 75. Comparison of health care standards in the five countries, 1960 and 1988.

	Costa Rica			Uruguay[a]			Mexico			Dominican Republic[a]			Peru		
	1960	1987	[b]	1965	1987	[b]	1960	1988	[b]	1960	1988	[b]	1960	1988	[b]
Infant mortality	68.6	17.8	−74	47.9	23.8	−50	74.2	46.0	−38	132.2	65.0	−50	140.9	86.0	−39
Life expectancy	60.2	74.7	24	68.4	71.0	4	56.3	68.9	22	51.0	65.9	29	48.0	62.0	29

Sources: Tables 35, 44, 69; World Bank, 1990.
[a]Data on infant mortality and life expectancy are the most favorable among various series available.
[b]Percentage change in period.

of data made it impossible to systematically compare the evolution of the pathological and morbidity profiles in those countries. The table shows that, in 1960, Uruguay had the lowest infant mortality rate and the highest life expectancy, followed in order by Costa Rica, Mexico, the Dominican Republic, and Peru. By 1988, Costa Rica had moved up to first place and Uruguay down to second; the other three countries remained in the same positions. These changes occurred because Costa Rica's reduction in infant mortality and increase in life expectancy occurred at a much quicker pace than Uruguay's. These comparisons should be taken with caution because we saw the contradictions in statistics related to these indicators in Uruguay and, particularly, in the Dominican Republic. For Table 75, we selected the most favorable series in each of these two countries, but the outcome would have been different if the least favorable series had been selected.

As a pioneer welfare state, Uruguay had achieved the highest health standards in the Region by the middle of the century, but stagnation of both its economy and public health expenditures induced a slowdown in the improvement of its health standards. In the meantime, other Latin American and Caribbean countries accelerated their health improvements and left Uruguay behind. Table 75 shows the period of slowdown in Uruguay's health standard improvement. Conversely, the table shows the period when Costa Rica accelerated the expansion of coverage of social security and launched health care programs that, combined with other variables, induced the rapid improvement of health standards. Although Peru and the Dominican Republic show significant improvements in both indicators in 1988, these were at similar levels to those of Costa Rica and Uruguay three decades earlier. Relatively rapid improvements in these two least developed countries are largely the result of massive prevention techniques, such as immunization. Health standards in the two most developed

countries, particularly Costa Rica, were already so high that it is increasingly difficult to reduce infant mortality and increase life expectancy; the easier improvements, such as those accomplished in Peru and the Dominican Republic, had already been achieved, and more sophisticated and costly techniques now have to be used.

Information on the causes of death in Costa Rica shows that in 1965, almost half of deaths were caused by "diseases of underdevelopment," such as contagious, intestinal, respiratory, and prenatal diseases, but the proportion declined to one-fourth in 1987, as "diseases of development," such as cardiovascular diseases, tumors, and accidents, caused more than half of the deaths. In Uruguay, the transformation of the epidemiological profile probably occurred in the 1940s and 1950s, and the available data for 1978 and 1987 do not indicate significant changes in that profile: in the two years, two-thirds of the causes of death were "diseases of development," while "diseases of underdevelopment" caused 8% and 7% of deaths. Both countries dramatically reduced deaths in children younger than 1 year caused by intestinal and respiratory diseases and malnutrition (11% in Costa Rica and 14% in Uruguay in 1987). Widespread vaccination also has practically eliminated or significantly reduced immunopreventable diseases. Conversely, Peru and the Dominican Republic have not yet transformed their pathological and morbidity profiles; for instance, in the latter, 38% of deaths of children younger than 1 year were caused by diarrhea and intestinal infections, respiratory diseases, and malnutrition. Hence, there is still considerable room in those two countries to rapidly improve health standards with relatively simple and cheap techniques.

In view of the above, the heavy emphasis given to curative specialized medicine vis-a-vis preventive medicine in the most developed countries, such as Costa Rica and Uruguay, although not justifiable, makes more sense than those priorities in the least developed countries, such as the Dominican Republic and Peru, and even Mexico. An increase in resources devoted to prevention and targeted to the poor and other vulnerable groups would have a much greater impact in reducing diseases of underdevelopment and infant mortality.

In Costa Rica, there are indications that the Ministry of Health programs have had more impact (relative to its significantly lower share of resources) on rising health standards than the social insurance programs. Within the latter, funds invested in care for indigents, pregnant women, and infants, probably have been more beneficial than the more expensive programs geared to middle-income and productive-age groups. One study on the impact of the Ministry of Health programs for the rural poor in the 1970s found a positive correlation between the degree of coverage by county of such programs and increases in life expectancy. Another study covering the Ministry's programs for both rural and urban marginal populations showed that as the degree of coverage increased, infant mortality decreased. These programs also appeared to contribute to a reduction in inequalities in health standards among counties.

In Mexico, the impact of COPLAMAR on health standards of the rural poor is difficult to evaluate because: little information is available on the services transferred to the states; due to the economic crisis, the COPLAMAR budget was cut (per capita expenditures were halved in 1982–1986), inducing reductions in personnel and supplies; and COPLAMAR's success varies significantly among communities depending on geographical accessibility, previous living standards, ethnicity, local authority support, and skilled personnel. Clinic and hospital utilization and services increased in most communities, at least until the decentralization process began. There may have been a decline in population coverage in 1986–1988 when the decentralization process took place, but there was a later increase in both population coverage and facilities, at least in the two-thirds of the program retained by IMSS. Most services rates per 10,000 people covered increased substantially between 1980–1982 and 1986: from 50% to 370% in prevention/sanitation services, 50% to 100% in treatment of priority diseases, and 16% to 100% on all hospital services; rates of clinical services declined. Morbidity rates for 1983 and 1986–1987 need to be interpreted with caution, but indicate significant declines in practically all transmittable diseases (from 11% to 65%), such as influenza, enteritis, acute tonsillitis, and am-

ebiasis; only scabies rates increased. Rates of immunopreventable diseases such as polio, pertussis, meningitis, tetanus, measles, and tuberculosis also declined, from 29% to 83%; human rabies and typhoid rates increased. Although the decline in such rates cannot be assumed to be an exclusive result of COPLAMAR prevention/sanitation services, these played a part in reducing rural morbidity.

To further improve COPLAMAR's performance, that program's cut funds should be restored and certain changes should be introduced. Prevention and/or sanitation and local paramedic personnel should be further emphasized over curative medicine and physicians; the program's single health model should diversify in order to address specific features and needs of different villages; the community's participation through health committees should be strengthened. Moreover, physicians should be trained before being assigned, and they should spend at least three years in a rural post to be able to learn from the community and be accepted by it; and qualified clinic assistants must be given increasing responsibility and training to perform more important tasks, while the number and roles of health volunteers should be expanded and their stipends raised. Finally, community work done in exchange for health services, should be specified and tailored to a given community's needs, resources, and interests. Whether decentralization should continue or the current fragmentation of this program between IMSS and the states be terminated and all its parts placed under one single authority (be it the Ministry of Health or social insurance) is currently being debated. Before making such an important decision, there needs to be better data to evaluate the performance of both IMSS-COPLAMAR and the decentralized state services.

In 1975–1986, the Dominican Republic received $US39 million from different international agencies primarily to develop health care coverage and prevention, particularly among the rural and marginally urban poor. Concrete objectives involved the improvement of nutritional levels and of access to potable water through hand pumps and to excreta disposal through building latrines, the reduction of immunopreventable diseases and infant deaths caused by diarrhea and parasites through rehydration and antiparasitic campaigns, the improvement of the health care of the infant-maternal group, and the creation of a system of medicine supply at low cost. The overall expected outcomes were a reduction in infant mortality and an increase in life expectancy and other health standards. Apparently, no comprehensive evaluation of the impact of these programs has been done. Nevertheless, a study of one rural community found that, despite the great investment in infrastructure and operational costs, the Ministry's services were of poor quality, and, because of that, two-thirds of the community's out of pocket expenses for health care went to private services. The reasons found to explain the poor quality of services included: *pasantes* spent only one year in the community and did not develop any interest in it, promoters were not well trained and did not receive proper guidance, *pasantes* spent minimal time on outpatient consultations, medicine supply was quite irregular, and maintenance was poor.

Yet, there have been some clear positive outcomes from those programs. In a short period of time, there was a three-fold increase in rural clinics and new urban clinics were introduced, the Program of Essential Medicines was established and began to supply medicines, although the supply is still quite irregular, and thousands of health promoters were trained. A lack of data and contradictory opinions among experts have made these programs extremely difficult to evaluate. It has been seen, however, that there has been no expansion of the poor population covered; in fact, there may even have been a decline due to the poor quality of public services. Furthermore, the number of hospital beds declined. Even the most favorable series on infant mortality and life expectancy show that in 1975–1985, the period when the programs were in operation, there was either stagnation or deceleration in the rate of improvement of such indicators. Information on immunization, antiparasitic and rehydration campaigns, and expansion of latrines and hand pumps is so scattered and contradictory that any serious evaluation of these programs is impossible. While the economic crisis of the 1980s undoubtedly contributed to the deterioration of health care, the Ministry's programs began in the mid-1970s and the crisis did not hit the country until 1982. To summarize, it appears that abundant resources were wasted through inefficiency and mismanagement, and that most of the programs were not successful.

Income Distribution

In 1982, surveys on the impact of state subsidies on income distribution were conducted in Costa Rica, the Dominican Republic, and Uruguay; social expenditures included health care, pensions, education, water and sewage, and housing. The public health sector was basically represented by the Ministry of Health, but also included social insurance sickness-maternity programs, the armed forces (except in Costa Rica), and other public providers (IAMCs in Uruguay were excluded). In all countries, the subsidies to health care had the highest degree of progressiveness among all social expenditures, and in the Dominican Republic, health subsidies were the only ones that were progressive.

Within the health sector, the highest degree of progressiveness was found in the subsidy to the Ministry of Health. In Uruguay, the subsidy to the social insurance maternity program ranked second in progressiveness, but the subsidy to the sickness insurance program was the least progressive; it should be recalled that the maternity program targets lower income groups and the country's interior, whereas the sickness program aims at middle-income groups and Montevideo. In Costa Rica, 89% of the subsidy went to curative medicine, with only 11% going to preventive medicine; however, the latter had a much more progressive effect than the former. The share of the subsidy assigned to rural areas, which have a higher poverty incidence, was usually smaller than the share allocated to urban areas.

Last, but not least, the share of the subsidy assigned to health care was smaller than the share of all other social services. Therefore, health subsidies had the highest degree of progressiveness, but because of the smaller proportion of funds allocated to them vis-a-vis other services, the actual impact of health subsidies in reducing income inequality was lower than that of other subsidies. This was also the case regarding rural versus urban subsidies and preventive versus hospitalization subsidies. The highest impact of the subsidy in reducing income distribution was found in Costa Rica, followed by Uruguay; the least impact was registered in the Dominican Republic.

A reallocation of the state subsidy that increased the share of public health—and within it, the shares of the Ministry of Health, preventive services, and rural areas—would raise the redistributive impact of the subsidy. Cuts in the Ministry of Health budget in the 1980s, therefore, should have reduced the progressiveness of state subsidies, while increases in the budget, such as were seen in Uruguay in the second half of the 1980s, should have increased such progressiveness. An expansion of health care coverage to low-income groups (Uruguay since 1985) and, particularly, to the poor and indigents (Costa Rica since the 1970s), must have had a significant progressive impact on distribution. Finally, a shift from state subsidies away from social insurance, if that program covers middle-income groups and excludes the poor, should also have a progressive impact.

FINANCIAL VIABILITY OF SOCIAL INSURANCE AND/OR THE PUBLIC SECTOR TO PROTECT THE POOR

In Costa Rica, the combined resources of social insurance and the Ministry of Health are sufficient and financially capable of maintaining current coverage of the poor and improving their care at higher levels of attention, but the serious disequilibrium of the pension program needs to be urgently corrected in order to avoid a collapse of the entire social security system. In Uruguay, neither social insurance nor the IAMCs appear capable of expanding coverage to the small group of uncovered poor without a substantial increase of an already burdensome state subsidy; conversely, the Ministry of Health has enough resources to undertake this task, but needs to improve the quality of its services and its administrative efficiency. In Mexico, COPLAMAR has been successful in extending primary health care coverage to most rural poor, but this has required substantial investment from the Federal Government and social insurance support; conversely, social insurance has failed to extend coverage to the informal sector, and because of its financial deterioration in the 1980s, it does not appear to be a feasible instrument for achieving this goal, unless it undergoes a significant reform. This is also the case of the Ministry of Health, which has suffered more from the crisis than social insurance. In Peru, the crisis that has afflicted social insurance since the early 1980s became even more acute in 1988, making it impossible to achieve the projected extension of coverage to the urban and rural poor; the Ministry of Health model of health care, although less expensive, is also currently unfeasible. Finally, in the Dominican Republic, social insurance is totally incapable of covering the poor; the Ministry of Health is besieged by enormous problems and inefficiency and also appears unable to achieve that task unless it is dramatically transformed.

In Costa Rica, there is virtually universal coverage of the poor through the combined health care services of social insurance and the Ministry of Health. If there are poor left unprotected, possibly at the secondary and tertiary level of care, they would be in the least developed, most isolated rural counties, and probably could be incorporated with the existing infrastructure and resources combined with an improved referral system and education. The question remains of whether the current system of health care is financially viable in the long run to maintain, and, one hopes, to improve, both universal coverage and the quality of services.

The social insurance sickness-maternity program spends three-fourths of total expenditures, and has ended in a deficit during most of 1975–1982. In terms of revenue, the deficit was caused by the huge state debt ($US61 million in 1987, 86% of which was in sickness-maternity due to state failure to reimburse the cost of indigent care); evasion and payment delays, mainly among the self-employed; and an insufficient percentage contribution to cover program expenditures. In terms of expenditures, the deficit resulted from overgenerous benefits, excessive personnel earning too high salaries, and some hospital inefficiencies. Since 1983, several of these problems have been corrected or ameliorated—the contribution was increased, a few generous benefits were eliminated, agreements were signed with the state to pay the debt in bonds, hospital efficiency was improved, and some employees were dismissed. As a result, since 1983 the sickness-maternity program has generated a surplus that is predicted to continue until 1998. And yet, the overall stability of the institution is threatened by a serious disequilibrium in its pension program, which is projected to go bankrupt by the year 2000 unless drastic measures are rapidly introduced. This crucial problem must be solved before any attempts can be made to improve high-level services for the rural poor and before a few sectors of uncovered informal workers, such as domestic servants, can be incorporated. A project to insure a portion of the self-employed who are currently treated as indigents has been halted due to administrative and financial difficulties.

In 1973–1987, Ministry of Health facilities in Costa Rica increased fivefold, mostly through additional health posts, while the social insurance growth was 55%, basically in clinics. The number of hospitals and beds per 1,000 slightly declined, but first level services greatly expanded. Table 76 shows that Ministry resources are insufficient compared with those of social insurance; for example, the latter's per capita expenditures are six times higher than the former's. These differences may be partly explained by the divergent nature of the services provided by each institution; social insurance offers curative intensive care, and the Ministry provides preventive primary health care. Still, the disparity between the allocation for preventive services and that for curative services is too great and should be reduced.

The Ministry's tiny share of hospital beds is due to the fact that all hospitals are operated by social insurance, and the Ministry only has a few beds in health centers—and these beds are only half utilized. Social insurance hospital occupancy is fairly high (79% and rising), and the average length of stay is reasonable (6.1 days) and declining. These statistics indicate that hospital facilities in Costa Rica are the most efficiently managed of the five countries. In summary, the social insurance public health system currently enjoys financial stability and enough resources to maintain current coverage of the poor and improve their protection at higher levels of care. However, social insurance must rapidly put the pension program on sound financial footing, in order to avoid bankruptcy of the entire health system in the medium term.

Uruguay's social insurance sickness and maternity programs have had a deficit since 1982, and it has increased from 5% to 32% of income, despite the 1986–1987 economic recovery. These programs also have taken a growing proportion of the overall institution deficit (27% in 1987), which in 1988 equaled 1.4% of the GDP and required a state subsidy of 2.7% of the GDP. The major causes of the deficit in terms of income are the twofold increase in population coverage in the second half of the 1980s, mainly to low-income groups that contribute less; in terms of expenditures, the growing health care costs at IAMCs are responsible. The growing disequilibrium of the sickness and maternity programs, combined with the huge imbalance of the pension program despite significant state subsidies, indicates the inability of social insurance to expand its coverage to the poor. Since 1977, IAMCs have faced increasing financial difficulties; bankruptcies have cut down their number 38%, and four-fifths of those remaining in operation face serious imbalances. Because of a rising premium, the number of IAMC affiliates first declined, but then increased with the expansion of social insurance coverage and economic recovery; still, by 1987, IAMC affiliation was under the 1984 peak. Due to the higher premium, the proportion of those covered by IAMC in the lowest income group has declined from 16% to 4%, obviously showing that IAMCs are not feasible vehicles to cover the poor.

The public health sector in Uruguay (Ministry of Health and University Hospital) has enough facilities and resources to expand coverage to any potential poor left unprotected. Table 76 shows that the public sector share of physicians and expenditures was proportional to its share of population, and its share of hospital beds was more than twice that of its population. While the private had a higher ratio of hospital beds per population covered than the public sector, and its expenditures per capita were twice as high, the IAMCs rated slightly better on physicians and expenditures. Nevertheless, Uruguay's Ministry resources compared quite well with those in the other four countries. Furthermore, in 1987 the Ministry's percentage of hospital occupancy was 60.9%, and, although it has been increasing since 1980, it was still low; in the country's interior, one-half of the installed hospital capacity was unused. In addition, the average length of stay was ten days and increasing; it was twice as high as the IAMCs average. A reduction of the hospital stay would leave even more unutilized capacity to cover the poor. Rather than quantity, the problem is one of quality, because public services are less good than those of the IAMCs and the private sector.

Due to budget cuts carried out under the military government, public hospitals (which were quite old) seriously deteriorated in their physical plant and equipment. Management has not been very efficient either, as the previous figures showed; there is too much centralization without adequate coordination and an excessive allocation of resources to the secondary and tertiary levels of care. Since 1986, the Ministry's budget has been increased and new hospitals have been built or are under construction. Given the excessive available capacity, however, such funds would have been better spent on repairs, remodeling, maintenance, and new equipment. Hopefully, the quality of public services will increase and reach all of the poor. Otherwise, serious consideration should be given to transferring a portion of the state subsidy away from social insurance (and IAMCs indirectly) and to the Ministry of Health.

Social insurance (IMSS) in Mexico has largely accomplished the goal of extending health care coverage to most of the rural poor, but it has failed to cover even a small proportion of the informal sector. In 1980–1987, IMSS generated a surplus, but as a percentage of income, it declined from 18% to 4%, while actuarial reserves decreased from 18% to 0.4%. Such reserves are inadequate to meet this institution's long-term obligations, which also recently faced a liquidity crisis. The main causes for the financial deterioration in terms of expenditures have been the deficit in the sickness-maternity program combined with very high administrative costs, and, in terms of revenues, an insufficient insured employer contribution, a cutback in government subsidies by half, and negative investment yields. Except for three years, the sickness-maternity program ended in a deficit between 1943 and 1988; this deficit was covered with transfers from other programs, particularly pensions, contributing to their decapitalization. As the pension program matured and its reserve decreased, its surplus declined, and so did the major source of financing for sickness-maternity. In 1989, this situation forced a 33% increase in the percentage contribution to the sickness-maternity program, but that contribution is still below the actuarial estimated level. IMSS administrative expenditures are among the highest in the Region, due to excessive personnel, high salaries, and overgenerous fringe benefits; despite the crisis, the ratio of employees to 1,000 insured kept growing, reaching a historical record in 1986. Since 1981, no information has been available on IMSS hospital efficiency, but it is probably low.

Currently, IMSS covers less than 1% of the informal sector, making it highly unlikely that it would be able to cover the remaining 99% with such a weak financial base and considering that sector's low income and the administrative difficulties inherent in that task. In order to achieve that goal, it would be necessary to either increase the percentage contribution to sickness-maternity again, or obtain a government subsidy (the IMSS project to expand coverage to the self-employed is based on 50% state financing). None of these options are feasible, because the current percentage contribution is the second highest in the Region, and the state has halved its support to IMSS. Better measures would be to cut administrative expenditures, increase efficiency, eliminate the salary contribution ceiling, and design a low-cost package of health care benefits. But, even with this approach, the expansion of coverage would still face serious difficulties. The incorporation of the informal sector (domestic servants and the self-employed) would increase IMSS current population coverage from 15% to 20%, but due to the crisis, that institution's per capita expenditures

and services have been cut. Social insurance officials realize that it is impossible to expand IMSS facilities under current conditions, and are considering the possibility of contracting private services.

The Social Solidarity-COPLAMAR model, financially viable in the 1970s, seems less feasible in the 1990s. These programs were launched at the time of the first oil boom, with substantial support from the Federal Government that supplied 60% of Social Solidarity costs and 100% of COPLAMAR costs. In addition, IMSS provided the remaining 40% for the first program and institutional support (estimated at as much as 50% of costs) in the second. With such abundant resources and dynamic leadership by IMSS, an impressive network of rural clinics and small hospitals was rapidly developed. But when the economic crisis forced a national adjustment program, the Federal Government decided to stop investing in these programs and to transfer the facilities to the states. Although only one-fourth of the facilities were transferred, and to the wealthier states, they lacked enough resources as IMSS support ceased. As a result, the quality of transferred services declined, and so did hospital occupancy.

To cope with these problems, the states began to charge user fees that probably reduced the poor's access and prompted protests; the transfer was stopped in 1988. And yet, Table 76 demonstrates that COPLAMAR is the least-expensive health care program in Mexico: its per capita expenditures are 11% that of IMSS, 17% that of the Ministry of Health, and 7% that of other social insurance programs. Hospital occupancy steadily rose to 83% in 1987, while the average length of stay declined to 3.5 days; although we lack comparable data for Mexico, COPLAMAR figures compare favorably with those of Costa Rica and Uruguay. Last, but not least, COPLAMAR appears to have had an impact on raising health standards among the rural poor. Consequently, COPLAMAR has been successful in expanding coverage with a low-cost package of benefits, but required substantial investment (particularly at its inception) from the Federal Government, as well as IMSS administrative and financial support.

A key aspect of Mexico's 1989–1994 National Development Plan is a National Solidarity Program that includes a strategy to expand health care coverage to the urban and rural poor through targeting, increased efficiency, emphasis on primary health care, and better coordination. These laudable goals, however, do not seem to be supported with the needed re-

Table 76. Comparison of health care facilities, expenditures, and efficiency in the five countries, 1985–1988.

	Percentage distributions				Per capita expenditures		Efficiency	
	Population covered	Hospital beds	Physi-cians	Expend-itures	$US	Ratio[a]	Hospital occupancy (%)	Days of stay ($\bar{X}$)
Costa Rica[b]	136	100	100	100	81	1.0	77.6	6.4
Social insurance	83	93	90	81	82	1.0	79.1	6.1
Ministry of Health	53	7	10	19	13	0.2	50.9	n.a.
Uruguay[c]	100	100	100	100	112	1.0	n.a.	n.a.
IAMCs/social insurance	52	18	63	60	131	1.2	n.a.	4.8
Ministry of Health	33	70	29	29	107	1.0	60.9	10.1
Armed forces	13	3	7	7	66	0.6	n.a.	n.a.
Private	2	9	1	4	186	1.7	n.a.	n.a.
Mexico[d]	100	100	100	100	n.a.	n.a.	n.a.	n.a.
Social insurance	73	n.a.	73	79	n.a.	n.a.	n.a.	n.a.
IMSS	48	n.a.	51	61	69	1.6	n.a.	4.2
Others	11	n.a.	18	16	115	2.6	n.a.	n.a.
COPLAMAR	14	n.a.	4	2	8	0.2	83.0	3.5
Ministry of Health	27	n.a.	27	21	44	1.0	n.a.	n.a.
Peru[e]	100	100	100	100	n.a.	n.a.	n.a.	n.a.
Social insurance	17	16	21	41	35	8.0	73.6	11.3
Ministry of Health	62	57	35	34	4	1.0	n.a.	n.a.
Armed forces	7	7	14	7	n.a.	n.a.	n.a.	n.a.
Private	14	20	30	18	n.a.	n.a.	n.a.	n.a.
Dominican Republic[f]	100	100	100	100	n.a.	n.a.	n.a.	n.a.
Social insurance	12	10	20	n.a.	46	5.1	51.7	10.4
Ministry of Health	54	34	25	n.a.	9	1.0	54.0	21.2
Armed forces	5	6	10	n.a.	n.a.	n.a.	n.a.	n.a.
Private	29	50	45	n.a.	28	3.1	n.a.	n.a.

Sources: Tables 33, 42, 53, 57, 63, 68.

[a]Based on national averages when available, otherwise on Ministry of Health's expenditures per capita.

[b]Due to overlap of services, the reported percentages add to 136%; based on the survey, they should be 95% in social insurances and 5% in the Ministry. Excludes the private sector which covers 5% of the population.

[c]Excludes a small proportion of public and charitable institutions.

[d]Excludes the armed forces, a few public providers, and the private sector (about 10% of the population). "Others" are civil servants and petroleum workers.

[e]Percentage distribution based on 1981, except per capita expenditures (1984).

[f]Santo Domingo.

sources and mainly rely on the public health sector. Table 76 shows that, with the exception of COPLAMAR, the Ministry of Health's share of hospital beds, physicians, and expenditures are proportionally lower than those of social insurances: the Ministry's per capita expenditures are one-half those of IMSS and one-third of wealthier social insurance programs that cover civil servants and petroleum workers. The impact of the economic crisis on the Ministry of Health has been more devastating than on IMSS: its population increased 27%, but its expenditures were cut 67%. Practically all Ministry services have declined since 1986. Obviously under the current critical conditions, the Ministry is not a viable vehicle to expand health care coverage to the urban poor.

In Peru, social insurance is in a worse financial situation than that of the previous three countries. In 1982–1988, there was an overall deficit, except for one year, and the disequilibrium worsened in 1988, forcing social insurance

to borrow and launch an emergency plan. The sickness-maternity program takes 58% of total expenditures and has ended in a deficit since 1977, becoming the main cause of the overall disequilibrium. Such deficits have been covered with loans and accounting transfers from the pension program, which has been gradually decapitalized and also faced a liquidity crisis in 1988. Causes of the deficit in terms of revenue have been the huge state debt (up to $US1.2 billion in 1979; its real value declined to $US49 million in 1988), very high evasions and payment delays, and negative investment yields that render the quite high percentage contribution insufficient. In terms of expenditures, the deficit has been caused by extremely high administrative costs (35% in 1988) due to an excessive bureaucracy, hospital inefficiency (hospital occupancy was 73.6% in 1986, but the average length of stay, 11.3 days, was the highest among all countries after the Dominican Republic); and expansion of coverage to dependents. Most of the 1988 emergency plan targets to tackle the social insurance crisis have not been fulfilled: evasion rapidly increased due to the termination of the program to computerize registration and collection combined with inflation rates nearing 3,000% that helped to virtually deplete reserves; the Government's promise to start paying the debt did not materialize; and the number of employees, rather than being cut, increased by 8% in 1989. The 1987 law mandated the extension of health care with full benefits to practically all the population including the two largest uncovered groups: the informal sector and peasants plus their dependents. The cost of such extension would have been $US746 million annually or twice the cost of the population already covered; with only primary health care, the cost would have been halved, but would still be completely out of reach. As these groups' income is quite low, the state was expected to contribute 1% of the national wage bill to facilitate the extension, but the crisis made that impossible.

Peru's Ministry of Health is expected to cover almost two-thirds of the population; at the beginning of the 1980s the Ministry's share of hospital beds appeared adequate, but its share of physicians and health expenditures were about one-half of what they ideally should be; the Ministry's per capita expenditures in 1987 were one-eighth of those of social insurance (see Table 76). The economic crisis of the 1980s has affected the Ministry less than social insurance, but both institutions have suffered sharp declines in expenditures, investment (paralyzed since 1988), supplies, and medicine. Although the Ministry's model of primary health care and sanitary posts would be considerably less expensive and, hence, more feasible than that of social insurance, the crisis has made the extension of coverage to the poor impossible even with that less costly model.

In the Dominican Republic, two-thirds of total social insurance expenditures go to the sickness-maternity program; this program usually ends in a deficit that is covered with declining surpluses of pension and employment-injury programs. The three schemes do not have separate accounts; since 1986, there have been virtually no reserves, accounting is chaotic, and there have been no actuarial balances for a very long time. The causes of the deficit in terms of revenue have been the cumulative state debt ($US95 million in 1980), from 30% to 35% evasion and payment delays, negative investment yields, and a very low percentage of contribution. The causes for the deficit in terms of

expenditures have been administrative expenditures as high as one-third of total expenditures, the highest in the Region (the ratio of 23 employees per 1,000 insured is a Regional record too); illegal free provision of 40% of health services to noninsured patients; and hospital inefficiency (in 1985, hospital occupancy was 51.7%, the lowest of the five countries, and the average length of stay was 10.4 days, the second highest). There is plenty of unutilized capacity, but population coverage is about 4%; the quality of services is so poor that a large proportion of insured is also covered by private insurance, and with such an expensive and inefficient program, universalization would cost 17% of GDP. Obviously, social insurance is totally unsuitable to extend coverage to the poor.

The situation is no better at the Ministry of Health, which was assessed in 1985 as "terrible" and "not working," and this was before the crisis worsened matters. Some of the numerous flaws found were excessive centralization without effective coordination—all personnel appointments, assignments, promotions, and salaries are centrally controlled without input from the local units; 90% of expenditures go to the tertiary level, but 90% of those services could be offered at lower levels if they were properly equipped, supplied, and managed; physicians work one-fourth of the legal schedule, are frequently absent, cannot be dismissed or disciplined by the Ministry, and often go on strike to get salary increases; from 75% to 90% of the equipment did not work in the mid-1980s, and in the first half of 1990 most operating rooms were shut down; in some hospitals, two patients often shared one bed, while other hospitals were empty; patients had to supply food, linen, medicine, and basic medical supplies; and in some facilities, appointments were sold. As in other countries, the problem is not one of insufficient quantity but of poor quality of services. In 1974–1985, there was an impressive expansion of facilities, particularly at the primary and secondary level, in both urban and rural areas, but only 25% to 35% of their outpatient services are utilized due to their poor quality. Table 76 suggests that the Ministry's share of hospitals and physicians is insufficient to serve the population it theoretically covers; furthermore, per capita expenditures are one-third those of private facilities and one-fifth of those in social insurance. However, note that hospital occupancy is 54%, dipping to a 3% low in some provinces, and the average length of stay is 21.2 days, twice as high as for social insurance and the averages of Uruguay and Peru, three times the average of Costa Rica, and five times that of Mexico. In 1981, public sector per capita expenditures were higher than those in more developed countries such as Argentina, Brazil, and Mexico. Drastic budget cuts occurred in the 1980s, but salaries were not affected, provoking a decline in all other budget lines. If the Ministry's facilities were efficiently used, would target the poor, would be less concentrated at the tertiary level, and their personnel were more productive, the quality of these services would improve significantly, and one-fourth of the poor would not need to buy services from the private sector.

User fees could be an alternative to improve coverage, services, and utilization in the public health sector; to that end, the experiences of the three largest hospitals in the capital and the National Laboratory were studied. This showed that revenues from user fees in the hospitals are utilized to fill crucial gaps created by the Ministry's shrinking funds, and, hence, they are instrumental in maintaining a minimum level of services and avoiding a total halt. However, due to the unfavorable administrative environment and the relatively small importance of the fees as a source of hospital revenue, such fees cannot improve the quality of services. Conversely, the National Laboratory has a good administrative environment, and fees generate about half of total revenues and have been used to hire managerial personnel, provide labor incentives and training, and give research opportunities to professionals. In this case, the fees have induced a significant improvement in the quality of services. For the National Laboratory model to work, however, important changes should be introduced in the Ministry of Health, such as hospitals should be allowed to hire, assign, pay basic salaries, and promote key personnel who should be in turn stimulated with revenues from fees. Furthermore, hospitals need to improve their efficiency and standardize the means test applied to patients. Currently, such tests are informal, and decisions to waive or reduce fees are not actually based on income, but are arbitrarily taken based on other criteria. It is not clear that all the poor are exempt: in the National Laboratory all users pay, although half of them pay a reduced fee; in the three hospitals, only from 1% to 36% of fees are waived. The current test also is inefficient in identifying who can pay a full fee, and those who benefit are not necessarily the neediest. Although user fees are substantially lower than private prices for the same services, there is no standardized method to set the fees; they should be set on real costs plus a surcharge. The application of these reforms would improve the quality of services and prevent anyone from being denied access because of a lack of means.

PRIVATE ALTERNATIVES TO EXPAND HEALTH CARE COVERAGE OF THE POOR AND IMPROVE QUALITY AND/OR EFFICIENCY OF SERVICES

The private health sector embraces different types of providers that can be divided into two broad categories: for-profit organizations, which include prepaid plans (individual and group insurance, employers plans, medical cooperatives) and private hospitals, clinics, physicians, and traditional doctors; and nonprofit NGOs, such as religious and charitable organizations, development institutions, and cooperative and community associations.

The size of the private sector, measured by the percentage of the population it covers, varies significantly among the five countries, and is inversely related to the size of the social insurance and public health sectors: 2% in Uruguay, if IAMCs are included, the proportion increases to one-third or more; 5% in Costa Rica; 10% in Mexico; and from 15% to 30% in the Dominican Republic and Peru. According to survey information, 7% of the poor in Costa Rica and more than one-fourth of the poor in Uruguay and the Dominican Republic purchase private services at significant personal cost. In Peru, the poor (both in the Andean highlands and in urban marginal towns) often borrow from friends and relatives when they have no other option but the private sector. Similar measures, as well as selling of possessions, are reported in Mexico and the Dominican Republic. In these three countries, many poor in rural and urban areas resort to traditional doctors (curanderos) to whom they may pay in kind or cash.

In Uruguay, a few groups of low-income workers are organized in associations, unions, or cooperatives to obtain supplementary coverage of their families and better health services. Groups of informal workers in Mexico also have become associated and signed prepaid agreements with private clinics. Peruvian street vendors and other informal workers use a rudimentary solidarity fund (junta) that is awarded, in turn, to those contributors who suffer accidents or serious illness. Charitable and religious clinics (the old *beneficencias*) and physicians enrolled by churches also provide health services to the urban poor.

Most NGOs that help microenterprises and other groups of informal employers and workers provide them with credit and training, but very few offer health services. In Lima, out of 200 NGOs engaged in development, two were identified as providing health services: IDESI, through a contract with an insurance company, offers "popular family insurance" to its 50,000 members that covers pregnancy care and accidents but no sickness; and PRODESE, which manages a clinic in a poor neighborhood of Lima, 40% of whose inhabitants are informal workers, that offers prevention, outpatient consultation, laboratory tests, infant-maternal care, control and treatment of some contagious diseases, and medicine.

In this section, the findings and lessons of five private alternatives to extend coverage or improve the quality/efficiency of health services to the poor are summarized.

Costa Rica: Social Insurance Collaboration with the Private Sector

In the 1980s, the Costa Rican Social Security Fund (CCSS) developed three programs with the private sector as a way to cut costs and increase the efficiency and quality of health services: enterprise physicians, mixed medicine, and a health cooperative. The first two programs do not help the poor directly, but strengthen CCSS both financially and in the quality of its services, and these improvements increase the capacity of social insurance to maintain free health services for the poor at the secondary and tertiary levels.

Through enterprise physicians, 630 private enterprises hire and pay a doctor and provide an office and a nurse to care for their employees, while CCSS contributes laboratory and other diagnostic services and medicines. Under the mixed medicine program, the insured at CCSS select a physician from those enrolled in the program, and pay for the services, while CCSS provides diagnostic support and medicine. These two programs combined serve 7% of the population covered by CCSS, and provide per capita consultations to the insured at a lower cost.

The health cooperative, organized in 1988, has received a fully equipped clinic from CCSS,

plus monthly sums per user; in exchange, the cooperative provides prevention services, antiparasitical treatment, curative medicine, diagnostic services, dental care, medicine, etc. Indigents are entitled to use these services and may freely select a physician from the cooperative. If successful, this experiment could take advantage of the surplus of physicians in Costa Rica to expand services to marginal urban areas.

Uruguay: A Worker's Cooperative Clinic

The cooperative, COTER, is one of the few successful self-managed enterprises in Montevideo, and since 1985 it has operated a clinic for the workers and their families, covering more than 600 people. The clinic's building and equipment were purchased with IAF grants; the cooperative employs and pays a few medical professionals and has an agreement with an IAMC to provide supplementary curative services. Reportedly, COTER members are in the upper level of the third lowest income bracket of the population, and are not covered by social insurance; and most of them cannot pay the IAMC premium. Before the clinic was established, the workers either had to pay user fees for poor quality services in the Ministry of Health or pay higher prices to get better private services; if the needed treatment was expensive, the cooperative paid part of the cost. Some of the clinic services are free, others charge small user fees (one-fifth of market prices). COTER pays half of the IAMC premium for supplementary family coverage, and the other half is paid by the workers. Services include prevention, outpatient consultation, infant-maternal care, minor surgery and emergencies, dental care, laboratory tests, and medicine. Users report that the quality of services is high, there are no waiting lines, and they have closer contact with medical personnel. The entire package saves the workers 30% of the average cost of similar services available elsewhere, a price they could not afford. In exchange for the IAF grants, COTER made a commitment to extend the clinic primary health care services to workers in six other factories located in the neighborhood, as well as to poor residents in a nearby slum. By the end of 1989, the expected extension of services had not begun and without pressure from IAF, they may not materialize.

One might think that the COTER model would have to be an economically successful cooperative committed to the welfare of its members and to have external aid in order to be duplicated. However, external aid to COTER was modest—less than $US34,000, a sum similar to the annual costs of COTER health services. Furthermore, the per capita annual cost of the entire package is $US90, one-half of the IAMC average per capita and 16% of the Ministry of Health per capita, an indication of the efficiency of the COTER program. Hence, it is possible that other enterprises, not only cooperatives, could develop a similar program. In view of IAMC rising premiums, the COTER model makes sense. The modest external aid investment in this project has resulted in high social dividends and should be expanded.

Mexico: Institutionalized Traditional Medicine for the Poor

The Mexican Institute of Traditional Medicine "Tlahuilli" was established in the state of Morelos in 1984 by a group of physicians who believe that traditional medicine is effective, inexpensive, and accepted by poor communities that basically lack access to modern medicine. The Institute has trained more than 200 health promoters, most of them *curanderos*, midwives, and herbal doctors who are members of the communities, with rudimentary knowledge on modern medicine. About 20 outpatient consultation posts and four clinics are attended by promoters, managed by health committees, and supervised by the physicians; they serve approximately 100,000 people in twelve poor communities. These communities range in size from 300 to 50,000 inhabitants, and include *ejidos*, rural villages, small towns, and shantytowns in small cities; their populations are blue-collar and informal workers, rural peasants, and indigenous groups, practically all of them poor. Most of these communities have no health services, or if they do, they are grossly insufficient. The Institute's services concentrate on the ten most common diseases such as gastroenteritis, parasites, and bronchitis. It provides curative services, herbal medicines, and steam baths for very low fees; promoters are expected to cultivate herbal gardens, prepare medicine, and collaborate on local campaigns for vaccination, disease control, and sanitation.

The Institute has received financial support from a Dutch foundation and a $US104,000 grant from IAF that ended in 1989; the IAF funds were used to build one of the headquarters buildings, buy land or buildings for some facilities, as well as equipment, salaries for part of the personnel, and the production of educational materials. Communities are expected to maintain the facilities, which are to be self-financed through user fees. The Institute generates revenues through fees for training courses and profits from an annual medicinal plant festival. The annual budget, when outside funding was available, averaged $US187,000, 38% of which came from external aid, 43% was expected to come from the communities, and the rest from the Institute. Currently, the Institute generates $US12,000; revenues from the community are small, and a minimum of $US60,000 is needed to continue all operations. The average expenditure per person covered was $US1.88 in 1987, about one-fourth of the COPLAMAR per capita, the lowest in Mexico.

In addition to the above-mentioned accomplishments, the Institute has been successful on several fronts: it launched a successful campaign against a dengue epidemic based on a natural medicine treatment discovered by the Institute that was more effective and faster than modern medicine; it organized a successful anti-parasitical campaign based on herbal medicine; it holds an annual well attended medicinal plant festival; and it published four issues of an annual bulletin on traditional and herbal medicine.

In addition to the funding cuts, which have forced a reduction in physicians and activities, the Institute confronts several problems. Most promoters, who are volunteers, spend little time at the Institute facilities, instead operating independently from their homes for a profit. The health committees have had a decline in membership, and they are not generating the expected contribution to the program. Some communal activities, such as the construction of latrines and cultivation of herb gardens, have not been as successful as the anti-dengue campaign. The Institute's facilities are underutilized in some communities, and their planned expansion has been halted. Patients who do not respond to the traditional medicinal treatment are not always referred to modern-medicine facilities by the promoters. The initial leadership of the Institute, although dynamic and successful, did not allow full participation of the communities; current leaders are more open to consultation, criticism, and community participation.

Some changes are needed to improve the Institute's performance. Emphasis should be placed on training promoters and insisting on the need for transfers when necessary. The promoters' independent operation should not be discouraged, because they need an incentive to continue their useful services. An evaluation should be conducted on whether to continue or to close facilities with low utilization rates and that are not self-financed. Physicians should devote more of their time to train, supervise, and counsel promoters. A study of the health needs of the population served and an evaluation of the Institute's performance in meeting such needs should be conducted. Effective consultation and participation of the community should be expanded. The cumulative experience and knowledge on herbal and therapeutic medicine, as well as on campaigns to fight diseases, should be systematized and published as a manual on how to treat the ten most common diseases that afflict the poor population. New sources of revenue should be explored, such as more and better courses; the sale of the recommended manual; and the establishment of a center for the wholesale, collection, and sale of inputs for traditional medicine. External aid should be made available to facilitate the Institute's transformation into an even more effective vehicle for helping the poor.

Peru: Community Mobilization for Primary Health Care in Villa El Salvador

As a result of one of the fastest rates of urbanization in Latin America and the Caribbean, hundreds of shantytowns (*pueblos jóvenes*) have boomed in Peru in the last two decades. Villa El Salvador is a remarkable ''young town'' that has successfully mobilized to provide, among other things, primary health care to its inhabitants. Established in 1971, the town is based on a self-government structure (CUAVES) and community participation at all levels. In 1988, there were 250,000 inhabitants in Villa El Salvador, and projections for the year 2000 are as high as 600,000. Despite significant improvements in living standards, one-fourth of the population is still indigent, and an unknown proportion is poor. One-fifth of the *families* earn one-fourth of the national *per capita* income. Most of the people work in the informal sector as street vendors, self-employed, and employees of microenterprises. The most common diseases are those typical of underdevelopment.

There are neither secondary nor tertiary level facilities in the community. The Ministry of Health has four primary health care centers and one health post, but these services are insuffi-

cient; basic services such as child delivery are not provided, so patients must go to a hospital in another city. The municipality manages three health posts that offer preventive services only, and there are no social insurance facilities in the town. The most important health services are organized by CUAVES through 35 modules, originally financed by UNICEF, that provide primary health care and target the infant-maternal group. Specific services are immunization, control of child malnutrition, treatment of diarrhea and respiratory diseases, and attention to pregnant women, mostly by midwives. Medical personnel in the modules are mainly supplied by various NGOs. One of these, the Institute for Support of Popular Health, was selected for study. Under CUAVES leadership, a United Health Plan integrated all health care services in town and involved the community. A census taken in the mid-1980s classified the households into three groups of health risks and based on that data, special programs targeted the most vulnerable groups (children and pregnant women) and common diseases. Because of its uniqueness and success, Villa El Salvador has attracted external financing from many international agencies and charitable institutions.

The Villa El Salvador experience proves that relatively few health resources supplied by multiple providers can be successfully integrated to maximize their use by targeting the groups with the highest health risks and by emphasizing primary care. Proportionally, the community's resources are roughly one-third of those available to the population served by the Ministry of Health and one-fifth those of social insurance. And yet, 60% to 70% of Villa El Salvador's children under 5 years of age are immunized, the vast majority of pregnant women receive care, and the incidence of common diseases, such as acute diarrhea, has been significantly reduced through a powdered milk supply, increasing the use of boiled water to prepare the formula, and oral rehydration. Unfortunately, there are no sound data to do a serious evaluation of the impact of these programs on the population health standards.

Villa El Salvador is not exempt from problems, such as conflicts among political ideologies and different health philosophies of providers, lack of secondary and tertiary level services, insufficient or not well-qualified personnel at some NGOs, reluctance of some groups to fully integrate with the Unified Health Plan, and flaws in community participation. Even after fully considering these problems, Villa El Salvador is worthy of replication elsewhere, because it offers a successful model of community mobilization to provide minimal health care to the urban poor.

Dominican Republic: Health Care for "Subsistence" Microenterprises Through Igualas

The poor quality of public health services forces the poor to buy private services at great sacrifices. Three-fourths of the health insurance market in the Dominican Republic is controlled by *igualas* (HMOs) that are extremely competitive, and provide comprehensive health care to subscribers for a monthly premium. Currently, there are 20 *igualas* in the nation which cover 450,000 people. To qualify for a plan, *igualas* require a minimum of 15 to 50 employees, and that minimum is rapidly rising; the monthly premium range is between $US5 and $US10 per person. Most employers of mid-size enterprises cover 75% of the premium and the rest is paid by the workers, most of whom earn from $US79 to $US90 monthly. In 1989, the poverty line for a family of five was estimated at $US115; hence, without the substantial employer contribution, many of those workers could not afford *iguala* coverage. Still, these income levels and standards are too high for the urban poor.

In 1988, there were 145,000 microenterprises that employed 400,000 workers and none of them were covered by *igualas*. The reason is that the average number of employees in these microenterprises is fewer than 3, far below the minimum number required to enter an *iguala*. And yet, there are indicators that both employers and employees of these enterprises want to join *igualas*. The grouping mechanism can be provided by associations of microenterprises that already have a network of salaried promoters who negotiate loans and collect monthly payments from the employers. Two of these associations, with a potential market of 100,000 people, are willing to provide the necessary grouping mechanism and collect the premium from the joining microenterprises. Most relevant to the poor is ADOPEM, an association of "subsistence" microenterprises, actually small groups of women vendors of foodstuffs and clothing. The plan would offer a reduced package of benefits for $US0.80 to $US1.50 monthly, 15% of average premium of a standard *iguala* package; half of the premium would be paid by the enterprises, which would discount the other half from employees who want to join.

Services would be limited to basic curative care, routine diagnostic tests, infant-maternal care, essential medicine, and preventive services such as immunization and treatment of diarrhea and parasites. ADOPEM would collect the premiums from the enterprises and the *iguala* would contract with clinics located in impoverished areas, which, in turn, would provide the plan services.

In order for this project to be feasible, financial assistance, probably from USAID, is needed to train ADOPEM personnel in the required administrative skills to run the plan and for *igualas* to improve their efficiency and add preventive services not currently provided by their benefit packages. If this plan materializes and is successful, it should rapidly expand throughout the informal sector helping to solve the serious lack of health care access by the urban poor.

FINAL POLICY RECOMMENDATIONS

Throughout this study, and particularly in this last chapter, a series of concrete policy recommendations have been made. Herein, the most important policy issues are summarized and consolidated.

General Anti-Poverty Policies

Policies to provide health care for the poor should be framed within a general strategy to fight poverty, articulated on two fronts—growth and distribution. The promotion of economic growth should be based on increasing savings and improving efficiency in resource allocation, and should ultimately aim at expanding productive employment opportunities for the poor and at raising their incomes. But economic growth *per se* does not guarantee those results, so the government should apply redistributive policies, through taxes and transfers, to ensure that the poor benefit from the economic expansion. Furthermore, adjustment policies advocated by international agencies, although they might be beneficial in the long run, have brought on negative social effects in the short and medium term, making it necessary to protect the indigent and to create a safety net for the poor. The redistributive goals could be achieved through the direct provision of basic social services targeted to the poor, such as primary health care, sanitation, family planning, nutrition, primary education, and basic housing. Specific policies for the informal sector should include the legalization of the informal economy and the elimination of barriers to its development, as well as the provision of credit and training; policies for the rural poor should focus on eliminating or, at least, reducing the physical and cultural isolation of this group. To maximize their effects, all these policies should be properly integrated.

Traditional redistributive policies such as labor legislation and social insurance not only have missed the poor—because they are outside of the formal sector which is the principal beneficiary of such conventional policies—but often have worsened their situation due to the negative effects they have had on employment. New redistributive policies should target the poor and should avoid, as much as possible, the pervasive effects on job creation. An important aspect of this new approach should be to shift away from generalized indiscriminate state subsidies granted to the overall population, moving instead towards subsidies targeted to the poor. State revenues, mostly from indirect taxes, used to finance generalized subsidies are usually regressive because they impose a burden on the poor who seldom benefit from the subsidies. Conversely, targeting subsidies to the most vulnerable groups and programs would bring about a progressive redistributive effect and would minimize leaks to unintended beneficiaries (free riders). As has been seen, state subsidies to health care had the highest degree of progressiveness among all social services in three countries, but little progressive impact due to the relatively small share assigned to that sector; an increase of that share would strengthen the subsidy's impact.

A major concern with a targeted policy is how to reduce administrative complexity and related costs. However, some experts believe that a full-blown social bureaucracy is unnecessary, if some simple guidelines are used to determine which groups and/or programs to target. For example, in terms of geography, it is known that the poor live in well defined areas such as urban slums and impoverished countryside; regarding age, children under 5 years of age and pregnant mothers are particularly vulnerable groups; and concerning health programs, preference should be given to preventive over curative medicine, and the most common diseases of underdevelopment such as parasites, diarrhea, respiratory infections, contagious diseases, and malnutrition should be targeted. By combining various targeting mechanisms their benefits for

the poor will be maximized. The experience of three countries shows that by reallocating the state subsidy to health care and by increasing the shares of the Ministry of Health, preventive services, and rural areas, the redistributive impact of the subsidy can be enhanced (Musgrove, 1987; World Bank, 1987, 1990; Pfeffermann and Griffin, 1989; Psacharopoulos, 1989; Mesa-Lago, 1990a).

The Region's economic crisis in the 1980s has both increased destitution and made it more urgent, and more difficult, to fight poverty and to provide health care to the poor. The crisis brought on a reduction in public health care expenditures (although Uruguay saw an increase in the second half of the 1980s); a paralysis or drastic cutback in investment in physical plant, equipment, and maintenance; a slowdown or decline in population coverage by the social insurance sickness-maternity program and an aggravation of its traditional deficit (although Costa Rica experienced a noticeable improvement); and a stagnation, fragmentation, or decline in programs of extension to rural and urban marginal areas (although at the turn of the decade, Costa Rica and Mexico showed signs of improvement). The crisis also has led to a growth of the informal sector, unemployment, and poverty, increasing the demand for welfare and/or public health services at a time when its funding was being cut.

Although most of the countries studied have not yet experienced a marked overall decline in health standards (partly because of the previous development of the health infrastructure), if these previous trends are not rapidly reversed, negative effects may be visible in the 1990s in the Dominican Republic and Peru, and perhaps in Mexico. The economic crisis has been a serious obstacle for reaching the goal of health care for all by the year 2000, but it also has raised the pressure to implement effective reforms. Solving the Region's economic crisis calls for international cooperation in order to alleviate the burden of the debt service and to reactivate external aid and credit. A vigorous economic recovery would generate productive employment, renew the growth of the formal sector, increase real salaries, and reduce unemployment, all of which, in turn, would help the health sector.

Unfortunately, most experts agree that a vigorous expansion is not likely to occur in Latin America and the Caribbean in the 1990s. In the fall of 1990, the Persian Gulf crisis and the danger of a recession in the United States worsened matters for most of the Region's countries. Consequently, it is illusory to expect that the solution of the problem lies in economic recuperation in the medium term, and, the longer the proper action is postponed, the more costly the remedy will be. In this context, government commitment to anti-poverty policies, combined with support from international financial agencies, is fundamental to push and facilitate the reforms suggested below.

Specific Health Policies for the Poor

In the past three decades, international or regional specialized agencies and experts have produced and reiterated a series of general recommendations for coping with the Region's existing health care problems, including the universalization of coverage. With very few exceptions, however, that advice has been ignored or the needed action postponed by establishing study commissions; in other cases, recommendations apparently have been pursued through inoperative legislation. Although this study supports the general advice, the analysis of five cases demonstrates that countries have significant differences in terms of general factors, current coverage of the poor, viability of social insurance and/or the public sector to protect the poor, and private alternatives, which make it impossible to issue a single general prescription to reach universalization of coverage; the general advice must be tailored to each country's reality.

This study also has shown the enormous vacuum of data on fundamental aspects of poverty and health care in Latin America and the Caribbean. It is important to better identify and quantify poverty groups and their characteristics, such as their income, occupation, health standards, and access/utilization of health services. We need data on actual coverage by the Ministry of Health, disaggregated social insurance statistics by urban-rural location and by occupational groups, and information on health protection of the poor by NGOs. The dire need for more precise information, nevertheless, should not excuse postponing action—this study provides a fair diagnosis of the problem and suggests alternative policies to deal with it. Furthermore, relatively simple targeting techniques such as those listed in the previous section should reduce the need for information. Actually, much more important than additional data is the national political commitment required to implement the necessary reforms.

Improvements in Organization

The public health sector is usually included in national plans, but this rarely is the case with social insurance, and even when the latter is considered, there are no effective measures to coordinate the health policies of the two main institutions. A plan for extending coverage to the poor, even in the most developed countries with the best social security systems, requires a clear determination of priorities on the groups to be covered and the benefits to be granted. A first step, therefore, should be to elaborate a health plan or program incorporating the two major health institutions, with concrete policies, a master financial plan, the identification of concrete goals, and an assessment of costs and needed resources (WHO, 1987). Ideally, the plan should coordinate health policies with nutrition, employment, distribution, and education policies. The achievement of key goals such as protection of the poor, integration or coordination of health services, and allocation of resources according to the most pressing needs will require a concentrated national effort, the establishment of priorities, and technical decision-making that can only succeed within a planning framework.

A key target should be the integration or a high degree of coordination of services provided by the ministries of health and by social insurances. New terms invented to mollify this problem will not solve it. As a PAHO expert has noted, it is time to transform into policy, through specific programs, the theory elaborated in the ·three previous decades (Castellanos, 1985). The crux is how to functionally and progressively integrate the existing resources and services of both institutions in a given geographical area, and how to plan integrated resources and services for the future. To that end, it is crucial to design joint basic units for the administration of health care (WHO, 1987). The increasing cooperation among international and regional agencies for coordinating services of the two institutions is laudable, but ultimately, the problem must be solved by each nation's political commitment. The fact that all five countries have laws that aim at such coordination, but only Costa Rica actually has achieved it, attests to both the practical difficulties involved in that task and its feasibility where political commitment exists.

Of equal significance is the need to achieve a better balance between preventive and curative services and among the three levels of care and a more rational allocation of health resources between the Ministry of Health and social insurance, as well as the application of those resources according to the country's morbidity and pathological profiles. In most countries, those policies should result in more resources assigned to primary health care, potable water supply, excreta disposal systems, immunization, care of the infant-maternal group, nutritional supplements, health education, and the ministries of health.

In recent years, there has been a trend towards the decentralization of health care administration, because the collection of revenue and the provision of services is often better when it is closer to the users and more adjusted to their resources and needs. Although this clearly is a positive move, it should not be used as a way to cut resources to health care. Moreover, decentralization could expand inequalities between the most and least developed regions, which, respectively, have the best and worst health services; therefore, part of the health resources must remain centralized to help the least developed regions (World Bank, 1987; Musgrove, 1987).

Expansion of Coverage to the Poor

The five cases offer diverse models and levels of health care coverage of the poor. In Costa Rica, all the poor are covered and receive full health care treatment without discrimination through a highly coordinated health system. This model, however, is relatively expensive, and would be difficult to replicate in the three countries that do not enjoy Costa Rica's advantages.

In Uruguay, the large majority of the poor are covered, but there is a multiplicity of institutions and a stratified health system, and the services available to the poor are of much lower quality than those enjoyed by higher income groups. This system is as expensive as Costa Rica's, but considerably less efficient and in much need of coordination. A reallocation of state subsidies from social insurance to the Ministry of Health, combined with a significant improvement of efficiency in the latter, could lead to the universalization of coverage and higher quality of services and utilization.

Mexico's health system also is characterized by multiplicity, stratification, and a lack of coordination; COPLAMAR provides primary health care to the majority of the rural population with a more limited but cheaper benefit package, but a similar protective mechanism has not been developed for the urban poor. The COPLAMAR model appears more financially feasible for less developed countries such as Peru and the Do-

minican Republic than does Costa Rica's model. And yet, Mexico's abundant resources allowed the launching of COPLAMAR, but the economic crisis has affected its evolution and impeded the expansion of that model to the urban sector. Countries with fewer resources than Mexico might find, therefore, that the COPLAMAR model is too expensive.

Finally, in Peru and the Dominican Republic, the vast majority of the poor is not covered and the two countries also exhibit multiplicity of institutions, stratification, and lack of coordination. In both countries, the Ministry of Health and social insurance seem incapable, under their current organizations, to extend coverage to the poor, leaving communal and private approaches as the only apparent alternatives.

The less developed countries in the Region confront a situation similar to that of Peru and the Dominican Republic. The issue is whether it is possible to drastically reorganize the public and social insurance sectors in those countries in order to expand coverage and incorporate the poor. This would require a triage approach: in a context of very limited resources, the one alternative that would serve more people and save more lives should be selected (McGreevey et al, 1984). This would constitute an administratively rational, economically viable, and socially equitable solution, but one that would be politically difficult to implement. Under this approach, integrated resources of the two main health institutions, with improved organization and efficiency, would concentrate on basic but universal benefits founded on the principle of solidarity among income strata.

The poor would then have access to adequate primary health care, and the population with more resources would be able to buy supplementary or better care from the private sector, but using their own means rather than public subsidies. Actually, in the Dominican Republic, social insurance services are of such poor quality that many within the insured minority do not utilize such services and pay duplicate coverage in the private sector. In Peru, however, social insurance services are slightly better, and a larger proportion of the population utilizes them. It has been argued that concentrating resources on primary health care would deprive the population of adequate care at higher levels of attention (''hospitals cannot be eliminated''), and that those covered at the primary level would eventually claim care at secondary and tertiary levels (Musgrove, 1989; Tamburi, 1990). However, under the current situation, the majority of the population in these countries either does not have access to health care at all or, due to the poor quality of available services, their level of utilization is very low. The proposed approach does not advocate eliminating public secondary and tertiary level facilities, but rather concentrating scarce resources on primary health care. After all the population is assured care at that level, the public sector could gradually improve services at the higher levels according to the availability of resources, either directly or by contracting private services. Finally, a vigorous private sector should be able to provide specialized, complex medicine for those who can afford it.

Where the basic universal care model is not politically feasible, a dual-care model might be. In countries such as Mexico, the extent of coverage and quality of care offered by social insurance is considerably higher than in the Dominican Republic and Peru. Therefore, the Mexican middle-income group does use such services and would resist an attempt to incorporate the poor if it meant a reduction in the quality of care. The dual system is, therefore, a result of both the degree of social insurance development and of political resistance. Those already covered would maintain full-care services, while the poor would be incorporated with a more limited benefits package (COPLAMAR). Although this approach provides minimal care to those who previously lacked all protection, it does not correct the regressivity of state subsidies to middle-income groups.

If none of the two previous models is viable, the only alternatives left in less developed countries are to be found in the private sector. We have seen successful examples of this in Villa El Salvador's community mobilization, in flourishing *igualas* in the Dominican Republic, and in improved traditional medicine in Mexico. In all these cases, there has been external financial aid in varying degrees. In absence of that aid, the government should provide minimal financial support to those initiatives when they emerge from nonprofit organizations (Akin et al, 1987; Musgrove, 1989).

Financing Health Protection for the Poor

In the model of basic universal care and social solidarity, coverage of the informal and rural poor could be partially financed through taxes and/or transfers from the urban-formal sector and/or higher income groups. This could also be applied to the dual-care model. In both models, state subsidies should be reserved for extending and/or improving care to the poor.

If the social insurance sickness-maternity program is the viable mechanism to protect the poor, it is imperative that the entire institution be put on solid financial footing. This implies an elimination of transfers from other programs to cover the deficit in sickness-maternity, which should become self-financed through increased revenues and/or reduced expenditures.

An initial step for raising revenue should be to improve detection, registration, inspection, collection, and auditing, in order to reduce evasion and payment delays. Computerization, a single national identification card for all financing purposes, fixing of interest plus fines at a higher rate than both inflation and commercial bank rates, prosecution of delinquents, and managerial improvements are some measures to achieve those goals. And yet, while these actions are relatively easy to adopt in the urban and formal sectors they are much more difficult to carry out when attempting to enforce mandatory coverage of the informal and rural sectors. For the latter, it is advisable to determine if such controls are administratively feasible and financially profitable, otherwise, it would be better to stimulate voluntary affiliation, combined with a welfare program for indigents where it is economically possible. All the remuneration should be subject to social insurance taxes, except for poor groups, and contribution ceilings for entry and payment should be eliminated. If there is a state debt, it should be renegotiated to index it to inflation or to avoid its devaluation. Investment yields are not important in a sickness-maternity program because it operates without reserves or with a small contingency fund.

If all of these measures fail to achieve a financial balance, the percentage of contribution should be raised. Because the insured's contribution is approximately one-third of the total and a raise in the already high employer contribution could potentially damage the generation of employment, preference should be given to increasing the insured's contribution, particularly in those countries where it is at a relatively low level. Finally, new sources of financing should be explored, particularly those that have a neutral effect on employment, such as the income tax and the value-added tax (VAT).

The previous measures could eliminate the deficit, but would rarely generate enough of a surplus to finance the incorporation of the poor, which would require state subsidies. Contributions from the self-employed, except for those with high income, should not be set by trying to compensate for the absence of an employer, because the resulting contribution would be unrealistically high. It is more reasonable to set a lower contribution and adjust benefits accordingly, or to subsidize coverage of the group through state subsidies. The same is true for other informal and rural groups.

If the Ministry of Health is to be considered as the viable institution for incorporating the poor, it should have adequate facilities and funding for that task. And yet, we have seen that in several countries, the ministry has adequate resources but needs to improve its efficiency and quality of services. It follows that investment of resources should not always go to the expansion of facilities, but to remodeling, re-equipping, maintenance, and hiring of competent managerial personnel. As has been analyzed in the Dominican Republic's case, user fees can be a significant source of revenue and a mechanism for improving the efficiency and quality of services in those countries or programs where the proper administrative environment exists (Akin et al, 1987; Musgrove, 1989; La Forgia, 1989). The poor should be exempt from paying user fees or the fees should be lowered to a level that would not impede this group's access to services. For reasons of equity and for economic sense, it is important to improve the means test used to waive user fees charged by the ministry and to provide indigents free access to social insurance services. The test should be standardized and humanized to ascertain that those who can pay are not exempt and to avoid denial of services to the truly poor.

Reducing Costs and Improving Efficiency

In most countries, the universalization of coverage based on social insurance, even with increased revenues, would be financially unfeasible under the current structure and the current level and quality of benefits available for the insured minority, because costs would be prohibitive (17% of GDP in the Dominican Republic and Peru). In the relatively more advanced countries, such as Costa Rica, the elimination of overgenerous benefits has resulted in significant savings. But, as has already been discussed, in most countries the overall level of benefits would have to be substantially cut down, either for the entire population (in the basic-universal care model) or for the poor under special programs (in the dual-care model).

Administrative expenditures must be drastically reduced in all countries, but particularly in the Dominican Republic, Mexico, and Peru. Emergency plans to cut expenditures often have

frozen jobs, but only temporarily; dismissals of redundant and incompetent employees are politically difficult to carry out, but absolutely necessary to achieve financial balance.

Changing the philosophy of care to emphasize lower-cost preventive medicine rather than the more expensive curative medicine through such measures as a reduction of uneconomical outpatient consultation at the tertiary level, should diminish costs and improve efficiency. The wholesale purchase and distribution of drugs and medical supplies could generate some savings, although the experience of the Program of Essential Medicines in the Dominican Republic is not convincing.

Low hospital occupancy and long length of stay are typical of most countries, but were found to be particularly serious in the Dominican Republic and Uruguay. An improvement in the quality of services, combined with education, could increase efficiency and utilization, and could reduce hospital costs. Similar results could be achieved through the proper cooperation of social insurance with the private sector, as has been done in Costa Rica.

Finally, a high percentage of government expenditures in health care does not always result in increased protection of the poor or higher overall health standards. Costa Rica has slightly lower health per capita expenditures than Uruguay, but ranks higher than the latter on both counts; Mexico and the Dominican Republic proportionally spend similar amounts, but the former is clearly well above the latter. The way that resources are spent and their efficiency and targeting explain the divergent performance among these countries.

The Politics of Reform

Opposition to the policies discussed above is inevitable, because protecting the poor requires resources that must be drawn from other programs and groups that usually are better organized than the poor. For instance, the shift of state subsidies from middle-income groups to the poor or from social insurance to the Ministry of Health is bound to generate antagonism, although in some cases, political coalitions are feasible; for example, expansion of health services to the poor might provide jobs for middle-income medical personnel and pharmaceutical producers. However, the reform may alienate some of those groups—physicians who have multiple employment may oppose the integration of services of social insurance and the Ministry of Health, and bureaucrats also may oppose integration because it could lead to job reductions. Middle-class insured who use social insurance health services may reject the incorporation of the poor if they fear it would downgrade the services. Personal and political conflicts between the minister of health and the director of social insurance are common and have often impeded the integration of their services. These experiences indicate the need for a firm commitment from the government to elaborate and implement the reform, and for education and political mobilization of the poor to support such action (Pfeffermann and Griffin, 1989; World Bank, 1990; Guerra de Macedo, 1990).

Associations of informal workers, peasants, and other poor groups should be encouraged and their leaders educated on the need to elaborate long-term plans of action with concrete objectives, and these associations should engage in negotiations with the government and with political parties. For example, in Peru, the various associations of street vendors should join to request that taxes collected from them by municipalities are actually employed in providing health care to them.

Finally, the public must be educated to change the current negative attitude toward some poor groups such as street vendors and peasants; bureaucrats must be made to treat indigents with dignity; and the poor themselves must be instructed on their rights, benefits to which they are entitled, and the importance of using health services.

The Role of International Aid

There are many examples of successful international programs that have extended health services to the poor, such as immunization, oral hydration, and sanitation campaigns and programs to control contagious diseases. External aid is needed not only for the less developed countries in the Region, which obviously should have priority, but also for the relatively more developed countries that are role models and struggle to maintain or improve successful programs in the midst of the economic crisis.

Foreign aid such as World Bank structural adjustment loans, USAID loans for health care, and IDB loans to build health facilities should be tied to national efforts to reduce poverty and to provide health care to the poor. In addition, international and regional agencies should donate moderate sums to vulnerable poor groups and programs, such as rural clinics that serve the poor, immunization and nutrition programs for children, efforts to establish nonprofit medical cooperatives and to train associations of informal workers, and for microentrepreneurs to develop mutual-aid societies or to become effective intermediaries in dealing with HMOs and insurance companies that offer low-cost packages of health benefits.

This study has shown that sometimes large programs with substantial external funding have failed due to inefficient bureaucracies, waste, and lack of effective supervision. Conversely, we have given several examples of small projects that, with modest external support, have been successful. These should be used as models to be replicated elsewhere with international aid. Bureaucratic programs elaborated without consultation with the poor run the risk of expending considerable sums in employing unnecessary personnel, being inadequate to the poor's needs, and, consequently, possibly being rejected by them. Programs that effectively engage the poor and respond to their interests are more likely to succeed in meeting their most urgent health needs and in eliciting their support.

BIBLIOGRAPHY AND FURTHER READING

Acuña Ulate, José A., "Propuesta de reforma al Reglamento de Trabajadores Independientes," San José, February 1988.

Acuña, Jorge, et al., "Perfil del sector salud de la República Oriental del Uruguay: su financiamiento y problemas," Brasília, Seminario Financiamiento del Sector Salud en América Latina, World Bank-PAHO, October 1987.

Aguirre, Rosario, and Méndez, Estela, "El trabajo informal urbano en Uruguay," *Suma*, 3:4 (April 1988): 89–103.

Ahmad, Ehtisham, and Dréze, Jean, eds., *Social Security in Developing Countries*, London, STICERD at London School of Economics and WIDER, 1990.

Akin, John; Birdsall, Nancy; and de Ferrante, David, *Financing Health Services in Developing Countries: An Agenda for Reform*, Washington, D.C., World Bank Policy Study, 1987.

Altimir, Oscar, *The Extent of Poverty in Latin America*, Washington, D.C., World Bank Staff Working Paper no. 552, 1982.

—————, "Poverty, Income Distribution and Child Welfare in Latin America," *World Development*, 12:3 (1984): 261–282.

Annis, Sheldon, and Franks, Jeffrey, "The Idea, Ideology and Economics of the Informal Sector: The Case of Peru," *Grassroots Development*, 13:1 (1989): 9–22.

Apezechea, Héctor; Prates, Susana; and Franco, Rolando, *Elementos para un diagnóstico social del Uruguay*, Montevideo, UNICEF/CIESU/ILPES, 1984.

Arán, Adrián (Ministerio de Salud Pública, Costa Rica), Interview, San José, December 15, 1989.

Arán, Daniel, "Financiamiento del sector salud en Uruguay," Montevideo, CELADU, February 1986.

Arellano, José Pablo, "Gasto público en salud y distribución del ingreso," in *Salud pública y bienestar social*, Livingston and Racynski, eds., Santiago, Centro de Estudios de Planificación Nacional (CIEPLAN), 1976.

—————, "The Impact of Social Security on Savings and Development," in Mesa-Lago, 1985b, chapter 7.

—————, *Políticas sociales y desarrollo: Chile 1924–1984*, Santiago, CIEPLAN, 1985.

—————, *La salud en los años 80: análisis desde la economía*, Santiago, CIEPLAN, 1987.

Arroba, Gonzalo, "La financiación de la seguridad social en los países en desarrollo," *Estudios de la Seguridad Social*, 29 (1979): 5–31.

Banco de Previsión Social (BPS), Asesoría Económica y Actuarial, "Seguros de enfermedad: cobertura y evolución," Montevideo, 1987.

―――――, "La evasión de los aportes al Banco de Previsión Social," "La evasión de los aportes de Industria y Comercio," "Evasión de los aportes rurales," Montevideo, n/d.

―――――, "Seguros de enfermedad: cobertura y evolución," Montevideo, n/d(a).

―――――, *Boletín Estadístico*, nos. 31–33, 1988–1989.

Barranzuela, Roel (General Secretary, Comunidad Urbana Autogestionaria [CUAVES], Villa El Salvador), Interview, May 6, 1988.

Barreiro, Norma, "Informe de la Evaluación del Projecto de Medicina Tradicional del Instituto Mexicano Tlahuilli A.C.," December 4, 1989.

―――――, Interview in Mexico City, December 13, 1989a.

Barrig, Maruja, and Fort, Amelia, "La ciudad de las mujeres: pobladores y servicios, el caso de El Agustino," Lima, draft, 1987.

Bartlett, Lawrence, "Financial Analysis" and "Financial Management Systems within SESPAS," Santo Domingo, USAID, August 1983.

Beirano, Luis; Luyo, Fernando; and Vicuña, Irene (Instituto de Salud Hugo Pesce [INSAHP], Villa El Salvador), Interviews, September 24, 1988.

Beirute, Luis Asís, "Extensión del seguro social a la zona rural en Costa Rica," in *Seguridad social, atención médica y políticas de salud en América Latina*, Buenos Aires, ISSA-Oficina Regional para las Americas, Serie Actas no. 9, 1988.

Betances, Luis, "Seguridad social y la medicina privada en la República Dominicana," Buenos Aires, Asociación Nacional de Clínicas y Hospitales Privados, April 1986.

Bitran, Ricardo, *Household Demand for Medical Care in Santo Domingo, Dominican Republic*, Stony Brook, USAID/HCF/LAC, no. 9, March 1989.

Bolaños Mesen, Víctor M., "Protección social de grupos marginados urbanos en Costa Rica," IMSS-AISS, *Memoria Reunión sobre la Protección Social a los Grupos Marginados Urbanos*, Mexico City, 1988.

Borzutzky, Silvia, "Politics and Social Security Reform" in Mesa-Lago, 1985b, chapter 9.

Briceño, Edgar, and Méndez, Eduardo, "Salud pública y distribución del ingreso en Costa Rica," *Revista Ciencias Económicas*, 1:2, 2:1–2 (1982): 49–69.

Caja Costarricense de Seguro Social (CCSS), *Memoria 1983* and *1987*, San José, 1983 to 1988.

―――――, *Anuario Estadístico 1981* to *1987*, San José, 1982 to 1988a.

―――――, "Informe que estudia el aseguramiento obligatorio de los trabajadores independientes y temporarios," San José, April 1988b.

―――――, *Seguro Enfermedad y Maternidad: Programa 2000 Anuario 1988*, San José, 1989.

―――――, "Evaluación actuarial del Seguro de Vejez, Invalidez y Muerte," San José, 1990.

Calventi, V. (Director, Hospital Ntra. Sra. Altagracia), Interview, Santo Domingo, June 16, 1986.

Carbonetto, Daniel, "La medición del empleo en Lima," in *El sector informal urbano en los países andinos*, Carbonetto et al., eds., Quito, ILDIS/CEPESIU, 1985.

—————, and Chávez, Eliana, "Sector informal urbano: heterogeneidad del capital y exedente bruto de trabajo," *Socialismo y Participación* (Lima) 26 (1984): 1–31.

Carvajal, Eloy, "Bancarrota de pensiones antes del 2000," *La República*, July 5, 1990, p. 3-A.

Castañeda, Tarsicio, "Contexto socioeconómico del descenso del la mortalidad en Chile," *Estudios Públicos*, 16 (1984): 5–56.

—————, "El sistema de salud chileno: organización, funcionamiento y financiamiento," *Boletín de la Oficina Sanitaria Panamericana*, 103:6 (1987): 544–570.

—————, "Innovative Social Policies for Reducing Poverty: Chile in the 1980s," Washington, D.C., World Bank, draft, August 1989.

Castellanos, Jorge, "La extensión de servicios de salud y la seguridad social," *Estudios de la Seguridad Social*, 27 (1978): 33–83.

—————, "Políticas y metas regionales de salud," 1982, and "Coordinación entre las entidades del sector público que prestan servicios de atención de salud," 1985, in PAHO-ILO-CPISS, 1986.

—————, "La atención de salud en áreas urbanas," IMSS-AISS, *Memoria reunión sobre la protección social a los grupos marginados urbanos*, Mexico City, 1988.

Centro Interamericano de Estudios de Seguridad Social (CIESS), *Atención primaria en la seguridad social en México: la experiencia del Programa IMSS-COPLAMAR*, Geneva, ILO, 1987.

—————, *Problemas contemporáneos de la seguridad social*, Mexico City, CIESS, 1988.

Cobas, Eduardo, "Problemas estructurales y de la crisis económica en el desarrollo social del Uruguay...," Lima, ECLAC, November 25, 1986.

Comisión Americana Jurídico-Social, "Financiamiento y extensión de la. seguridad social," *Seguridad Social*, 129–130 (1981): 203–236.

Consejo Nacional de Población y Familia (CONAPOFA), *Población y sociedad (Seminario Nacional, 1983)*, Santo Domingo, Imp. Gerardo, 1985.

Conte Grand, Alfredo, "La seguridad social," *Revista de Ciencias Jurídicas*, 1:9 (May 1985): 271–276.

COPLAMAR, "Memoria de Actividades 1976–1982," Mexico City, Presidencia de la República, 1982.

—————, *Necesidades esenciales en México: situación actual y perspectivas al año 2000--Salud*, Mexico City, Siglo XXI, 1983.

Cortés, Fernando, "La informalidad del sector informal extralegal," Mexico City, draft, 1988.

CUAVES, "Plan Unico de Salud," Villa El Salvador, 1986.

Dávila, P. Alvaro, "Proyecciones financieras del seguro de vejez, invalidez y muerte para el año 2000," San José, CCSS, February 1988.

Davrieux, Hugo, *Papel de los gastos públicos en el Uruguay (1955–1984)*, Montevideo, Estudios CINVE no. 9, 1987.

De Ferranti, David, *Paying for Health Services in Developing Countries*, Washington, D.C., World Bank Staff Working Paper no. 721, 1985.

————, ''El pago por servicios de salud en los países en desarrollo: un enfoque realista,'' *Foro Mundial de la Salud*, 6 (1985a): 115–122.

De Geyndt, W., ''Chile SAL III: Health Sector,'' Washington, D.C., World Bank, August 1987.

Del Rosario, Gumersindo, and Gámez, Susana, *Privatización de los sistemas de salud*, Santo Domingo, Fundación Friedrich Ebert, 1988.

De Soto, Hernando, et al., *El otro sendero: la revolución industrial*, Lima, Casa Editorial el Barranco, 1986.

Development Technologies, Inc. (DETEC), *Costa Rica: análisis socio-económico del sector salud*, San José, draft, December 1987.

Diaz, Alejandro; Rojas, Horacio; Redondo, María (President, Vice-President, Nurse, and five promoters—IMMTTCA, Cuernavaca, Jujutla, Xoxocotla, and Barranca Honda), Interviews, December 11–12, 1989.

Diéguez, Héctor L., ''Social Consequences of the Economic Crisis: Mexico, the Facts,'' Washington, D.C., World Bank, draft, 1986.

————, and Giral-Bosca, Juan, *Uruguay, Inquiry into Social Security: Its Evolution, Current Problems and Prospects*, Washington, D.C., World Bank, June 1988.

Dirección General de Estadística y Censos (DGEC), *Anuario Estadístico Uruguay 1970–1978 to 1988*, Montevideo, 1981 to 1989.

————, *VI Censo de Población y IV de Viviendas*, Montevideo, 1989a.

————, and ECLAC, *Pobreza y necesidades básicas en el Uruguay: indicadores y resultados preliminares*, Montevideo, Arca, 1989.

Dirección General de la Seguridad Social (DGSS), *Boletín Estadístico* (Montevideo), nos. 22–30, 1986–1988.

Duarte, Isis, *Trabajadores urbanos: ensayos sobre fuerza laboral en República Dominicana*, Santo Domingo, Editora Universitaria, 1986.

————, Gómez, Carmen; La Forgia, Gerard; and Molina, Maritza, ''Los servicios de salud del distrito nacional por sectores, 1987: organización, cobertura, financiamiento y utilización,'' Santo Domingo, IEDP, 1989.

Durán, Valverde, ''Estudio y propuesta de una readecuación de contribuciones a los seguros sociales,'' San José, CCSS, February 1988.

Early, Lisa (Health Officer, USAID Santo Domingo), Interviews, June 12 and 20, 1986.

Economic Commission for Latin America and the Caribbean (ECLAC-CEPAL), *Desarrollo, transformación y equidad: la superación de la probreza*, Santiago, November 4, 1986.

————, ''El impacto de la crisis económica en el campo de la salud: problemas y alternativas en las Américas,'' Lima, November 1986a.

————, ''Reunión sobre crisis externa: proceso de ajuste y su impacto inmediato y de largo plazo en el desarrollo social,'' Lima, CEPAL-PNUD-UNICEF, November 1986b.

————, *Preliminary Overview of the Latin American Economy 1988* and *1989*, Santiago, December 1988 and 1989.

————, *Statistical Yearbook for Latin America and the Caribbean 1988*, Santiago, 1989a.

————, *Estudio Económico de América Latina y el Caribe*, República Dominicana, 1988a and 1989b.

————, *Magnitud de la pobreza en América Latina en los años ochenta*, Santiago, May 31, 1990.

————, ILPES and UNICEF, *Pobreza, necesidades básicas y desarrollo*, Santiago, 1982.

Equipo Técnico de la Municipalidad Villa El Salvador, "Villa El Salvador y su proyecto popular de desarrollo integral," Villa El Salvador, March 1988.

Fernández, Sonia, et al., "Proyección de la población económicamente activa para la República Mexicana: 1970–1985," Mexico City, Centro Nacional de Información y Estadísticas del Trabajo, 198?.

Fernández Campos, Luis, and Alfaro, Noemi (Chief, Department of Projects, and Vice-Director of Social Action, IMAS), Interview, May 10, 1988.

Ferrari, César, "Desarrollo social y pobreza en Perú; factores estructurales de la crisis externa; las políticas adoptadas para lograr el desarrollo económico y social," Lima, ECLAC, November 1986.

Fields, Gary S., "Employment and Economic Growth in Costa Rica," Washington, D.C., USAID, 1985.

Fortuna, Juan C., and Prates, Suzana, "Informal Sector Versus Informalized Labor Relations in Uruguay," in *The Informal Economy*, Portes et al., ed., 1989, pp. 78–94.

Galindo, Iginio (Director, Centro de Salud del MS Juan Pablo Segundo, Villa El Salvador), Interview, Lima, September 24, 1988.

Galván Ulloa, Adolfo, "Extensión del régimen del seguro social en los años recientes," *Cuestión Social*, 8 (Summer 1987): 3–6.

————, "Mecanismos innovadores de acceso a la seguridad social," Mexico City, draft, March 1988.

García, Alan, "Mensaje a la Nación del Presidente..," *La Crónica* (Lima), July 29, 1988: 19–21.

García Hernández, Carlos, "Extensión del régimen en el seguro social [IMSS]," Mexico City, draft, February 1987.

Gautreaux, Rafael (University Professor of Medicine), Interview, Santo Domingo, June 20, 1986.

Giral, Juan, et al., *Country Economic Memorandum on Uruguay*, two vols., Washington, D.C., World Bank-LACR, August 1986.

Gómez, Lilian, and Gross, Joselyn (PROMESE officials), Interview, Santo Domingo, June 17, 1986.

Gómez, Luis Carlos, *Household Survey of Health Services Consumption in Santo Domingo, Dominican Republic: Methodology and Preliminary Findings*, Stony Brook, USAID/HCF/LAC, no. 8, September 1988.

Gómez Ulloa, Mario, "El sistema de salud en la República Dominicana," Washington, D.C., PAHO/WHO, 1985.

González Gautreaux, Rafael (Director, Laboratorio Nacional), Interview, Santo Domingo, June 16, 1986.

Green, Dianne W., "Some Effects of Social Security Programs on the Distribution of Income in Costa Rica," Ph.D. Dissertation, University of Pittsburgh, 1977.

Grompone, Romeo, "Las políticas y programas para el mejoramiento de las condiciones de trabajo y bienestar de los trabajadores del SIU: el caso de Lima," ILO Report, Lima, 1987.

————, "Iniciativas populares en Lima," Lima, Instituto de Estudios Peruanos (IEP), draft, 1988.

————, and Tuesta, Fernando, Interview, Lima, May 3, 1988.

Guevara, José, *La pobreza en América Latina*, Stockholm, Institute of Latin American Studies, Report no. 32, September 1981.

Guzmán, Daniel (Under-Secretary of SESPAS), Interview, Santo Domingo, June 13, 1986.

Gwynne, Gretchen, ed., "Private Sector Care Alternatives for Agricultural Workers on the South Coast of Guatemala," Stony Brook, HCF/LAC, no. 7, August 1988.

————, and Zschock, Dieter, *Health Care Financing in Latin America and the Caribbean, 1985–1989: Findings and Recommendations*, Stony Brook, HCF/LAC, no. 10, September 1989.

Haan, Hans, *El sector informal en Centroamérica*, Santiago, Investigaciones sobre Empleo, no. 27, 1985.

Hernández Llamas, Héctor, "Algunas consideraciones sobre la historia del campo mexicano: la atención médica en el medio rural mexicano," in *La atención médica rural en México*, Héctor Hernández Llamas, ed., Mexico City, IMSS, 1986.

Injarte, Julio, and Sattin, Guido (Physicians of Municipio Villa El Salvador), Interview, May 6, 1988.

Instituto de Libertad y Democracia (ILD), "Compendio técnico y estadístico de 'El otro sendero'," 2 vols., Lima, October and November 1986.

Instituto Dominicano de Seguros Sociales (IDSS), "Estimados actuariales definitivos del Anteproyecto de Ley sobre el nuevo régimen de seguridad social," August 1983.

————, *Informe Estadístico* (different titles), Santo Domingo, 1984–1985.

————, *Boletín Estadístico 1986*, Santo Domingo, 1987.

Instituto Guatemalteco de Seguridad Social (IGSS), "Comisión...de la extensión del programa...enfermedad y maternidad a la costa suroccidental del pais," Guatemala City, April 1988.

Instituto Mexicano de Medicina Tradicional Tlahuilli C.A. (IMMTTCA), *Medicina Alternativa* (Cuernavaca), no. 1 (1985), no. 2 (1986), no. 3 (1987), no. 4 (1988).

Instituto Mexicano de Seguro Social (IMSS), *Diagnóstico de salud en las zonas marginadas rurales de México*, Mexico City, IMSS, 1983.

————, *Memoria Estadística 1986*, Mexico City, October 1987.

————, "Informe Mensual de la Población Derechohabiente," Mexico City, December and May 1987a, 1988.

—————, ''Proyecto de Decreto para incorporación voluntaria al régimen obligatorio del seguro social a los trabajadores independientes,'' Mexico City, draft, June 1987b.

—————, *Ley de Seguro Social*, Mexico City, 1987c.

—————, and COPLAMAR, *Memoria: Primera reunión anual de análisis del desarrollo del programa IMSS-COPLAMAR*, Mexico City, IMSS, 1981.

—————, and COPLAMAR, Budget Summaries, Mexico City, IMSS-COPLAMAR, 1983–1987.

—————, and COPLAMAR, *Anuario Estadístico* (1982–1986), Mexico City, IMSS-COPLAMAR, Coordinación Médica, 1987a.

—————, and COPLAMAR, ''Estudio de opinión sobre la calidad de los servicios y la participación de la población como respuesta a las acciones de salud del programa IMSS-COPLAMAR,'' Mexico City, IMSS-COPLAMAR, mimeographed document 1987.

—————, and COPLAMAR, ''El Programa Nacional de Solidaridad Social por Cooperación Comunitaria (IMSS-COPLAMAR),'' Managua, II Simposio Internacional de Extensión de Seguridad Social al Campo, February-March 1988.

—————, and COPLAMAR, ''Anexos del Documento Básica,'' Managua, 1988a.

—————, and International Social Security Association (ISSA-AISS), *Reunión sobre la protección social a los grupos marginados urbanos*, Mexico City, June 1988.

Instituto Nacional de Estadística (INE), *Encuesta nacional de hogares sobre medición de niveles de vida (1985–1986)*, Lima, 1988.

—————, *Perú: Compendio estadístico 1988*, Lima, May 1988a.

Instituto Nacional de Estadística, Geografía e Informática (INEGI), *Agenda Estadística 1986*, Mexico City, Secretaría de Planificación y Presupuesto (SPP), 1987.

Instituto Peruano de Seguridad Social (IPSS), ''Metas de extensión de cobertura,'' Lima, 1985 and 1987.

—————, ''Proyecto de Reglamento [a Ley 24,645 de 18–12–1986] de Incorporación de Trabajadores del Campo a la Seguridad Social,'' Lima, 1987a.

—————, ''Proyecto de Reglamento de Incorporación de Nuevos Asegurados [Eventuales, Informales, etc.] a la Ley no. 24,620 de 26–12–86,'' Lima, 1987b.

—————, *Estimados de la Dirección de Estadística*, Lima, 1988.

Inter-American Development Bank (IDB-BID), *Economic and Social Progress in Latin America 1987, 1988*, and *1989*, Washington, D.C., 1987, 1988, and 1989.

Inter-American Foundation (IAF), ''Grant to Cooperativa de Producción del Termo (COTER),'' several documents, Washington, D.C., 1987.

—————, Project Records, Memoranda of Meetings, Field Reports, Grant Agreement and Review related to IMMTTAC, February 18, 23, 26, March 11, April 27, 1987, September 20, 1988.

International Labour Office (ILO-OIT), *Yearbook of Labour Statistics*, Geneva, 1981 to 1987.

—————, *The Cost of Social Security 1975–1977, 1978–1980*, and *1981– 1983*, and *Basic Tables*, Geneva, 1981a, 1985a, 1988.

————, *Introduction to Social Security*, Geneva, 1984.

International Social Security Association (ISSA-AISS), ''Financiamiento y control de los servicios de atención médica,'' *Estudios de la Seguridad Social*, 42 (1982): 5–21.

Isuani, Ernesto A., ''Social Security and Public Assistance'' in Mesa-Lago, 1985b, chapter 3.

————, ''Seguridad social y gasto social en la República Dominicana,'' Buenos Aires, May 1989.

————, and Mercer, Hugo, ''La fragmentación institucional del sector salud en la Argentina,'' *Boletín Informativo Techint*, no. 244, September-December 1986.

————, and Mesa-Lago, Carmelo, ''La seguridad social en Panamá: avances y problemas,'' Santiago, ILPES, 1981.

Jaramillo Antillón, Iván, and Miranda, Guido, *La integración de servicios de salud en Costa Rica*, San José, Ministerio de Salud, 1985.

Katz, Jorge, and Muñoz, Alberto, *Organización del sector salud: puja distributiva y equidad*, Buenos Aires, CEPAL, 1988.

Kleinekathoefer, Michael, *El sector informal, integración o transformación*, Santo Domingo, Fundación Friedrich Ebert, 1987.

Lacey, Robert, ''The Privatization of the Social Security System in Chile,'' Washington, D.C., World Bank, PSMU/PPD, February 1987.

La Forgia, Gerard M., ''El sector privado de salud en la República Dominicana,'' Santo Domingo, 1988.

————, ''User Fees, Quality of Care and the Poor: Lessons from the Dominican Republic,'' Washington, D.C., Inter-American Foundation, September 1989.

————, ''Challenging Health Service Stratification: Social Security-Health Ministry Integration in Panama, 1973–1986,'' Doctoral Dissertation, University of Pittsburgh, School of Public Health, 1990.

————, ''The Extension of Health Services to Low-income Families Through Private Pre-payment Plans: Assessment and Recommendations,'' Washington, D.C., The Urban Institute, June 1990a.

————, Interview, Pittsburgh, August 10, 1990b.

————, ''Health Services for Low-income Familes: Extending Coverage through Pre-payment Plans in the Dominican Republic,'' Washington, D.C., USAID HFS Technical Report no. 1, October 1990c.

''La seguridad social y el IPSS en la transición hacia el nuevo marco político,'' *Análisis Laboral*, 14:153 (March 1990): 3–5.

León, Francisco, ''Pobreza rural: realidades y perspectivas de política,'' in UN/ECLAC/UNDP, 1980.

Lewis, Maureen A., ''The Hospital User Fee Experience in the Dominican Republic,'' Washington, D.C., USAID-REACH, October 1987.

————; Sulvetta, Margaret; and La Forgia, Gerard, *Estimating Public Hospital Costs by Measuring Resource Use: A Dominican Case*, Washington, D.C., The Urban Institute, July 1990.

Lizardo, Sonia, "Comparative Study of Micro and Small Business as Poverty Alleviation Programs in the USA, Latin America and the Caribbean," Pittsburgh, University of Pittsburgh, June 1990.

Llach, Juan; Diéguez, Héctor; and Petrecolla, Alberto, "El gasto social en la Argentina: una propuesta de estudio," Buenos Aires, Instituto Torcuato Di Tella y PNATSS, 1988.

López Acuña, Daniel, *La salud desigual en México*, Mexico City, Siglo XXI, 1980.

López Vargas, Luis G., "Estimación del costo financiero del subsidio en dinero para trabajadores independientes," San José, March 1988.

Lozoya, Xavier, and Zolla, Carlos, "Programa de interrelación de la medicina tradicional con las actividades del IMSS-COPLAMAR," Mexico City, IMSS, mimeographed document, 1983.

Macedo, Carlyle Guerra de, Notes on a Conference on Health Care in Latin America, Washington, D.C., PAHO, February 12, 1990.

Mackenzie, G.A., "Social Security Issues in Developing Countries: The Latin American Experience," *IMF Staff Papers*, 35:3 (September 1988): 496–522.

Mallet, Alfredo, "Social Protection of the Rural Population," *International Social Security Review*, 33:3–4 (1980): 359–393.

—————, "Problemas contemporáneos de la seguridad social," in CIESS, *Problemas contemporáneos de la seguridad social*, Mexico City, 1988.

Malloy, James, *The Politics of Social Security in Brazil*, Pittsburgh, University of Pittsburgh Press, 1979.

—————, and Borzutzky, Silvia, "Politics, Social Welfare Policy, and the Population Problem in Latin America," *International Journal of Health Services*, 12:1 (1982): 77–98.

Mares, Marco A., "El Programa IMSS-COPLAMAR, casi paralizado por la descentralización del sector salud," *Uno Más Uno*, Mexico City, July 7, 1986, p. 3.

Márquez, Patricio V., "Uruguay: Population, Health and Nutrition Sector Memorandum," Washington, D.C., World Bank, LA4, March 31, 1989.

Marx, Martita M., "The Effects of Medical Services on Health Status in a Developing Nation," Doctoral Dissertation, University of California—Los Angeles, 1978.

McGreevey, William, "The High Costs of Health Care in Brazil," *Bulletin of the Pan American Health Organization* 22:2 (1988): 145–166.

—————, "Do Public Social Spending and Social Security Protect the Poor in Latin America?," Washington, D.C., World Bank, HRD/LACTD, September 1988.

—————, *Social Security in Latin America: Issues and Options for the World Bank*, Washington, D.C., World Bank, LACRO, October 1990.

—————, et al., *Política e financiamento do sistema de saúde brasileiro: uma perspectiva internacional*, Brasília, IPEA, 1984.

—————, "Priorities for Reform of Health Care, Nutrition, and Social Security in Brazil," Washington, D.C., World Bank, PHND, January 1988.

—————, "Temas actuales de la seguridad social brasileña," in CIESS, 1988, pp. 157–165.

Meerhoff, Ricardo, "Financiamiento del sector salud en el Uruguay: modalidades, alternativas y problemas," Montevideo, March 1986.

Melgar, Alicia, "El mercado de trabajo en la coyuntura," *Suma*, 3:4, (April 1988): 25–41.

Mendoza, Hugo (Director, Hospital de Niños Robert Reid Cabral), Interview, Santo Domingo, June 16, 1986.

Mesa-Lago, Carmelo, *Social Security in Latin America: Pressure Groups, Stratification and Inequality*, Pittsburgh, University of Pittsburgh Press, 1978.

———, "Social Security and Extreme Poverty in Latin America," *Journal of Development Economics*, 12 (1983): 83–110.

———, "Financing Health Care in Latin America and the Caribbean with a Special Study of Costa Rica," Washington, D.C., World Bank, PHND, March 1983a.

———, "Social Security in Ecuador," Washington, D.C., World Bank, December 1984.

———, *La reforma de la seguridad social: Análisis comparativo del Perú dentro del contexto latino-americano*, Lima, Universidad del Pacífico-Fundación Friedrich Ebert, 1985.

———, *El desarrollo de la seguridad social en América Latina*, Santiago de Chile, Estudios e Informes de la CEPAL no. 43, 1985a.

———, ed., *The Crisis of Social Security and Health Care: Latin American Experiences and Lessons*, Pittsburgh, University of Pittsburgh, Latin American Monogr. and Doc. Series no. 9, 1985b.

———, "Comparative Study of the Development of Social Security in Latin America," *International Social Security Review*, 39:2 (1986): 127–133.

———, "Financiamiento de los programas de salud del Instituto Peruano de Seguridad Social," Lima, ANSSA-Perú, May 1986a.

———, "Exploratory Visit to the Dominican Republic to Review the Field and Identify Health Financing Studies," Stony Brook, State University of New York at Stony Brook, HCF/LAC, June 1986b.

———, "Atención de salud en Costa Rica: auge y crisis," *Boletín de la Oficina Sanitaria Panamericana*, 102:1 (1987): 1–18.

———, "Social Security in Bahamas, Barbados and Jamaica," Geneva, ILO, July 1987a.

———, "Medical Care Under Social Security: Costs, Coverage and Financing," in *Health Care in Peru*, D. K. Zschock, ed., 1988.

———, "Social Insurance: The Experience of Three Countries in the English-Speaking Caribbean," *International Labour Review*, 127:4 (1988a): 479–496.

———, "Análisis económico de los sistemas de pensiones en Costa Rica y recomendaciones para su reforma," Washington, D.C., Development Technologies, Inc., March 1988b.

———, "Informe económico sobre la extensión de la cobertura poblacional del programa de enfermedad-maternidad del IPSS" (IPSS-USAID), Stony Brook, State University of New York at Stony Brook, December 1988c.

———, *Financiamiento de la atención de la salud en América Latina y el Caribe con focalización en el seguro social*, Washington, D.C., World Bank, Institute of Economic Development, no. 42, 1989.

————, "Investment Portfolio of Social Insurance/Pension Funds in Latin America and the Caribbean: Significance, Composition and Performance," Washington, D.C., World Bank, LACTD, May 1989a.

————, "Financial and Economic Evaluation of Social Insurances (IESS) in Ecuador," Washington, D.C., World Bank, November 1989b.

————, *Ascent to Bankruptcy: Financing Social Security in Latin America*, Pittsburgh, University of Pittsburgh Press, 1989c.

————, "Economic and Financial Aspects of Social Security in Latin America and the Caribbean: Tendencies, Problems and Alternatives for the Year 2000," Washington, D.C., World Bank, LATD, May 1990.

————, *La seguridad social y el sector informal*, Santiago, PREALC, Investigaciones sobre Empleo no. 32, 1990a.

————, "Formal Social Security in Latin America and the Caribbean," in E. Ahmad and J. Dréze, eds., *Social Security in Developing Countries*, London, STICED, 1990b.

————, and De Geyndt, W., "Colombia: Social Security Review," Washington, D.C., World Bank, HRD, September 1987.

————; Cruz-Saco, Maria A.; and Zamalloa, Lorena, "Determinantes de los costos y la cobertura del seguro/seguridad social: una comparación internacional enfocada en América Latina," *El Trimestre Económico*, 158:1 (January-March 1990): 27–57.

Midgley, James, *Social Security, Inequality and the Third World*, New York, John Wiley and Sons, 1984.

Ministerio de Salud, "Mortalidad infantil por cantón de residencia en Costa Rica, 1985–1986," San José, November 1987.

Ministerio de Salud/Caja Costarricense de Seguro Social (MS/CCSS), "Projecto para la administración de los servicios de salud...por una cooperativa de autogestión," San José, August 1988.

Ministerio de Salud Pública, "Encuesta familiar de salud, 1982: informe general, sintesis," Montevideo, 1983.

————, "Principales indicadores de salud según departamento y región: año 1986," Montevideo, November 1987.

Ministerio de Trabajo y Promoción Social (MTPS)—Dirección General de Empleo (DGE), Questionnaire from the "Encuesta Nacional de Empleo y Seguridad Social," Lima, 1979.

————, Questionnaire from the "Encuesta de Niveles de Empleo," Lima, 1986.

Ministerio de Trabajo y Seguridad Social (MTSS), Dirección General de Estadística y Censo, *Encuesta nacional de hogares, empleo y desempleo*, San José, 1980 to 1986.

Miranda, Guido, "La salud y la seguridad social en Costa Rica," Lecture, Washington, D.C., PAHO, February 12, 1990.

Moles, Ricardo, "Contribuciones de la AISS al estudio de los problemas de financiamiento de la seguridad social en América Latina," *Seguridad Social*, 34:155–156 (1985): 151–161.

Molina, Luis Henry, *Nuevo sistema de seguridad social*, Santo Domingo, Instituto Nacional de Estudios Laborales, 1983.

Molina, Sergio, "La pobreza en América Latina: situación, evolución y orientaciones de política," in UN/ECLAC/UNDP, 1980.

Montaño, Jorge, "Barreras institucionales de entrada al sector informal en la Ciudad de México," Santiago, PREALC-ILO, March 1985.

Montes, Romero, "Privatización y obligatoriedad del seguro social," *Análisis Laboral*, 134 (August 1988): 9–10.

Moya Pons, Frank, ed., *Población y pobreza en la República Dominicana*, Santo Domingo, Forum, no. 2, 1984.

Musgrove, Philip, "The Impact of Social Security on Income Distribution," in Mesa-Lago, 1985b, chapter 6.

————, "Reflexiones sobre la demanda por salud en América Latina," *Cuadernos de Economía*, 66 (August 1985a): 293–305.

————, "The Economic Crisis and Its Impact on Health and Health Care in Latin America and the Caribbean," *Int J Health Serv*, 17:3 (1987): 411–441.

————, "Distribución del ingreso familiar en la República Dominicana, 1976–1977: la encuesta nacional de ingresos y gastos familiares," *El Trimestre Económico* 53:2 (1986a): 341–392.

————, ed., "Número especial sobre economía de la salud," *Boletín de la Oficina Sanitaria Panamericana*, 103:6 (December 1987).

————, ed., *Health Economics: Latin American Perspectives*, Washington, D.C., PAHO, Scientific Publication no. 517, 1989.

————, "Health, Debt and Disease: The Links Between Economics and Health," *The IDB*, December 1989a: 4–8.

Nadal, Pablo, "Nueva visión de la seguridad social," Santo Domingo, Instituto Nacional de Estudios Laborales, 1986.

Oficina Nacional de Estadística (ONE), *República Dominicana en Cifras 1965 to 1987*, Santo Domingo, 1965 to 1987.

————, *Censo nacional de población y vivienda 1981: resultados preliminares*, Santo Domingo, March 1983.

Oficina Nacional de Planificación (ONP), "Estudio de base del sector salud-nutrición-fármacos," Santo Domingo, November 1983.

Overholt, Catherine, et al., *Costa Rica: Health Sector Overview*, Boston, USAID, January 1986.

Pan American Health Organization-Organización Panamericana de la Salud (PAHO-OPS), *Extensión de la cobertura de servicios de salud con las estrategias de atención primaria*, Washington, D.C., Official Document no. 156, 1978.

————, "Coordinación entre los sistemas de seguridad social y la salud pública," Washington, D.C., 1981.

————, *Investigación operativa de los servicios de salud*, Santo Domingo, September 1983.

————, "Coordination of Social Security and Public Health Institutions," Washington, D.C., Document CE99/19, June 1987.

————, "Los sistemas de la seguridad social y la salud," Washington, D.C., November 1989.

————, "Round Table on Financing Health Services in Developing Countries: An Agenda for Reform (A World Bank Policy Study)," in Musgrove, 1989, pp. 145–191.

————, ILO, and Comité Permanente Interamericano de Seguridad Social (CPISS), *Atención primaria y estragias de salud en la seguridad social en América Latina*, Geneva, 1986.

————, UNDP, and UNICEF, "Nota del Representante Residente sobre el 4° Programa Nacional del PNUD para la República Dominicana," Santo Domingo, March 1986.

Pérez Montas, Hernando, "Plan de desarrollo de la seguridad social, 1974–1978," Santo Domingo, 1974.

Petrei, A. Humberto, *El gasto público social y sus efectos redistributivos: un examen comparativo de cinco países de América Latina*, Rio de Janeiro, ECIEL, no. 6, 1987.

Petrera Pavone, Margarita, "Eficacia y eficiencia de la seguridad social en relación con el ciclo económico: el caso peruano," *Boletín de la Oficina Sanitaria Panamericana*, 103:6 (1987): 620–634.

Pfeffermann, Guy, and Griffin, Charles, *Nutrition and Health Programs in Latin America: Targeting Social Expenditures*, Washington, D.C., World Bank, 1989.

Pinilla, Susana, "Concepción, características y promoción del sector informal urbano," Lima, Instituto de Desarrollo del Sector Informal (IDESI), September 1986.

————, *La mujer y el sector informal*, Lima, IDESI, 1987.

Piñera, Sebastián, "Definición, medición y análisis de la pobreza: aspectos conceptuales y metodológicos," Santiago, PPC/CDE, May 1978.

————, "Medición, análisis y descripción de la pobreza en algunos países latinoamericanos," Santiago, CEPAL, 1978a.

Poder Ejecutivo Federal, *Plan Nacional de Desarrollo: informe de ejecución 1989*, Mexico City, Presidencia de la República, 1990.

Pollack, Molly, and Ulhoff, A., *Costa Rica: evolución macroeconómica 1976–1983*, Santiago, PREALC, Demografía sobre Empleo no. 50, 1985.

Portes, Alejandro, *Latin America Class Structures: Their Composition and Change during the Last Decades*, Baltimore, Johns Hopkins University Press, Occasional Paper no. 3, 1984.

————; Blitzer, Silvia; and Curtis, John, "The Urban Informal Sector in Uruguay: Its Internal Structure, Characteristics, and Effects," *World Development*, 14:6 (1986): 727–741.

————; Castells, Manuel; and Benton, Lauren, eds., *The Informal Economy: Studies in Advanced and Less Developed Countries*, Baltimore, Johns Hopkins University Press, 1989.

Programa Regional de Empleo para América Latina y el Caribe (PREALC), *Sector informal: funcionamiento y políticas*, Santiago, 1981.

————, *Dinámica del subempleo en América Latina*, Santiago, Estudios Informes de la CEPAL no. 10, 1981a.

————, *Mercado de trabajo en cifras, 1950–1980*, Santiago, 1982.

————, *The Urban Informal Sector and Labour Market Information Systems*, Santiago, 1986.

—————, *Deuda social ¿Qué es, cuánto es, cómo se paga?*, Geneva, ILO, 1988.

Psacharopoulos, George, *Recovering Growth with Equity: World Bank Poverty Alleviation Activities in Latin America*, Washington, D.C., World Bank, HRD/LACR, April 1989.

—————, *A Bibliography on Poverty and Income Distribution in Latin America*, Washington, D.C., World Bank, HRD/LACR, November 1989a.

Puffert, Douglas J., and Jiménez, Emmanuel Y., "The Macroeconomics of Social Security in Brazil: Fiscal and Financial Considerations," Washington, D.C., World Bank, draft, October 1988.

Quirós Coronado, Roberto, "Síntesis de la labor de la Comisión que estudia el aseguramiento de trabajadores independientes y temporales," San José, September 3, 1987.

Raczinsky, Dagmar, *El sector informal urbano: interrogantes y controversias*, Santiago, Investigaciones sobre Empleo no. 3, 1977.

Reyes, Rolando, *Microenterprise and the Informal Sector in the Dominican Republic: Operation and Promotion Policy*, Washington, D.C., Commission for the Study of International Migration and Cooperative Economic Development, no. 47, July 1990.

Rezende, Fernando, "Redistribution of Income through Social Security: The Case of Brazil," 31st Congress of the Institute of Public Finance, 1974.

—————, *Financiamiento de las políticas sociales*, Santiago, ILPES-UNICEF, 1983.

—————, and Mahar, Dennis, "Salud y previsión social: un análisis económico," Rio de Janeiro, IPEA, 1974.

—————, et al., "Os custos da assistência médica e a crise financeira de previdência social," *Dados*, 25:1 (1982): 25–43.

Robinson, Eugene, "Upstart Shantytown of 1960s Now is a Major Peruvian City," *The Washington Post*, December 26, 1988, A33.

Rodríguez, Jorge, and Wurgaft, José, *La protección social a los desocupados en América Latina*, Geneva, PREALC-ILO, Investigaciones sobre Empleo no. 28, 1987.

Rodríguez, Renán, "Problemas contemporáneos de la seguridad social en Uruguay," en CIESS, 1988, pp. 43–58.

Rodríguez Cubero, Mario (Director of DESAF), Interview, San José, May 11, 1988.

Rodríguez Grossi, Jorge, "El acceso a la salud, la eficacia hospitalaria y la distribución de los beneficios de la salud pública," *Cuadernos de Economía*, 66 (August 1985): 267–291.

—————, "Public Spending on Social Programs [in the Dominican Republic]: Issues and Options," Washington, D.C., World Bank, 1989.

Rodríguez V., Adrián, "El gasto público en salud y su impacto en la distribución del ingreso familiar: Costa Rica 1982," San José, Universidad de Costa Rica, Instituto de Investigaciones en Ciencias Económicas, no. 100, December 1986.

Rojas Alba, Mario, "Situación de la población y recursos para la salud en el Estado de Morelos," *Medicina Alternativa*, no. 4 (May 1988).

Romero, Fredis Emilio, and Quesada, Ana Marta (Actuaries, IDSS), Interview, Santo Domingo, June 18, 1986.

Rossini, Renzo; Thomas, Jim; et al., *Los fundamentos estadísticos de 'El otro sendero': debate sobre el sector informal en el Perú*, Lima, Fundación Friedrich Ebert, 1987.

Roura, Carlos; Güida, Edgar; Lanza, Jorge; Roya, R.; and Ferolla, C. (Officials, Physicians, and Dentists of Cooperativa de Producción del Termo and Policlínico), Interviews, Montevideo, December 14 and 15, 1989.

Rovira Mas, Jorge, *Costa Rica en los años '80*, San José, FLACSO-Editorial Porvenir, 1988.

Saenz, Lenín, *Salud sin riqueza (El caso de Costa Rica)*, San José, 1985.

Saldaín, Rodolfo, ''Seguridad social y salud en Uruguay,'' *Seguridad social, atención médica y prácticas de salud en América Latina*, Buenos Aires, AISS, no. 9, 1988, 214–239.

————, ''Uruguay,'' *Social Welfare in Latin America*, J. Dixon and R. Schuerell, eds., London, Routledge, 1990, 249–274.

Salinas de Gortari, Carlos, *Primer Informe de Gobierno 1989: anexo*, Mexico City, Presidencia de la República, 1989.

Samaniego, Norma, ''Los efectos de la crisis de 1982–1986 en las condiciones de vida de la población en México,'' Lima, CEPAL, November 1986.

Saunders, Margaret K., ''Analysis and Summary of World Bank Activity in Health Insurance,'' Washington, D.C., World Bank-EDI, December 1989.

Scarpaci, Joseph L., *Primary Health Care in Chile: Accessibility Under Military Rule*, Pittsburgh, University of Pittsburgh Press, 1988.

Schulthess, Walter E., ''El sistema bolivano de seguridad social: pautas para su reforma,'' La Paz, Ediciones UDAPE, July 1988.

————, ''Bolivia: seguro social y servicios de la salud,'' Washington, D.C., World Bank, LATHR, 1989.

Secretaría de Estado de Salud Pública y Asistencia Social (SESPAS), *Estadísticas de Salud 1979* to *1985*, Santo Domingo, n/d.

————, ''El hospital dominicano dentro del contexto 'Salud para todos en el año 2000','' Santo Domingo, February-March 1984.

————, *Memoria 1983* to *1985*, Santo Domingo, 1983 to 1986.

————, Statistics on SESPAS Hospitals and Other Facilities by Region, Santo Domingo, 1986a.

Secretaría de Planificación y Presupuesto (SPP), *Plan Nacional de Desarrollo 1989–1994*, Mexico City, 1989.

Secretaría de Salud (SS), *Anuario Estadístico 1986*, Mexico City, 1986.

————, ''Población abierta 1985,'' Mexico City, 1986a.

————, ''Estadística trimestral de la prestación de servicios: acumulado anual 1987,'' Mexico City, April 1988.

Secretaría de Salud Pública (SSP) et al., *La ocupación informal en áreas urbanas 1976: encuesta complementaria a la encuesta continua sobre ocupación*, Mexico City, December 1979.

Secretaría de Trabajo y Previsión Social (STPS), *Características de la ocupación informal urbana*, 2nd ed., Mexico City, June 1985.

Secretaría Ejecutiva de Planificación Sectorial de Salud (SEPSS), *Estudio de organización y funcionamiento del sector salud*, San José, August 1984.

Selowsky, Marcelo, "Hacia la eliminación del deficit de satisfacción de necesidades básicas," in UN/ECLAC/UNDP, 1980.

Sherraden, Margaret S. "Primary Health Care for the Rural Poor in Mexico: The Case of IMSS-COPLAMAR (1979–1988)," St. Louis, Washington University, April 1989.

————, Letter to the author, June 20, 1989a.

Skolnik, Richard (HNPD-World Bank), Telephone interview, June 9, 1986.

Soberón, Guillermo; Kumate, Jesús; and Laguna, José, *La salud en México: testimonios 1988*, Mexico City, Fondo de Cultura Económica, 1988.

Suárez-Berenguela, Rubén, *Financing the Health Sector in Peru*, Washington, D.C., World Bank, LSMS Working Paper no. 31, April 1987.

Tamburi, Giovanni, "Valuación actuarial en las instituciones de seguridad social," XII Asamblea General de la Conferencia Interamericana de Seguridad Social, Santo Domingo, March 17–21, 1980.

————, "Evolución, tendencias y perspectivas de los sistemas de salud de la seguridad social en América Latina," in PAHO-ILO-CPISS, 1986.

————, "Social Security in Latin America: Principles, Current Issues and Trends" in Mesa-Lago, 1985b, chapter 2.

————, Discussion at PAHO, February 12, 1990.

Thullen, Peter, "Social Security Financing: Problems and Trends," in Mesa-Lago, 1985b, chapter 5.

Tokman, Víctor, "Pobreza urbana y empleo: líneas de acción," in UN/ECLAC/UNDP, 1980.

————, "Adjustment and Employment in Latin America," *International Labour Review*, 125:5 (1986): 535.

————, "El sector informal: quince años después," *El Trimestre Económico*, 54:3 (July-September 1987): 513–536.

————, "El imperativo de actuar: el sector informal hoy," *Nueva Sociedad*, 90, July-August 1987a.

Torres, Guillermo, PAHO/WHO Representative in the Dominican Republic, Interview, Santo Domingo, June 16, 1986.

Ugalde, Antonio, "Where There Is a Doctor: Strategies to Increase Productivity at Lower Costs; the Economics of Rural Health Care in the Dominican Republic," *Social Science and Medicine*, 19:4 (1984): 441–450.

————, ed., "Health and Social Science in Latin America," *Social Science and Medicine*, 21:1 (1985).

—————, "The Integration of Health Programs into a National Health Service," in Mesa-Lago, 1985b, chapter 4.

—————, and Homedes, Nuria, "Toward a Rural Health Corps Concept: Lessons from the Dominican Republic," *Journal of Rural Health*, 4:1 (January 1988): 41–58.

United Nations, *U.N. Demographic Yearbook 1980 to 1987*, 1980 to 1987.

—————, Economic Commission for Latin America and the Caribbean, and U.N. Development Program (UN/ECLAC/UNDP), *¿Se puede superar la pobreza?: Realidad y perspectivas en América Latina*, Santiago, ECLAC, 1980.

—————, and UNICEF, *The State of the World's Children, 1988*, New Delhi, 1988.

USAID Mission to the Dominican Republic, "Health Sector Assessment for the Dominican Republic," February 1975.

United States Social Security Administration (US-SSA), *Social Security Programs Throughout the World 1987*, Washington, D.C., DHHS, 1987.

Vásquez Córdoba, Sergio, et al., "Estructura y evolución del presupuesto programático ejercido por las instituciones que conforman el sector salud," *Higiene*, 37:1 (1987): 22–25.

Vedova, Mario A., "Economic Recession in Costa Rica and the Consequences on the Poor," Washington, D.C., World Bank, 1986.

Velázquez Díaz, Georgina, Interview, Mexico City, May 19, 1988.

—————, "Diez años de IMSS-COPLAMAR," *Cuestión Social*, 15 (Summer-Fall 1989): 11–14.

Vereda, Antonio, "Alternativas a la economía informal," Lima, draft, 1988.

Weber, Ron, "IAF Support for the ILD and Villa El Salvador," *Grassroots Development*, 13:1 (1990): 18.

Wilkie, James W., "Social Security in Mexico," Washington, D.C., World Bank, 1990.

Wilson, Richard, "The Impact of Social Security on Employment," in Mesa-Lago, 1985b, chapter 8.

World Bank, *Poverty in Latin America: The Impact of Depression*, Washington, D.C., September 1986.

—————, "Argentina: Population, Health and Nutrition Sector Review," Washington, D.C., 1987a.

—————, "Argentina: Social Sectors in Crisis," Washington, D.C., 1988.

—————, *World Development Report 1988* and *1989*, Washington, D.C., Oxford University Press, 1988a and 1989.

—————, *Poverty: World Development Report 1990*, Oxford, Oxford University Press, 1990.

World Health Organization (WHO-OMS), *Primary Health Care: Report of the International Conference on Primary Health Care, Alma-Ata, USSR, 6–12 September 1978*, Geneva, 1978.

—————, *Economic Support for National Health for All Strategies: 40th World Health Assembly*, Geneva, May 1987.

Zolla, Carlos, "Medicina tradicional y sistemas de atención a la salud," in CIESS, *El futuro de la medicina tradicional en la atención a la salud de los paises Latinoamericanos*, Mexico City, CIESS, 1987.

Zschock, Dieter K., *Health Care Financing in Developing Countries*, Washington, D.C., American Public Health Association, International Health Programs, Monograph Series, no. 1, 1979.

—————, "Medical Care Under Social Insurance in Latin America," *Latin American Research Review*, 21:1 (1986): 99–122.

—————, ed., *Health Care in Peru: Resources and Policy*, Boulder, Westview Press, 1988.

☆U.S. GOVERNMENT PRINTING OFFICE: 1992-330-011